Vasculitis

Editors

ELI M. MILOSLAVSKY
ANISHA B. DUA

RHEUMATIC DISEASE CLINICS OF NORTH AMERICA

www.rheumatic.theclinics.com

Consulting Editor
MICHAEL H. WEISMAN

August 2023 • Volume 49 • Number 3

ELSEVIER

1600 John F. Kennedy Boulevard • Suite 1800 • Philadelphia, Pennsylvania, 19103-2899
http://www.theclinics.com

RHEUMATIC DISEASE CLINICS OF NORTH AMERICA Volume 49, Number 3
August 2023 ISSN 0889-857X, ISBN 13: 978-0-323-93869-3

Editor: Joanna Gascoine
Developmental Editor: Karen Justine S. Dino

Rheumatic Disease Clinics of North America (ISSN 0889-857X) is published quarterly by Elsevier Inc., 360 Park Avenue South, New York, NY 10010-1710. Months of issue are February, May, August, and November. Business and editorial offices: 1600 John F. Kennedy Boulevard, Suite 1800, Philadelphia, PA 19103-2899. Periodicals postage paid at New York, NY and additional mailing offices. Subscription prices are USD 377.00 per year for US individuals, USD 865.00 per year for US institutions, USD 100.00 per year for US students and residents, USD 444.00 per year for Canadian individuals, USD 1081.00 per year for Canadian institutions, USD 100.00 per year for Canadian students/residents, USD 484.00 per year for international individuals, USD 1081.00 per year for international institutions, and USD 230.00 per year for foreign students/residents. To receive student/ resident rate, orders must be accompanied by name of affiliated institution, date of term, and the *signature* of program/residency coordinator on institution letterhead. Orders will be billed at individual rate until proof of status received. Foreign air speed delivery is included in all *Clinics* subscription prices. All prices are subject to change without notice. **POSTMASTER:** Send address changes to *Rheumatic Disease Clinics of North America,* Elsevier Health Sciences Division, Subscription Customer Service, 3251 Riverport Lane, Maryland Heights, MO 63043. **Customer Service: 1-800-654-2452 (US and Canada). From outside of the US and Canada: 314-447-8871. Fax: 314-447-8029. For print support, e-mail: JournalsCustomerService-usa@elsevier.com. For online support, e-mail: JournalsOnlineSupport-usa@elsevier.com.**

Reprints. For copies of 100 or more of articles in this publication, please contact the Commercial Reprints Department, Elsevier Inc., 360 Park Avenue South, New York, New York, 10010-1710; Tel.: +1-212-633-3874, Fax: +1-212-633-3820, and E-mail: reprints@elsevier.com.

Rheumatic Disease Clinics of North America is covered in *MEDLINE/PubMed (Index Medicus), Current Contents/Clinical Medicine, Science Citation Index, ISI/BIOMED,* and *EMBASE/Excerpta Medica.*

Contributors

CONSULTING EDITOR

MICHAEL H. WEISMAN, MD
Adjunct Professor of Medicine, Stanford University, Distinguished Professor of Medicine Emeritus, David Geffen School of Medicine at UCLA, Professor of Medicine Emeritus, Cedars-Sinai Medical Center, Los Angeles, California, USA

EDITORS

ELI M. MILOSLAVSKY, MD
Associate Professor of Medicine, Department of Medicine, Division of Rheumatology, Allergy and Immunology, Massachusetts General Hospital and Harvard Medical School, Boston, Massachusetts, USA

ANISHA B. DUA, MD, MPH
Associate Professor of Medicine, Department of Medicine, Division of Rheumatology, Northwestern University Feinberg School of Medicine, Northwestern University Hospital, Chicago, Illinois, USA

AUTHORS

MOEIN AMIN, MD
Mellen Center for Multiple Sclerosis Treatment and Research, Neurological Institute, Cleveland Clinic, Cleveland, Ohio, USA

MOSHE ARDITI, MD
Division of Infectious Diseases and Immunology, Department of Pediatrics, Guerin Children's at Cedars-Sinai Medical Center, Department of Biomedical Sciences, Infectious and Immunologic Diseases Research Center (IIDRC), Cedars-Sinai Medical Center, Smidt Heart Institute, Cedars-Sinai Medical Center, Los Angeles, California, USA

BONNIE L. BERMAS, MD
Professor of Medicine, University of Texas Southwestern, Dallas, Texas, USA

ALVISE BERTI, MD, PhD
Center for Medical Sciences (CISMed), Department of Cellular, Computational and Integrative Biology (CIBIO), University of Trento, and Division of Rheumatology, Santa Chiara Hospital, APSS Trento, Italy

JESSICA L. BLOOM, MD, MSCS
Assistant Professor, Section of Rheumatology, Department of Pediatrics, University of Colorado School of Medicine, Aurora, Colorado, USA

KEVIN BYRAM, MD
Associate Professor of Medicine, Division of Rheumatology and Immunology, Vanderbilt University Medical Center, Nashville, Tennessee, USA

DIVYA A. CHARI, MD
Assistant Professor of Otolaryngology, Department of Otolaryngology, Massachusetts Eye and Ear Infirmary, Harvard Medical School, Boston, Massachusetts, USA; Department of Otolaryngology, University of Massachusetts Memorial Health Center, Worcester, Massachusetts, USA

MEGAN E.B. CLOWSE, MD, MPH
Associate Professor of Medicine, Division of Rheumatology and Immunology, Duke University, Durham, North Carolina, USA

DIVI CORNEC, MD, PhD
Rheumatology Department, INSERM UMR1227 LBAI, Lymphocytes B, Autoimmunité et Immunothérapies, University of Brest, National Reference Center for Rare Systemic Autoimmune Diseases CERAINO, CHRU Brest, Brest, France

MARISSA DALE, MD
Department of Pediatrics, Columbia University Medical Center, Morgan Stanley Children's Hospital, New York, New York, USA

ANISHA B. DUA, MD, MPH
Associate Professor of Medicine, Department of Medicine, Division of Rheumatology, Northwestern University Feinberg School of Medicine, Northwestern University Hospital, Chicago, Illinois, USA

LINDSY J. FORBESS, MD, MSc
Assistant Professor, Division of Rheumatology, Cedars-Sinai Medical Center, Los Angeles, California, USA

MARK GORELIK, MD
Division of Allergy, Immunology, and Rheumatology, Department of Pediatrics, Columbia University Medical Center, College of Physicians and Surgeons Building, New York, New York, USA

STACEY T. GRAY, MD
Associate Professor of Otolaryngology–Head and Neck Surgery, Department of Otolaryngology, Massachusetts Eye and Ear Infirmary, Harvard Medical School, Boston, Massachusetts, USA

RULA A. HAJJ-ALI, MD
Cleveland Clinic Center for Vasculitis Care and Research, Cleveland Clinic, Cleveland, Ohio, USA

GÜLEN HATEMI, MD
Division of Rheumatology, Department of Internal Medicine, Behçet's Disease Research Center, Istanbul University–Cerrahpasa, Istanbul Turkey

AUDRA HOROMANSKI, MD
Assistant Professor, Division of Immunology and Rheumatology, Stanford University, Palo Alto, California, USA

TANAZ A. KERMANI, MD, MS
Associate Clinical Professor of Medicine, Division of Rheumatology, University of California Los Angeles, Santa Monica, California, USA

CAROL A. LANGFORD, MD, MHS
Professor of Medicine, Department of Rheumatic and Immunologic Diseases, Cleveland Clinic, Cleveland, Ohio, USA

ELI M. MILOSLAVSKY, MD
Associate Professor of Medicine, Division of Rheumatology, Allergy and Immunology, Department of Medicine, Massachusetts General Hospital, Harvard Medical School, Boston, Massachusetts, USA

PAUL A. MONACH, MD, PhD
Rheumatology Section, VA Boston Healthcare System, Associate Professor, Harvard Medical School, Boston, Massachusetts, USA

MATTHEW R. NAUNHEIM, MD
Assistant Professor in Otolaryngology–Head and Neck Surgery, Department of Otolaryngology, Massachusetts Eye and Ear Infirmary, Harvard Medical School, Boston, Massachusetts, USA

DESH NEPAL, MD
Department of Medicine, Division of Rheumatology, Hub for Collaborative Medicine, Medical College of Wisconsin, Milwaukee, Wisconsin, USA

MAGALI NOVAL RIVAS, PhD
Division of Infectious Diseases and Immunology, Department of Pediatrics, Guerin Children's at Cedars-Sinai Medical Center, Department of Biomedical Sciences, Infectious and Immunologic Diseases Research Center (IIDRC), Cedars-Sinai Medical Center, Los Angeles, California, USA

MICHAEL PUTMAN, MD, MS
Department of Medicine, Division of Rheumatology, Hub for Collaborative Medicine, Medical College of Wisconsin, Milwaukee, Wisconsin, USA

LAUREN AMBLER ROBINSON, MD
Department of Medicine, Pediatric Rheumatology, Hospital for Special Surgery, Department of Pediatric Rheumatology, New York, New York, USA

SEBASTIAN E. SATTUI, MD, MS
Division of Rheumatology and Clinical Immunology, University of Pittsburgh, Pittsburgh, Pennsylvania, USA

CATHERINE A. SIMS, MD
Division of Rheumatology, Duke University, Durham, North Carolina, USA

JASON M. SPRINGER, MD, MS
Associate Professor, Vanderbilt University Medical Center, Nashville, Tennessee, USA

DIDAR UÇAR, MD
Department of Ophthalmology, Behçet's Disease Research Center, Istanbul University–Cerrahpasa, Istanbul Turkey

KEN UCHINO, MD
Cerebrovascular Center, Cleveland Clinic, Cleveland, Ohio, USA

SEBASTIAN UNIZONY, MD
Massachusetts General Hospital, Vasculitis and Glomerulonephritis Center, Harvard Medical School, Boston, Massachusetts, USA

UĞUR UYGUNOĞLU, MD
Department of Neurology, School of Medicine, Istanbul University–Cerrahpasa, Istanbul, Turkey

ALEXANDRA VILLA-FORTE, MD, MPH
Associate Professor, Cleveland Clinic, Cleveland, Ohio, USA

ZACHARY S. WALLACE, MD, MSc
Harvard Medical School, Clinical Epidemiology Program, Mongan Institute, Massachusetts General Hospital, Division of Rheumatology, Allergy, and Immunology, Department of Medicine, Massachusetts General Hospital, Boston, Massachusetts, USA

ISAAC WASSERMAN, MD
Resident in Otolaryngology, Department of Otolaryngology, Massachusetts Eye and Ear Infirmary, Harvard Medical School, Boston, Massachusetts, USA

MICHAEL E. WECHSLER, MD, MMSc
Professor of Medicine, Division of Pulmonary, Critical Care, and Sleep Medicine, Department of Medicine, National Jewish Health, Denver, Colorado, USA

HASAN YAZICI, MD
Rheumatology, Academic Hospital, Istanbul, Turkey

YUSUF YAZICI, MD
Division of Rheumatology, New York University School of Medicine, New York, New York, USA

Contents

Technological advances and increased recognition of the prevalence and implications of large vessel vasculitis have led to robust research into various imaging techniques. Although there is still debate about which modality to choose in specific clinical scenarios, Ultrasound, PET/CT, MRI/A, and CT/A offer complementary information regarding diagnosis, disease activity, and vascular complication monitoring. Recognition of the strengths and limitations of each technique is important for appropriate application in clinical practice.

Prolonged glucocorticoid tapers have been the standard of care for giant cell arteritis (GCA) and polymyalgia rheumatica (PMR), but recent advancements have improved outcomes for patients with GCA while reducing glucocorticoid-related toxicities. Many patients with GCA and PMR still experience persistent or relapsing disease, and cumulative exposure to glucocorticoids for both diseases remains high. The objective of this review is to define current treatment approaches as well as new therapeutic targets and strategies. Studies investigating inhibition of cytokine pathways, including interleukin-6, interleukin-17, interleukin-23, granulocyte-macrophage colony-stimulating factor, Janus kinase–signal transduction and activator of transcription, and others, will be reviewed.

The finding of aortitis, often incidentally noted on surgical resection, should prompt evaluation for secondary causes including large-vessel vasculitis. In a large proportion of cases, no other inflammatory cause is identified and the diagnosis of clinically isolated aortitis is made. It is unknown whether this entity represents a more localized form of large-vessel vasculitis. The need for immunosuppressive therapy in patients with clinically isolated aortitis remains unclear. Patients with clinically isolated aortitis warrant imaging of the entire aorta at baseline and regular intervals because a significant proportion of patients have or develop abnormalities in other vascular beds.

We have made significant headway in our ability to induce and maintain remission in patients with granulomatosis with polyangiitis and microscopic
polyangiitis. With increased understanding of the pathogenesis of antineutrophilic cytoplasmic antibody–associated vasculitides (AAV), therapeutic
targets have been identified and studied in clinical trials. From initial induction strategies including glucocorticoids and cyclophosphamide, we have
discovered effective induction regimens with rituximab and complement
inhibition that can significantly decrease the glucocorticoid cumulative
doses in patients with AAV. There are many trials underway evaluating
management strategies for refractory patients and exploring new and
old therapies that may help to continuously improve outcomes for patients
with AAV.

Eosinophilic granulomatosis with polyangiitis (EGPA) is an eosinophilic
vasculitis that affects a variety of organ systems. Historically, glucocorticoids and a variety of other immunosuppressants were used to abrogate
the inflammation and tissue injury associated with EGPA. The management of EGPA has evolved greatly during the last decade with the development of novel targeted therapeutics that have resulted in significantly
improved outcomes for these patients including therapies that target B
cells or modulate eosinophils; many more novel targeted therapies are
emerging.

Behçet's syndrome is a systemic vasculitis affecting arteries and veins of
all sizes as well as recurrent oral, genital, and intestinal ulcers, skin lesions,
predominantly posterior uveitis, and parenchymal brain lesions. These can
be present in various combinations and sequences over time and diagnosis is made by recognizing the manifestations, as there are no diagnostic
biomarkers or genetic tests. Treatment modalities include immunomodulatory agents, immunosuppressives and biologics, tailored according to
prognostic factors, disease activity, severity, and patients' preferences.

Central nervous system vasculitis (CNSV) is a group of disorders leading to
inflammatory vasculopathy within the brain, spinal cord, and leptomeninges. CNSV is divided into primary angiitis of the central nervous system
(PACNS) and secondary CNSV based on the underlying etiology. PACNS
is a rare inflammatory disorder with poorly understood pathophysiology
and heterogeneous and highly variable clinical features. The diagnosis depends on a combination of clinical and laboratory variables, multimodal

imaging, and histopathological examination as well as exclusion of mimics. Several systemic vasculitides, infectious etiologies and connective tissue disorders have been shown to cause secondary CNSV and require prompt recognition.

The approach to diagnosis of primary systemic vasculitis can be challenging, often requiring consideration of important secondary causes of vasculitis and non-inflammatory mimics. An atypical pattern of vascular involvement and/or atypical features of primary vasculitis (eg, cytopenia, lymphadenopathy) should prompt a more thorough investigation into other diseases. Herein, we review selected mimics organized by the size of blood vessels typically affected.

Auricular, nasal, and laryngeal manifestations occur frequently in rheumatic diseases. Inflammatory ear, nose, and throat (ENT) processes often result in organ damage and have profound effects on quality of life. Herein, we review the otologic, nasal, and laryngeal involvement of rheumatic diseases, focusing on their clinical presentation and diagnosis. ENT manifestations generally respond to treatment of the systemic disease, which is outside the scope of this review; however, adjunctive topical and surgical treatment approaches, as well as treatment of idiopathic inflammatory ENT manifestations will be reviewed.

Multisystem inflammatory syndrome in children (MIS-C) is a delayed postinflammatory disorder associated with the previous infection with severe acute respiratory syndrome coronavirus 2 (SARS-CoV-2). Initially, MIS-C was described as highly similar to Kawasaki disease (KD), a pediatric febrile systemic vasculitis that can lead to the development of coronary artery aneurysms (CAAs). While KD and MIS-C are both inflammatory disorders, the 2 entities differ in their epidemiological, clinical, immunological, and pathological features. MIS-C clinical and laboratory characteristics are more closely related to toxic shock syndrome (TSS) than KD, which informs the understanding of pathogenesis and potential therapeutic approaches.

Kawasaki disease and multisystem inflammatory syndrome in children are hyperinflammatory conditions that share similar emerging pathophysiology hypotheses, clinical features, treatment strategies, and outcomes. Although both conditions have key differences, growing evidence suggests that both conditions might be closely related on a larger spectrum of postinfectious autoimmune responses.

RHEUMATIC DISEASE CLINICS OF NORTH AMERICA

SERIES OF RELATED INTEREST

Emergency Medicine Clinics
Available at: https://www.emed.theclinics.com/
Neurologic Clinics
Available at: https://www.neurologic.theclinics.com/

THE CLINICS ARE AVAILABLE ONLINE!
Access your subscription at:
www.theclinics.com

Foreword

Vasculitis

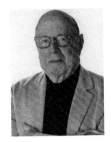

Michael H. Weisman, MD
Consulting Editor

When asked to create an issue on Vasculitis, Anisha Dua and Eli Miloslavsky not only jumped on the topic with great energy and enthusiasm but also essentially created a masterpiece ahead of schedule! The field is changing rapidly, and the importance of getting this information out is critical. We are especially indebted to our contributors, who have delivered an unbelievably well-documented and scholarly set of reviews addressing the various challenges in diagnosing and managing patients with vasculitis.

Large-vessel arteritis is wonderfully treated in several of our articles, emphasizing not only diagnosis with advanced imaging but also management options that have grown in importance over the past few years. Kawasaki disease and multisystem inflammatory syndrome in children not only are challenging from a diagnostic standpoint but also offer a glimpse into environmental triggers that need further characterization and explanation. Nowhere has the future been brighter for early diagnosis and effective management than in the granulomatous forms of vasculitis—we address this in several articles. COVID-19–related challenges in vasculitis as well as vasculitis mimics are particularly important in today's world of aggressive approaches to diagnosis and management; these articles are very well organized and complete. The complicated story of reproductive health issues is extremely well done, and new advances in epidemiology, pathogenesis, and management of Behcet syndrome are presented. What appear to be isolated forms of vasculitis in the central nervous system, the aorta, as well as otologic, sinus, and airway involvement are especially challenging situations; our editors and contributors have provided state-of-the-art scholarly work on these subjects. Our final article addresses the importance of research and clinical advancement in the field—what do we need to do to move forward with particular emphasis on

Rheum Dis Clin N Am 49 (2023) xiii–xiv
https://doi.org/10.1016/j.rdc.2023.04.002

the challenges of clinical trials, financial support, and regulatory approval. This is a landmark issue, and Anisha and Eli outdid themselves.

Michael H. Weisman, MD
Adjunct Professor of Medicine
Stanford University
10800 Wilshire Boulevard, #404
Los Angeles, CA 90024, USA

E-mail address:
michael.weisman@cshs.org

Preface

Emerging Concepts in the Diagnosis and Treatment of Systemic Vasculitis

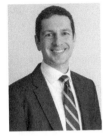 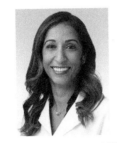

Eli M. Miloslavsky, MD   Anisha B. Dua, MD, MPH
Editors

Systemic vasculitides are a group of heterogenous conditions that share a predilection for angiocentric inflammation of large, medium, and small vessels. Early recognition and treatment have the potential to decrease the morbidity and mortality associated with vasculitis. Recent advances in the diagnosis and treatment of these conditions hold significant promise for our patients.

In this issue of the *Rheumatic Disease Clinics of North America*, we highlight the latest developments in our understanding of the pathophysiology, approach to diagnosis, and treatment of large, medium, and small vessel vasculitis. Specifically, we highlight advances in the use of imaging to diagnose large vessel vasculitis and emerging treatment approaches in giant cell arteritis/polymyalgia rheumatica as well as isolated aortitis. Perhaps the most significant advances in treatment paradigms have been made in ANCA-associated vasculitis, which we focus on in two articles on granulomatosis with polyangiitis/microscopic polyangiitis and eosinophilic granulomatosis with polyangiitis. This issue includes updates on Behcet disease, central nervous system vasculitis, and vasculitis mimics, which can be particularly difficult to diagnose and treat. The emergence of multisystem inflammatory syndrome in children associated with COVID-19 has shed new light onto the pathogenesis and treatment of Kawasaki disease, which we spotlight in two viewpoints. Because vasculitis frequently involves the skin as well as the ear, nose, and throat (ENT) systems, reviews on cutaneous vasculitis and its mimickers as well as ENT manifestations of systemic vasculitis highlight the challenges and pearls in the diagnosis and treatment of these organs. Finally, we focus on the challenges of vasculitis treatment as it relates to pregnancy and

Rheum Dis Clin N Am 49 (2023) xv–xvi
https://doi.org/10.1016/j.rdc.2023.04.001

COVID-19 and conclude with a look ahead to the future of vasculitis diagnosis, treatment, and research.

Eli M. Miloslavsky, MD
Department of Medicine
Division of Rheumatology, Allergy
and Immunology
Massachusetts General Hospital and
Harvard Medical School
Yawkey Center for Outpatient Care, Suite 4B
55 Fruit Street
Boston, MA 02114, USA

Anisha B. Dua, MD, MPH
Department of Medicine
Division of Rheumatology
Northwestern University
Feinberg School of Medicine
Northwestern University Hospital
Galter Pavilion
675 North St Clair Street, Suite 1400
Chicago, IL 60611, USA

E-mail addresses:
emiloslavsky@mgh.harvard.edu (E.M. Miloslavsky)
Anisha.dua@northwestern.edu (A.B. Dua)

The Role of Imaging in Diagnosis and Monitoring of Large Vessel Vasculitis

Audra Horomanski, MD[a],*, Lindsy J. Forbess, MD, MSc[b]

KEYWORDS

- Large vessel vasculitis • Giant cell arteritis • Takayasu's arteritis • Ultrasound
- 18F-FDG PET/CT • MRI • CT

KEY POINTS

- Imaging plays a critical role in the diagnosis of both cranial and large vessel involvement in patients with GCA.
- PET, MRI, and CT offer a comprehensive assessment of the extent of large vessel disease in both GCA and TAK, each with various strengths and limitations.
- Available imaging techniques offer complementary information that can be useful in determining disease activity and monitoring for progression of vascular damage.

INTRODUCTION

Over the past 20 years, there has been a dramatic expansion in the investigation and use of various imaging techniques in the diagnosis and monitoring of large vessel vasculitis (LVV). Although large vessel involvement can occur in numerous rheumatic diseases, the main focus has centered around 2 primary systemic vasculitides: Giant Cell Arteritis (GCA) and Takayasu's Arteritis (TAK). Although histologically similar, GCA and TAK are distinguished by age of onset (GCA incidence increases with age after 50 years, TAK is most commonly diagnosed in the third decade of life) and by vascular distribution.[1,2] TAK primarily affects the vessels of the aortic arch and spares the temporal arteries. While GCA is traditionally thought of as affecting the cranial arteries (the common superficial temporal artery and its branches), there has been greater recognition of the burden of large vessel involvement and isolated large vessel disease. Studies of newly diagnosed patients with GCA have shown that large vessel involvement is present in over 60% at diagnosis, with the majority of these patients lacking associated claudication symptoms or physical examination findings to indicate vascular

a Division of Immunology & Rheumatology, Stanford University, 300 Pasteur Drive, East Pavilion, Floor 3, Room H335, Palo Alto, CA 94304-5755, USA; b Division of Rheumatology, Cedars-Sinai Medical Center, 8700 Beverly Boulevard, Suite B131, Los Angeles, CA 90048, USA
* Corresponding author.
E-mail address: ahoroman@stanford.edu

Rheum Dis Clin N Am 49 (2023) 489–504
https://doi.org/10.1016/j.rdc.2023.03.001
0889-857X/23/© 2023 Elsevier Inc. All rights reserved.

abnormalities to the clinician.[3–5] Furthermore, while large vessel disease in patients with GCA has been associated with a decreased risk of cranial ischemia, it has also been linked with an increased risk of relapse and higher glucocorticoid requirements.[6,7] These clinical and prognostic implications of large vessel involvement in GCA has led to increased use of imaging in both diagnosis and monitoring of the disease.

While the diagnosis of TAK has always depended on imaging due to the lack of an easily accessible biopsy target, temporal artery biopsy (TAB) has been the presumed gold standard for the diagnosis for GCA. However, many studies have highlighted the pitfalls of TAB, namely the declining sensitivity, differences in sampling techniques, the impact of glucocorticoid duration prior to biopsy, and the increased awareness of large vessel involvement that is not assessed by TAB.[8–10] Furthermore, the majority of patients with a negative TAB are continued on immunosuppressive therapy on the basis of clinical presentation, suggesting that TAB has limited impact on clinical management.[11,12] In recently updated guidelines, both the American College of Rheumatology (ACR) and the European Alliance of Associations for Rheumatology (EULAR) have emphasized the importance of confirming a suspected diagnosis of GCA through imaging or histology.[13,14] With the known challenges of TAB, clinicians are increasingly relying on imaging for diagnosis, as well as for monitoring of disease progression and its known associated vascular complications over time.

This review will discuss the use of various imaging techniques in the diagnosis and management of GCA and TAK, including ultrasound, ^{18}F-flurodeoxyglucose (FDG) positron emission tomography (PET), magnetic resonance imaging (MRI), and computed tomography (CT). Although historically relevant, catheter-based angiography has fallen out of favor due to the higher risk of complication and is no longer recommended for routine use in LVV.[13,14]

ULTRASOUND
Ultrasound for Giant Cell Arteritis

Giant cell arteritis diagnosis

Launched by the seminal publication by Schmidt and colleagues in 1997, data supporting the use of ultrasound in the diagnosis and monitoring of LVV have grown exponentially.[15] Improvements in ultrasound technology and the use of high-frequency transducers (>15 MHz) have improved resolution and allowed for greater visualization of the intima-media complex (IMC) and associated vasculitic changes. Color Doppler is typically used to highlight the demarcation between the vessel wall and lumen. Granulomatous inflammation of the vessel wall causes edema and visible thickening of the IMC. The most common findings of GCA on cranial artery US include the halo sign, defined as "homogenous, hypoechoic wall thickening, well delineated toward the luminal side, visible both in longitudinal and transverse planes, most commonly concentric in transverse scans" and the compression sign, defined as when the "thickened arterial wall remains visible upon compression; hypoechoic vasculitic vessel wall thickening contrasts with the mid-echoic to hyperechogenic surrounding tissue" (**Fig. 1**).[16,17] While the halo sign can be observed in all arteries, compression ability remains limited to the superficial vessels. The intima-media thickness (IMT) can also be measured to further confirm vessel wall edema. In a control group of 70-year-old patients, the mean IMT of the temporal and axillary arteries measured 0.2 mm and 0.6 mm respectively. To maximize sensitivity and specificity, cutoffs of 0.4 mm for the temporal arteries and 1.0 mm for the axillary arteries are used to distinguish vasculitic changes from normal vessels.[18,19] Other findings reported in GCA include stenosis, occlusion, and transition points whereby a thickened vessel wall gradually

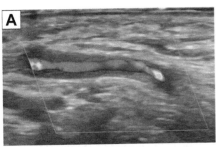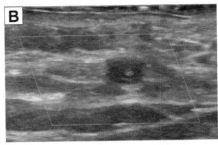

Fig. 1. Ultrasound of the common superficial temporal artery in longitudinal (*A*) and transverse (*B*) views demonstrating the halo sign in a patient with newly diagnosed GCA. (*Courtesy of* C Ponte, MD, PhD, Lisbon, Portugal.)

slopes down to a normal level (termed the "slope sign"), although these are not included in the diagnostic framework.[16,20]

A meta-analysis of the diagnostic performance of US in GCA found a pooled sensitivity of 77% and specificity of 96%.[21] When compared with a clinical diagnosis of GCA, the sensitivity was found to be 86% to 89%.[21] US also had high inter- and intra-rater agreement (91%–99%) with mean kappa values of 0.83 to 0.98 in the OMERACT US working group.[16] The TABUL study which compared US to TAB in the diagnosis of GCA found that the interclass correlation coefficient was similar between sonographers reviewing US images to pathologists reviewing biopsies (0.61 and 0.62 respectively).[9]

These promising findings have led to the development of GCA fast-track clinics in which patients with suspected GCA are evaluated with US, typically within 24 hours. The timing of evaluation is important due to a gradual decrease in US findings after glucocorticoid treatment is initiated. While many patients will have persistent vessel wall edema for months after starting treatment, some patients will have the resolution of findings within several days which can decrease the sensitivity of the exam.[9] The temporal artery halos have been shown to resolve more quickly compared with the large extracranial vessels which can be found even years after diagnosis.[22,23] Likely due to this slower resolution, the inclusion of the bilateral axillary arteries in addition to the common superficial temporal artery and the frontal and parietal branches improves diagnostic accuracy and is common practice in fast-track clinics.[24] In cases whereby there is uncertainty, the examination can be expanded to include the subclavian, carotid, facial, and vertebral arteries which can all show vessel wall inflammation. Several studies have shown that the implementation of fast-track clinics reduced the risk of permanent visual impairment in patients seen at the respective institutions.[25,26] Based on these data, the 2018 EULAR recommendations include temporal and axillary US evaluation as the first imaging modality recommended for the diagnosis of new-onset GCA. They acknowledge that an additional imaging modality or TAB may be needed if the diagnosis is unclear.[27] The 2021 ACR/Vasculitis Foundation guidelines recommended TAB over ultrasound due to less experience with the US in the United States compared with Europe, but note that it can be used as a complementary tool in centers whereby there is appropriate training and expertise.[13]

Giant cell arteritis monitoring

As previously noted, vessel wall edema represented as the halo sign gradually decreases after the initiation of therapy, more quickly in the temporal arteries compared with the extracranial arteries.[22] Ponte and colleagues similarly noted a gradual decrease in the number of segments with a halo sign as well as the sum of the halo IMT in their prospective study of newly diagnosed patients with GCA. They also observed an increase in the halo IMT in all assessed patients with disease flares compared with the previous US assessment.[23] This finding is supported by several other studies suggesting that the US may be sensitive to changes in disease activity, although the interval and extent of repeated assessments require further investigation.[28]

Ultrasound for Takayasu's Arteritis

Similar findings to GCA are seen in patients with TAK, although with some differences in vascular distribution. Increased IMT can be seen in the branches of the aortic arch, particularly the common carotid, axillary, and subclavian arteries. This was originally termed the "macaroni sign" in 1991, but is the same pathology represented by the halo sign as described above.[29] Although there are fewer studies compared with GCA, a meta-analysis found that the pooled sensitivity for diagnosis of TAK by US was 81% and that US detected more abnormal lesions compared with catheter-based angiography.[30]

Given the need for regular and repeated imaging in patients with TAK, there has also been interest in the use of US in disease monitoring. Svensson and colleagues showed that the IMT decreased significantly in newly diagnosis patients after the initiation of treatment. They also noted an increase in IMT in all five patients who had clinical and/or laboratory signs of relapse during the study.[31] In association with clinical symptoms, US can be a useful tool in diagnosis and monitoring, although frequently additional cross-sectional imaging is needed for assessment of the thoracic aorta which cannot be adequately evaluated by US (**Table 1**).

^{18}F-FLURODEOXYGLUCOSE POSITRON EMISSION TOMOGRAPHY/COMPUTED TOMOGRAPHY

Positron Emission Tomography for Large Vessel Vasculitis Diagnosis

Traditionally utilized in the field of oncology, PET/CT has gained expanded indications as technology and clinical experience have advanced. As a functional imaging technique, FDG-PET/CT detects elevated glucose uptake from the high glycolytic activity of inflammatory cells, such as those present in the vessel walls of patients with arteritis (**Fig. 2**).[32] In cases of suspected GCA, PET/CT has shown high diagnostic accuracy for both large vessel and cranial disease. A prospective study of patients with suspected new-onset GCA found that PET/CT had a sensitivity of 92% and specificity of 85% when compared with TAB and a sensitivity of 71% and specificity of 91% when compared with clinical diagnosis.[33] A meta-analysis of 8 studies on the diagnosis of LVV (both GCA and TAK) found that the pooled sensitivity and specificity of PET/CT were 75.9% and 93.0%, respectively.[34] When limiting to the 3 studies that included only GCA, the pooled sensitivity and specificity of PET/CT were 83.3% and 89.6%, respectively.[34] Another useful aspect of PET/CT is the ability to also assess for alternative diagnoses, particularly in patients with nonspecific symptoms. In patients with fever of unknown origin (FUO) or inflammation of unknown origin (IUO), PET/CT has been shown to identify malignancies, infections, and other noninfectious inflammatory disorders in addition to LVV.[35]

One significant limitation of PET/CT is the impact of glucocorticoids on sensitivity. In a study of newly diagnosed patients with GCA with confirmed large vessel involvement, PET/CT showed decreased uptake after 3 days of high-dose glucocorticoids, but still accurately diagnosed 10/10 patients. However, after 10 days of treatment, only 5/14 patients continued to have uptake consistent with LVV.[36] Other limitations

Table 1
Comparison of imaging techniques in patients with large vessel vasculitis imaging technique

	Findings	Advantages	Limitations	Primary Application
Ultrasound	• Wall thickening (halo, compression sign) • Vessel wall edema (IMT 0.4 mm for temporal arteries; 1.0 mm for axillary arteries)	• No radiation • Inexpensive	• Cannot image thoracic aorta • Requires training and expertise	• Diagnosis of GCA
18F-FDG PET/CT	• 18F-FDG metabolism reflecting increased glucose metabolism	• Assessment of alternate diagnoses (ie, malignancies, infections) • Whole body assessment	• Cost • Availability • Radiation • Variations in imaging protocol • Decreased sensitivity with glucocorticoid use	• Diagnosis of LVV • Assessment of LVV disease activity
MRI/A	• Wall thickening • Mural contrast enhancement • Luminal abnormalities (stenosis, occlusion, aneurysm)	• No radiation • Detection of active inflammation and structural lesions simultaneously • Cranial and body arterial assessment	• Cost • Availability • Time-consuming • Findings may not be specific to vasculitis (ie, atherosclerosis) • Not feasible with some metal devices • Claustrophobia • Contraindication for contrast in setting of renal insufficiency	• Diagnosis of LVV • Monitoring of LVV complications
CT/A	• Circumferential wall thickening with enhancement ("double ring sign")	• Shorter scanning time • Detects structural lesions with high resolution (preferred to monitor aneurysms)	• Radiation • Iodine-based contrast medium (limits those with allergy or renal insufficiency)	• Diagnosis of LVV • Monitoring of LVV complications

(continued on next page)

Table 1
(continued)

	Findings	Advantages	Limitations	Primary Application
	• Luminal abnormalities (stenosis, occlusion, aneurysm)	• Best to distinguish atheroma from vasculitis		
Angiography	• Stenoses and aneurysms can be seen	• Guides interventional procedures	• No signs of early vasculitis able to be detected (ie, wall thickening) • Radiation • Requires invasive cannulation via femoral access	• Recommended for use during interventional procedures

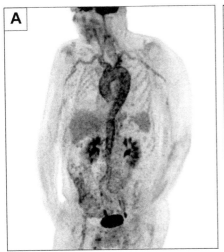 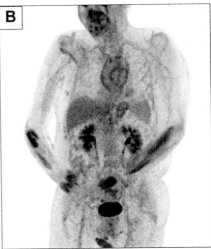

Fig. 2. 70 y/o male with biopsy-proven giant cell arteritis with initial FDG-PET scan (*A*) showing diffuse vascular FDG uptake throughout the aorta and subclavian arteries. The patient was treated with glucocorticoids and tocilizumab and repeat FDG-PET scan 6 months later (*B*) shows significant reduction in vascular FDG uptake. (*Courtesy of* Kaitlin A. Quinn, MD on behalf of the NIAMS Vasculitis Translational Research Program, Bethesda, MD.)

of PET/CT include cost, availability, radiation exposure, and variations in imaging protocol (see **Table 1**). In particular, the timing of imaging after FDG injection appears to affect the sensitivity for active vasculitis. In sequential assessments of the same patients, Quinn and colleagues found that a higher proportion of studies were interpreted as active vasculitis 2 hours after FDG injection compared to 1 hour: 77% versus 56% respectively.[37]

Positron Emission Tomography for Large Vessel Vasculitis Monitoring

Monitoring of disease activity in patients with LVV can be challenging, particularly in those receiving tocilizumab where inflammatory markers are no longer reliable. Banerjee and colleagues found that disease activity in patients with GCA and TAK as measured by the PETVAS (PET Vascular Activity Score) composite summary score decreased in patients where therapy was increased and increased when therapy was tapered. Notably, while FDG-PET avidity decreased from baseline, rarely did they find that the assessment returned to normal.[38] Supporting these findings, a meta-analysis of longitudinal studies in patients with LVV found consistently that FDG uptake decreases with treatment-induced remission, although not all returned to normal.[39] It has been suggested that this residual signal may be due to either smoldering inflammation or vascular remodeling, as can be seen in patients with atherosclerosis.[40] The extent of FDG-PET avidity at diagnosis has not been shown to correlate with the risk of relapse or refractory disease, although higher levels of FDG-PET activity during times of clinical remission have been associated with higher risk of future relapse.[3,41]

Another area of interest is whether FDG-PET activity at baseline can predict future angiographic damage. In a longitudinal study of 70 patients with GCA or TAK, Quinn and colleagues found that over 1.5 to 1.8 years of follow-up, only 1% of arterial territories developed new angiographic damage, and only in patients with TAK. However, of those areas that did have angiographic progression, 80% had baseline FDG-PET activity, which yielded nearly 20 times increased odds of future damage compared to an area without FDG-PET activity at baseline.[42]

MAGNETIC RESONANCE IMAGING AND MR ANGIOGRAPHY
Magnetic Resonance Imaging for Giant Cell Arteritis Diagnosis

Cranial giant cell arteritis

As noted above, EULAR recommends temporal artery ultrasound ($\pm$ axillary arteries) as the first imaging modality in those with suspected cranial GCA.[27] If ultrasound is not available or inconclusive, high-resolution MRI of the cranial arteries can be used to investigate mural inflammation and to assist with the diagnosis of GCA. In a prospective multicenter trial of 185 patients with GCA with clinical diagnosis serving as the gold standard (53% with TAB), the sensitivity of high-resolution MRI of the cranial arteries was 78.4% and the specificity was 90.4%, with the sensitivity decreasing after more than 5 days of systemic corticosteroid use.[43] The sensitivity and specificity of high-resolution MRI and color-coded duplex US of the temporal arteries in detecting mural inflammation in cranial GCA are comparable.[44] In a metanalysis of 39 GCA studies that were used to inform the recent EULAR guidelines, MRI of the cranial arteries and US ("halo sign") of the temporal arteries yielded pooled sensitivities of 73% and 77%, respectively, compared with a clinical diagnosis of GCA. Corresponding pooled specificities were 88% and 96%. When TAB was used as the reference standard, MRI of cranial arteries yielded a pooled sensitivity of 93% and specificity of 81%.[21]

An MRI scanner with a high magnetic field strength of preferably 3 T should be used with an 8-channel head-coil, and a Gd contrast-enhanced T1-weighted spin echo sequence with fat saturation gives the best results for the diagnosis of cranial GCA.[45,46] T2-weighted turbo spin sequences are significantly less sensitive to detect edema in mural inflammation and are more prone to artifact.[45] Depiction of mural inflammation in the superficial temporal arteries is shown with wall thickening, and mural contrast enhancement that is pronounced in active disease but decreases with corticosteroid treatment (**Fig. 3**) (see **Table 1**).[47]

Whether or not MRI is an acceptable surrogate for TAB in GCA remains controversial.[48] Based on studies where patients with GCA underwent MRI using TAB as the diagnostic gold standard, a normal temporal artery by high-resolution MR correlates closely with a negative TAB.[48] Rhéaume and colleagues demonstrated in 171 patients with GCA using TAB as the gold standard that high resolution MRI of the cranial arteries had a negative predictive value of 98.2%.[49] This suggests that TAB may be potentially avoided in those with normal scalp MRIs.[48] This study also found 2 suspected patients with GCA with isolated occipital artery abnormalities on MRI, only one of which had a positive TAB.[49] Therefore, while cases of sole inflammation of the superficial occipital arteries have been identified by this technique, their diagnostic and clinical implications need further study.[46,50] The ACR/VF guidelines acknowledge the limited applicability of MRI of the cranial vessels as a replacement for TAB due to the lack of technical expertise with this modality in the US.[13] While availability of MRI for cranial artery assessment is limited because

only a few centers provide the technical expertise and/or equipment, body MRI for large vessel assessment is more widely available.[51]

Extracranial Giant Cell Arteritis

MRI can be used to detect mural inflammation and/or luminal changes in extracranial arteries to support the diagnosis of LV GCA. Literature regarding the diagnostic performance of MRA for LVV diagnosis is limited. Using clinical diagnosis as the gold

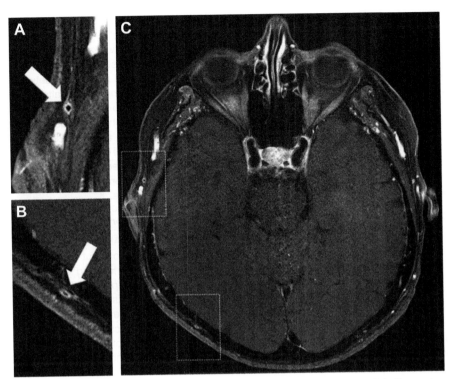

Fig. 3. High-resolution cranial 3 T MRI of a 72-year-old lady with GCA reveals inflammatory mural thickening and contrast enhancement of the right superficial temporal artery (*white arrow* in enlargement A) and right superficial occipital artery (*white arrow* in enlargement B). By depicting the entire cranial circumference the superficial temporal and occipital arteries and their branches can be assessed with one single scan (*C*). (Image courtesy of Dr. T. A. Bley.)

standard, Adler and colleagues demonstrated a sensitivity of 79% and specificity of 96% for MRA to detect inflammatory aortic involvement in GCA.[52] MR combined with MR angiography (MRA) enables assessment of the majority of the body's vasculature and allows the evaluation of vessel walls and lumens, as well as surrounding tissue simultaneously.[45] A 3.0 T MRI scanner with an 8-channel head and neck coil and a 16-channel body coil are used preferentially.[45] Edema, thickening, and contrast enhancement of vessel walls on MRI are suggestive of active vasculitis and a fair agreement with PET findings in large arteries has been reported.[51] When comparing MRI to PET in LVV, a study by Quinn and colleagues that evaluated 35 GCA and 30 patients with TAK revealed that MRA was better at capturing disease extent, whereas PET was better at assessing vascular activity.[53] A contrast-enhanced, fat-suppressed, high-resolution T1-weighted spin echo sequence is the most valuable sequence for detecting mural inflammation in MR imaging.[45] Luminal abnormalities (stenosis, occlusion and aneurysm) can be evaluated by MRA and provide information regarding disease extent and damage (see **Table 1**).[51]

Magnetic Resonance Imaging for Takayasu's Arteritis Diagnosis

MRI is the imaging test of choice to make a diagnosis of TAK.[27] A metanalysis by Barra and colleagues showed that MRA had a higher pooled sensitivity of 92% compared with ultrasound of 81% and both had high pooled specificities of greater than 90% for TAK diagnosis.[30] Another study investigated MRA for the diagnosis of TAK using conventional angiography as the reference standard and found a sensitivity and specificity of 100%.[54] Although fewer studies investigated CTA, the pooled sensitivity, and specificity for TAK diagnosis was high (>90%) and there is generally good agreement between CTA and FDG-PET.[30] Therefore, CTA, US, and FDG-PET/CT may be used as alternative imaging modalities to MRI in patients with suspected TAK. Due to its invasiveness and lack of adequate vessel wall imaging, conventional angiography has been mostly replaced by these less invasive imaging techniques.[45] With MRI/A, a generalized arterial survey can be done in Takayasu's and the entire aorta and its wall can be seen without radiation, which is important for young patients who will likely require repeat studies over their disease course (see **Table 1**). Vessel wall edema, contrast enhancement, and/or wall thickening are characteristic findings in active disease.[55]

Magnetic Resonance Imaging for Large Vessel Vasculitis Monitoring

The role of MRI/MRA in the monitoring of disease activity in TAK is still a matter of further research. MRI findings diminish after immunosuppression, but inflammatory changes may persist despite clinical remission. Vascular remodeling may cause increased mural contrast enhancement and thus lead to false-positive MRI results. There is limited predictive power for the development of new vascular lesions as patients with TAK may have no disease progression despite persistent vessel wall edema, and some may develop new lesions at sites without vessel wall edema.[56,57] The metanalysis previously described by Barra and colleagues of imaging modalities for TAK showed that the utility of vessel wall thickening and enhancement by MRA (and CTA) to predict disease activity varied across studies.[30] MRA is good for the initial diagnosis of aortitis and to monitor for future aneurysm formation or arterial stenoses (see **Table 1**). In recent EULAR guidelines, repeat imaging for patients with TAK in clinical remission was not routinely recommended.[27] In contrast, the ACR/VF guidelines recommend regularly scheduled non-invasive imaging in TAK in addition to routine clinical assessment for long-term monitoring of structural damage. However, the optimal interval between imaging was not well established (every 3–6 months or longer).[13] EULAR and ACR/VF guidelines both acknowledge that imaging in patients with large vessel involvement (GCA or TAK) may be used for long-term monitoring of structural damage (stenosis, occlusion, dilation, and/or aneurysm), but the choice of imaging modalities and frequency of screening has yet to be defined and is left up to individual discretion.[13,27]

The advantages of MRI are the absence of radiation and the contemporaneous detection of structural lesions (vessel wall thickening, luminal stenosis/occlusion) and contrast-enhancement of the arterial wall which is presumed to reflect active inflammation.[27] Limitations of MRI include claustrophobia and patients with certain metal implants (cardiac pacemakers and defibrillators) cannot undergo this type of imaging. In addition, renal insufficiency may be a relative contra-indication for Gd-based contrast agents due to the risk of nephrogenic systemic fibrosis. MRI is expensive and may not be readily available everywhere. It is also time-consuming and results may not always be specific to vasculitis (see **Table 1**). For example, it may be difficult to differentiate vasculitis from atherosclerosis on imaging such as MRI. Long, smooth stenoses that symmetrically affect the vessel wall, along with a marked increase in vessel wall thickening on imaging can point toward vasculitis, whereas asymmetric and patchy lesions, particularly if associated with calcifications can suggest atherosclerosis.[55] Atherosclerotic lesions also do not typically show contrast enhancement in the wall, and wall thickening is usually eccentric and focal.[58] Further imaging studies are needed to include more quantified and standardized parameters to distinguish atheromatous plaques from vasculitis.

PET/MRI is a relatively new hybrid imaging modality that can allow comprehensive analysis of vascular wall inflammation and the vascular lumen and limit radiation exposure as compared with PET/CT, which is crucial for young patients with TAK.[59] Further studies regarding its clinical value for diagnosis and use in monitoring and assessing disease activity are necessary.

COMPUTED TOMOGRAPHY AND COMPUTED TOMOGRAPHY ANGIOGRAPHY
Diagnosis of Large Vessel Vasculitis

Like MRI, vessel wall edema and mural enhancement on CT are signs of active vasculitis.[55] Circumferential wall thickening with enhancement and the so called "double ring sign," or edematous inner wall with enhancing outer wall on delayed contrast-enhanced images, are also suggestive of active inflammation (see **Table 1**).[60]

CT can be used as an alternative imaging modality to MRI for the initial imaging test for TAK. One study examined the role of CTA compared with angiography and reported a sensitivity and specificity of 100%.[61] If there is a question of coronary involvement, coronary artery CTA can be acquired.[62] Kang and colleagues demonstrated that 52% of 111 patients with TAK had coronary artery lesions regardless of symptoms and disease activity.[63] Pulmonary arteries are also well visualized on CTA.[60]

CT can also be used to detect mural inflammation and/or luminal changes in extracranial arteries to support the diagnosis of LV GCA. In a study by Prieto-González et al. where CTA was performed on 40 patients with newly diagnosed biopsy-proven GCA who were treatment naïve (corticosteroids <3 days), LVV was detected in 27 patients (67.5%) at the time of diagnosis and aortic dilation was already present in 15%.[5] CTA is a commonly used imaging modality to detect large vessel involvement in GCA and the ACR/VF guidelines recommend obtaining vascular imaging (with CTA or MRI) in all patients with newly diagnosed GCA to evaluate for baseline large vessel involvement.[13]

Monitoring of Large Vessel Vasculitis

CT is useful in assessing complications of vasculitis and monitoring structural damage (stenosis, occlusion, dilation, and/or aneurysms).[27] Mural enhancement usually resolves or markedly improves with treatment, although its improvement may lag behind clinical and laboratory improvement.[55] Prieto-González et al. repeated CTAs on 40 biopsy-proven patients with GCA 1 year after treatment with corticosteroids and demonstrated that while contrast enhancement resolved in the majority of patients, vessel wall thickening persisted in two-thirds despite clinical remission.[64] Albeit, the number of affected aortic segments as well as aortic wall thickness significantly decreased, and there was no new involvement of previously spared segments. This may indicate that persistent vascular wall thickening represents fibrosis and vascular remodeling rather than major persistent inflammation.[64] After ≥ 5 years in chronic cases, calcification can develop in the vessel wall and CTA is a technique that can easily detect mural calcification and allow the distinction between focal thickening associated with atheroma and concentric thickening suggestive of vasculitis (see **Table 1**).[62]

The advantages of CT are its non-invasiveness compared with conventional catheter-based angiography and its ability to detect structural lesions with a higher resolution and shorter scanning time than MRA, allowing for more arterial regions to be evaluated in one session.[48] It is also the preferred method to monitor changes in aortic aneurysm morphology over time.[53] A major advantage of CTA is its ability to differentiate atherosclerosis from vasculitis, which is particularly important in LV GCA whereby atherosclerotic disease is common due to the age of the affected population. Limitations of CT include its exposure to a significant amount of ionizing radiation which limits its repeated use in young individuals, and its use of iodine-based contrast medium injections in patients who have an iodine allergy or severe kidney dysfunction (see **Table 1**).[62]

ANGIOGRAPHY

Conventional angiography is no longer recommended in the diagnosis and monitoring of LVV.[45] It cannot show early vasculitis lesions such as thickening of the vessel wall and therefore noninvasive imaging is recommended over catheter-based dye angiography to assess disease activity (see **Table 1**).[13] Its role is primarily in guiding interventional procedures, but it involves exposure to ionizing radiation, requires invasive cannulation via femoral access, and carries a risk of complications, including allergic reactions, hematoma, iatrogenic embolization resulting in permanent stroke, and arterial dissection.[27,55] If obtained in the setting of interventional procedures, vascular complications such as stenoses or aneurysms can be ascertained.

SUMMARY

Technological advances and increased recognition of the prevalence and implications of LVV have led to robust research into many imaging techniques. Although there is still debate about which modality to choose in various clinical scenarios, clinicians now have numerous options that are safe and noninvasive. Ultrasound, PET/CT, MR/A, and CT/A offer complementary information regarding diagnosis and disease activity. Future investigations will continue to highlight the strengths and limitations of each technique in the diagnosis and management of large vessel vasculitis.

CLINICS CARE POINTS

- Large vessel involvement is present at diagnosis in over 60% of patients with GCA. Imaging (MRA, PET/CT, or CTA) is important for initial detection as well as monitoring over the course of the disease as most patients lack indicative symptoms or physical examination findings.
- When used for diagnosis of GCA, imaging should be performed within 3 days of steroid initiation to maximize the sensitivity. If conducted later in the treatment course, the results of the study should be interpreted with this associated context.
- While no imaging modality is perfect for all clinical situations, ultrasound, PET/CT, MRA, and CT/A can be leveraged for their varying strengths and tailored to each individual patient with large vessel vasculitis.

DISCLOSURE

A. Horomanski and L.J. Forbess have no financial or nonfinancial disclosures relevant to the content of this article.

REFERENCES

1. Hunder GG, Bloch DA, Michel BA, et al. The American College of Rheumatology 1990 criteria for the classification of giant cell arteritis. Arthritis Rheum 1990; 33(8):1122–8.

2. Arend WP, Michel BA, Bloch DA, et al. The American College of Rheumatology 1990 criteria for the classification of Takayasu arteritis. Arthritis Rheum 1990; 33(8):1129–34.
3. Blockmans D, de Ceuninck L, Vanderschueren S, et al. Repetitive 18F-fluoro-deoxyglucose positron emission tomography in giant cell arteritis: a prospective study of 35 patients. Arthritis Rheum 2006;55(1):131–7.
4. Muratore F, Kermani TA, Crowson CS, et al. Large-vessel giant cell arteritis: a cohort study. Rheumatol Oxf Engl 2015;54(3):463–70.
5. Prieto-González S, Arguis P, García-Martínez A, et al. Large vessel involvement in biopsy-proven giant cell arteritis: prospective study in 40 newly diagnosed patients using CT angiography. Ann Rheum Dis 2012;71(7):1170–6.
6. van der Geest KSM, Sandovici M, van Sleen Y, et al. Review: What Is the Current Evidence for Disease Subsets in Giant Cell Arteritis? Arthritis Rheumatol Hoboken NJ 2018;70(9):1366–76.
7. Sugihara T, Hasegawa H, Uchida HA, et al. Associated factors of poor treatment outcomes in patients with giant cell arteritis: clinical implication of large vessel lesions. Arthritis Res Ther 2020;22(1):72.
8. Rubenstein E, Maldini C, Gonzalez-Chiappe S, et al. Sensitivity of temporal artery biopsy in the diagnosis of giant cell arteritis: a systematic literature review and meta-analysis. Rheumatol Oxf Engl 2020;59(5):1011–20.
9. Luqmani R, Lee E, Singh S, et al. The Role of Ultrasound Compared to Biopsy of Temporal Arteries in the Diagnosis and Treatment of Giant Cell Arteritis (TABUL): a diagnostic accuracy and cost-effectiveness study. Health Technol Assess 2016;20(90):1–238.
10. Narváez J, Bernad B, Roig-Vilaseca D, et al. Influence of Previous Corticosteroid Therapy on Temporal Artery Biopsy Yield in Giant Cell Arteritis. Semin Arthritis Rheum 2007;37(1):13–9.
11. Lenton J, Donnelly R, Nash JR. Does temporal artery biopsy influence the management of temporal arteritis? QJM Int J Med 2006;99(1):33–6.
12. Bowling K, Rait J, Atkinson J, et al. Temporal artery biopsy in the diagnosis of giant cell arteritis: Does the end justify the means? Ann Med Surg 2017;20:1–5.
13. Maz M, Chung SA, Abril A, et al. American College of Rheumatology/Vasculitis Foundation Guideline for the Management of Giant Cell Arteritis and Takayasu Arteritis. Arthritis Rheumatol 2021;73(8):1349–65.
14. Hellmich B, Agueda A, Monti S, et al. Update of the EULAR recommendations for the management of large vessel vasculitis. Ann Rheum Dis 2020;79(1):19–30.
15. Schmidt WA, Kraft HE, Vorpahl K, et al. Color duplex ultrasonography in the diagnosis of temporal arteritis. N Engl J Med 1997;337(19):1336–42.
16. Chrysidis S, Duftner C, Dejaco C, et al. Definitions and reliability assessment of elementary ultrasound lesions in giant cell arteritis: a study from the OMERACT Large Vessel Vasculitis Ultrasound Working Group. RMD Open 2018;4(1): e000598.
17. Aschwanden M, Daikeler T, Kesten F, et al. Temporal artery compression sign–a novel ultrasound finding for the diagnosis of giant cell arteritis. Ultraschall Med Stuttg Ger 1980 2013;34(1):47–50.
18. Ješe R, Ž Rotar, Tomšič M, et al. The cut-off values for the intima-media complex thickness assessed by colour Doppler sonography in seven cranial and aortic arch arteries. Rheumatol Oxf Engl 2021;60(3):1346–52.
19. Schäfer VS, Juche A, Ramiro S, et al. Ultrasound cut-off values for intima-media thickness of temporal, facial and axillary arteries in giant cell arteritis. Rheumatol Oxf Engl 2017;56(9):1479–83.

20. Dasgupta B, Smith K, Khan AAS, et al. Slope sign': a feature of large vessel vasculitis? Ann Rheum Dis 2019;78(12):1738.

21. Duftner C, Dejaco C, Sepriano A, et al. Imaging in diagnosis, outcome prediction and monitoring of large vessel vasculitis: a systematic literature review and meta-analysis informing the EULAR recommendations. RMD Open 2018;4(1):e000612.

22. Aschwanden M, Schegk E, Imfeld S, et al. Vessel wall plasticity in large vessel giant cell arteritis: an ultrasound follow-up study. Rheumatol Oxf Engl 2019; 58(5):792–7.

23. Ponte C, Monti S, Scirè CA, et al. Ultrasound halo sign as a potential monitoring tool for patients with giant cell arteritis: a prospective analysis. Ann Rheum Dis 2021;80(11):1475–82.

24. Hop H, Mulder DJ, Sandovici M, et al. Diagnostic value of axillary artery ultrasound in patients with suspected giant cell arteritis. Rheumatol Oxf Engl 2020; 59(12):3676–84.

25. Diamantopoulos AP, Haugeberg G, Lindland A, et al. The fast-track ultrasound clinic for early diagnosis of giant cell arteritis significantly reduces permanent visual impairment: towards a more effective strategy to improve clinical outcome in giant cell arteritis? Rheumatol Oxf Engl 2016;55(1):66–70.

26. Monti S, Bartoletti A, Bellis E, et al. Fast-Track Ultrasound Clinic for the Diagnosis of Giant Cell Arteritis Changes the Prognosis of the Disease but Not the Risk of Future Relapse. Front Med 2020;7:589794.

27. Dejaco C, Ramiro S, Duftner C, et al. EULAR recommendations for the use of imaging in large vessel vasculitis in clinical practice. Ann Rheum Dis 2018;77(5): 636–43.

28. Monti S, Floris A, Ponte CB, et al. The proposed role of ultrasound in the management of giant cell arteritis in routine clinical practice. Rheumatol Oxf Engl 2018; 57(1):112–9.

29. Maeda H, Handa N, Matsumoto M, et al. Carotid lesions detected by B-mode ultrasonography in Takayasu's arteritis: "macaroni sign" as an indicator of the disease. Ultrasound Med Biol 1991;17(7):695–701.

30. Barra L, Kanji T, Malette J, et al. Imaging modalities for the diagnosis and disease activity assessment of Takayasu's arteritis: A systematic review and meta-analysis. Autoimmun Rev 2018;17(2):175–87.

31. Svensson C, Eriksson P, Zachrisson H. Vascular ultrasound for monitoring of inflammatory activity in Takayasu arteritis. Clin Physiol Funct Imaging 2020;40(1): 37–45.

32. Slart RHJA, Slart RHJA, Glaudemans AWJM, et al. FDG-PET/CT(A) imaging in large vessel vasculitis and polymyalgia rheumatica: joint procedural recommendation of the EANM, SNMMI, and the PET Interest Group (PIG), and endorsed by the ASNC. Eur J Nucl Med Mol Imaging 2018;45(7):1250–69.

33. Sammel AM, Hsiao E, Schembri G, et al. Diagnostic Accuracy of Positron Emission Tomography/Computed Tomography of the Head, Neck, and Chest for Giant Cell Arteritis: A Prospective, Double-Blind, Cross-Sectional Study. Arthritis Rheumatol Hoboken NJ 2019;71(8):1319–28.

34. Lee YH, Choi SJ, Ji JD, et al. Diagnostic accuracy of 18F-FDG PET or PET/CT for large vessel vasculitis : A meta-analysis. Z Rheumatol 2016;75(9):924–31.

35. Schönau V, Vogel K, Englbrecht M, et al. The value of 18F-FDG-PET/CT in identifying the cause of fever of unknown origin (FUO) and inflammation of unknown origin (IUO): data from a prospective study. Ann Rheum Dis 2018;77(1):70–7.

36. Nielsen BD, Gormsen LC, Hansen IT, et al. Three days of high-dose glucocorticoid treatment attenuates large-vessel 18F-FDG uptake in large-vessel giant

cell arteritis but with a limited impact on diagnostic accuracy. Eur J Nucl Med Mol Imaging 2018;45(7):1119–28.

37. Quinn KA, Rosenblum JS, Rimland CA, et al. Imaging acquisition technique influences interpretation of positron emission tomography vascular activity in large-vessel vasculitis. Semin Arthritis Rheum 2020;50(1):71–6.

38. Banerjee S, Quinn KA, Gribbons KB, et al. Effect of Treatment on Imaging, Clinical, and Serologic Assessments of Disease Activity in Large-vessel Vasculitis. J Rheumatol 2020;47(1):99–107.

39. van der Geest KSM, Treglia G, Glaudemans AWJM, et al. Diagnostic value of [18F]FDG-PET/CT for treatment monitoring in large vessel vasculitis: a systematic review and meta-analysis. Eur J Nucl Med Mol Imaging 2021;48(12):3886–902.

40. Sadeghi MM. 18F-FDG PET and Vascular Inflammation; Time to Refine the Paradigm? J Nucl Cardiol Off Publ Am Soc Nucl Cardiol 2015;22(2):319–24.

41. Grayson PC, Alehashemi S, Bagheri AA, et al. 18 F-Fluorodeoxyglucose-Positron Emission Tomography As an Imaging Biomarker in a Prospective, Longitudinal Cohort of Patients With Large Vessel Vasculitis. Arthritis Rheumatol Hoboken NJ 2018;70(3):439–49.

42. Quinn KA, Ahlman MA, Alessi HD, et al. Association of 18F-Fluorodeoxyglucose Positron Emission Tomography and Angiographic Progression of Disease in Large-Vessel Vasculitis. Arthritis Rheumatol Hoboken NJ 2022. https://doi.org/10.1002/art.42290.

43. Klink T, Geiger J, Both M, et al. Giant cell arteritis: diagnostic accuracy of MR imaging of superficial cranial arteries in initial diagnosis-results from a multicenter trial. Radiology 2014;273(3):844–52.

44. Guggenberger KV, Bley TA. Magnetic resonance imaging and magnetic resonance angiography in large-vessel vasculitides. Clin Exp Rheumatol 2018; 36(Suppl 114):103–7.

45. Guggenberger KV, Bley TA. Imaging in Vasculitis. Curr Rheumatol Rep 2020; 22(8):34.

46. Blockmans D, Bley T, Schmidt W. Imaging for large-vessel vasculitis. Curr Opin Rheumatol 2009;21(1):19–28.

47. Blockmans D, Luqmani R, Spaggiari L, et al. Magnetic resonance angiography versus 18F-fluorodeoxyglucose positron emission tomography in large vessel vasculitis. Autoimmun Rev 2019;18(12):102405.

48. Quinn KA, Grayson PC. The Role of Vascular Imaging to Advance Clinical Care and Research in Large-Vessel Vasculitis. Curr Treat Options Rheumatol 2019; 5(1):20–35.

49. Rhéaume M, Rebello R, Pagnoux C, et al. High-Resolution Magnetic Resonance Imaging of Scalp Arteries for the Diagnosis of Giant Cell Arteritis: Results of a Prospective Cohort Study. Arthritis Rheumatol Hoboken NJ 2017;69(1):161–8.

50. Bley TA, Weiben O, Uhl M, et al. Assessment of the cranial involvement pattern of giant cell arteritis with 3T magnetic resonance imaging. Arthritis Rheum 2005; 52(8):2470–7.

51. Schmidt WA, Nielsen BD. Imaging in large-vessel vasculitis. Best Pract Res Clin Rheumatol 2020;34(6):101589.

52. Adler S, Sprecher M, Wermelinger F, et al. Diagnostic value of contrast-enhanced magnetic resonance angiography in large-vessel vasculitis. Swiss Med Wkly 2017;147:w14397.

53. Quinn KA, Ahlman MA, Malayeri AA, et al. Comparison of magnetic resonance angiography and 18F-fluorodeoxyglucose positron emission tomography in large-vessel vasculitis. Ann Rheum Dis 2018;77(8):1165–71.

54. Yamada I, Nakagawa T, Himeno Y, et al. Takayasu arteritis: diagnosis with breath-hold contrast-enhanced three-dimensional MR angiography. J Magn Reson Imaging JMRI 2000;11(5):481–7.

55. Pipitone N, Versari A, Hunder GG, et al. Role of imaging in the diagnosis of large and medium-sized vessel vasculitis. Rheum Dis Clin North Am 2013;39(3): 593–608.

56. Tso E, Flamm SD, White RD, et al. Takayasu arteritis: utility and limitations of magnetic resonance imaging in diagnosis and treatment. Arthritis Rheum 2002;46(6): 1634–42.

57. Eshet Y, Pauzner R, Goitein O, et al. The limited role of MRI in long-term follow-up of patients with Takayasu's arteritis. Autoimmun Rev 2011;11(2):132–6.

58. Nienhuis PH, van Praagh GD, Glaudemans AWJM, et al. A Review on the Value of Imaging in Differentiating between Large Vessel Vasculitis and Atherosclerosis. J Pers Med 2021;11(3):236.

59. Laurent C, Ricard L, Fain O, et al. PET/MRI in large-vessel vasculitis: clinical value for diagnosis and assessment of disease activity. Sci Rep 2019;9(1):12388.

60. Poyyamoli S, Swamiappan E, Gandhi J, et al. Non-aortic vascular findings on chest CT angiogram: including arch vessels and bronchial arteries. Cardiovasc Diagn Ther 2019;9(Suppl 1):S59–73.

61. Sun Y, Ma L, Ji Z, et al. Value of whole-body contrast-enhanced magnetic resonance angiography with vessel wall imaging in quantitative assessment of disease activity and follow-up examination in Takayasu's arteritis. Clin Rheumatol 2016;35(3):685–93.

62. Aghayev A. Multimodality Imaging of Large-Vessel Vasculitis, From the AJR Special Series on Inflammation. Am J Roentgenol 2022;218(2):213–22.

63. Kang EJ, Kim SM, Choe YH, et al. Takayasu arteritis: assessment of coronary arterial abnormalities with 128-section dual-source CT angiography of the coronary arteries and aorta. Radiology 2014;270(1):74–81.

64. Prieto-González S, García-Martínez A, Tavera-Bahillo I, et al. Effect of Glucocorticoid Treatment on Computed Tomography Angiography Detected Large-Vessel Inflammation in Giant-Cell Arteritis. A Prospective, Longitudinal Study. Medicine (Baltim) 2015;94(5):e486.

Giant Cell Arteritis and Polymyalgia Rheumatica
Treatment Approaches and New Targets

Desh Nepal, MD[a],*, Michael Putman, MD, MS[a],
Sebastian Unizony, MD[b]

KEYWORDS

- Giant cell arteritis • Polymyalgia rheumatica • Tocilizumab • Glucocorticoids
- Mavrilimumab • Secukinumab • Abatacept • Guselkumab

KEY POINTS

- Treatment with tocilizumab has substantially reduced glucocorticoid toxicity for patients with giant cell arteritis (GCA) and has become the standard of care.
- Many patients with GCA still relapse despite this approach, and additional therapies are being studied, including mavrilimumab, secukinumab, guselkumab, abatacept, and upadacitinib.
- Fewer options have been studied for patients with polymyalgia rheumatica, but trials of tocilizumab, sarilumab, and rituximab have recently been completed or are underway.

INTRODUCTION

Giant cell arteritis (GCA) and polymyalgia rheumatica (PMR) are systemic inflammatory conditions that affect people aged 50 years and older.[1] GCA is a granulomatous large-vessel vasculitis involving the aorta and its major branches.[2] It often presents with constitutional symptoms (fever, fatigue, weight loss), jaw pain upon mastication (ie, jaw claudication), new-onset headache,[3] scalp tenderness, and visual symptoms (eg, diplopia, amaurosis fugax, and transient blurred vision).[4] Permanent vision loss, most commonly due to anterior ischemic optic neuropathy (AION), is the most feared complication and occurs in 15% to 20% of patients.[4] Approximately half of the patients with GCA report PMR symptoms defined as pain and stiffness involving the shoulder and hip girdles that develop after periods of immobilization (eg, early morning) and improve with activities. PMR can also be seen in the absence of other GCA

[a] Department of Medicine, Division of Rheumatology, Hub for Collaborative Medicine, Medical College of Wisconsin, 8701 Watertown Plank Road, Rheumatology, 6th Floor, Milwaukee, WI 53226, USA; [b] Massachusetts General Hospital, Vasculitis and Glomerulonephritis Center, Harvard Medical School, 55 Fruit Street, Yawkey 4B, Boston, MA 02114, USA
* Corresponding author.
E-mail address: dnepal@mcw.edu

Rheum Dis Clin N Am 49 (2023) 505–521
https://doi.org/10.1016/j.rdc.2023.03.005
0889-857X/23/© 2023 Elsevier Inc. All rights reserved.

rheumatic.theclinics.com

manifestations in a condition called primary PMR, which is 3 times more frequent than GCA.[3–7]

The vascular inflammation in GCA is predominantly composed of CD4$^+$ T cells and macrophages. The classic pathology finding of multinucleated giant cells can also be seen in roughly half of temporal artery biopsy specimens and likely reflect the highly inflammatory nature of the vascular infiltrate.[8] Studies suggest that the inflammatory process is driven by T helper (Th)17 and Th1 CD4$^+$ cells and that regulatory T cells demonstrate an inflammatory phenotype and have an impaired suppressive function.[9–14] Substantial progress has been made in the treatment of patients affected by GCA, but many individuals receiving standard of care treatment continue to demonstrate residual arterial inflammation, have vascular imaging changes raising the concern for possible ongoing disease activity (vs vascular wall remodeling), and develop clinical relapses.[13,15]

In this review, we elaborate on the established and novel treatment approaches for GCA and PMR and discuss future therapeutic perspectives for these disorders.

CURRENT TREATMENT APPROACHES FOR GIANT CELL ARTERITIS AND POLYMYALGIA RHEUMATICA
Glucocorticoids for Giant Cell Arteritis

Glucocorticoids (eg, prednisone) have been the mainstay of treatment for GCA for decades and continue to be required upfront to establish disease control (ie, induction of remission) and prevent irreversible sight loss. Glucocorticoids affect both the innate and the adaptive immune systems, which include suppression of Th17 cells and macrophages. However, reports suggest that these agents may incompletely suppress the Th1 pathway,[16] which could explain the high relapse rate of GCA patients receiving glucocorticoid monotherapy.[17–19]

High-quality evidence to inform recommendations for glucocorticoid administration and initial dosing is not available, but observational studies have described better visual outcomes with the early use of glucocorticoids.[20–22] Based on lower-quality evidence and consensus of expert opinions, the 2021 American College of Rheumatology (ACR)/Vasculitis Foundation (VF)[23] and the 2018 European Alliance of Associations for Rheumatology (EULAR)[24] GCA guidelines recommend high-dose oral glucocorticoids when GCA is diagnosed or suspected. While the ACR/VF recommends an initial dose of 1 mg/kg/d (up to 80 mg) of prednisone or equivalent, EULAR recommends a dose of 40 to 60 mg/d.[24]

The efficacy of intravenous (IV) pulse glucocorticoids for the treatment or prevention of visual ischemia has not been formally tested in randomized controlled trials (RCTs), and low-quality evidence has shown conflicting results regarding the value of initial treatment with IV pulse glucocorticoids versus oral glucocorticoids in terms of visual recovery in GCA patients presenting with visual impairment. That said, given the catastrophic consequences of ocular ischemia in GCA, both ACR/VF and EULAR recommend IV pulse glucocorticoids for those patients with threatened (eg, amaurosis fugax and episodic blurred vision) or new-onset vision loss (ACR/VF: methylprednisolone 0.5–1 g for 3–5 days; EULAR: methylprednisolone 0.25–1 g for up to 3 days).

The duration of the glucocorticoid therapy in GCA can be variable depending on the occurrence of relapse, the presence of comorbidities, and whether a glucocorticoid-sparing medication is concomitantly used. In the absence of relapse, glucocorticoids are generally tapered within 12 to 24 months when they are used in monotherapy and approximately within 6 months when they are administered in combination with a glucocorticoid-sparing medication. When used in monotherapy, approximately 65%

of the patients relapse when relapse is defined as the reoccurrence of characteristic GCA clinical manifestations regardless of the level of inflammatory markers.[17] Relapses mostly occur when the daily doses of prednisone fall below 10 mg.[25] A phase 3 open-label RCT to directly compare a 28-week versus a 52-week prednisone taper (CORTODOSE) is underway (ClinicalTrials.gov identifier: NCT04012905).

Glucocorticoids for Polymyalgia Rheumatica

Similar to GCA, no high-quality evidence exists to guide the glucocorticoid therapy for patients with primary PMR. A systematic review of studies comparing various prednisone starting doses concluded that the dose of 15 mg/d is effective in the great majority of the cases, with less than 1% of patients requiring an increase of the initial dose to control the PMR symptoms.[26] Similar rates of remission were observed among patients randomized to receive oral prednisone at 15 mg/d versus intramuscular (IM) methylprednisolone given at a dose of 120 mg every 3 weeks for 12 weeks[27] although the use of IM methylprednisolone has not been widely adopted in cases of PMR. In a more recent open-label study, 78% of patients starting prednisone 12.5 mg/d reported symptomatic improvement.[28] Current expert recommendations propose an initial daily dose between 12.5 mg and 25 mg of prednisone or equivalent.[3,29] The optimal duration of glucocorticoid taper in PMR has not been well defined, but experts recommend slow dose reductions over 12 to 18 months. A common practice is to taper the initial dose by 2.5 mg every 2 to 4 weeks until the dose of 10 mg daily is reached and then further decrease the daily dose by 1 mg every 2 to 4 weeks until discontinuation. Slower tapers have been proposed by some authors.[26] Regardless of the specific glucocorticoid reduction strategy, over half of patients with primary PMR may ultimately require glucocorticoid therapy for 2 years or more,[26] and over 50% of them relapse at some point during the prednisone taper.[30]

Glucocorticoid Toxicity

The toxicity burden of glucocorticoid exposure, especially among patients with GCA, can be high. Observational studies have observed mean cumulative doses of nearly 10 g.[31] Substantial morbidity is associated with such glucocorticoid exposure, which is compounded by the older age and comorbidities of patients with GCA. Short-term side effects can include anxiety, sleeplessness, infection, and hyperglycemia. Longer-term side effects can be devastating and include diabetes, hypertension, cardiovascular disease, osteoporosis, fractures, and cataracts. The rate of these adverse events is as high as 86% in patients with GCA, including fractures (38%), infections (31%), hypertension (22%), diabetes (9%), and cataract formation (41%).[31]

Accurately defining glucocorticoid toxicity as an outcome measure has historically been difficult.[32] Recently a validated measure of glucocorticoid toxicity, the Glucocorticoid Toxicity Index (GTI), has been developed.[33] The GTI has two components, the composite GTI and specific list. The composite GTI measures potential glucocorticoid toxicity in nine domains (body mass Index, glucose tolerance, blood pressure, lipids, bone density, steroid myopathy, skin toxicity, neuropsychiatric toxicity, infections), which when measured at study initiation and at 3-month intervals can be used to calculate a total score and a domain-specific score.[33] Important and often severe glucocorticoid-related toxicities (eg, hypertensive emergency, severe steroid-induced myopathy, severe skin toxicity, bowel perforation, adrenal insufficiency, etc.) that are not scored as a part of the composite GTI are included in a specific list, which assesses eleven domains and 23 individual items. It is hoped that the use of the GTI will improve reporting of glucocorticoid toxicity in clinical trials and provide clinicians with a more effective means to balance the risks and benefits of glucocorticoid therapy.

Interleukin-6 Blockade Therapy

Tocilizumab for giant cell arteritis

Substantial progress in reducing glucocorticoid exposure has been made in the last decade, during which interleukin (IL)-6 receptor blockade therapy with tocilizumab has become the standard of care for most patients with GCA in developed countries. The clinical utility of IL-6 inhibition for GCA was confirmed in a phase 3 RCT known as Giant Cell Arteritis Actemra trial (GiACTA).[34] In GiACTA, 251 patients were randomized into groups that received tocilizumab (weekly or every other week) plus a 26-week prednisone taper or a prednisone taper over 26 or 52 weeks in combination with placebo. The trial met its primary outcome measure, which was the rate of sustained glucocorticoid-free remission at week 52. Patients were significantly more likely to be in remission if randomized to tocilizumab (53%–56%) than to placebo (14%–18%). The study also showed that tocilizumab was overall well tolerated, led to reduced cumulative prednisone exposure, and improved health-related quality-of-life measures.[35] Considering these data, the US Food and Drug Administration (FDA) and the European Medicines Agency approved its use in GCA. The ACR/VF guidelines[23] recommend tocilizumab for all patients with newly diagnosed disease and for most patients with disease relapse, while the EULAR guidelines[24] recommend tocilizumab for patients with relapse or patients with new-onset disease if there is occurrence or increased risk of glucocorticoid-related adverse events.

Despite the progress made with the introduction of tocilizumab for the treatment of GCA, multiple important management questions remain unanswered. First, the optimal duration of treatment with tocilizumab has not been defined, and long-term outcome data after treatment discontinuation are scarce.[36] Second, the effects of tocilizumab on vascular inflammation and risk of long-term arterial complications (eg, aortic thoracic aneurysm) are largely unknown.[37] This gap in the current knowledge is especially important given that similar to glucocorticoids, IL-6 signaling blockade may preferentially target the Th17 pathway,[10] possibly leaving residual Th1 immune response activity that could manifest in the long term as slowly progressive structural arterial damage. Third, very few patients in the GiACTA studies experienced vision loss, which is likely due to selection bias from the patients enrolled into the trial. Therefore, the efficacy of tocilizumab in patients with ocular ischemia is unclear. Uncontrolled observational studies, however, have reported low rates of vision loss.[38] Finally, and perhaps most importantly, roughly 30% of patients fail treatment with tocilizumab due to refractory disease or disease relapse, and 5% to 10% of subjects must discontinue therapy due to adverse events.[34,38,39] Thus, even though IL-6 inhibition represents a substantial advancement in the treatment of GCA, more treatment options are needed.

IL-6 blockade therapy for polymyalgia rheumatica

A phase 2/3 RCT demonstrated efficacy of tocilizumab for primary PMR. In this study, 36 subjects were randomized to receive 11 weeks of prednisone in combination with tocilizumab or placebo. The patients assigned to tocilizumab demonstrated better remission rates at 16 weeks (63% vs 12% placebo; $P < .05$) and 24 weeks (58% vs 18% placebo; $P < .05$) and required less prednisone than the patients assigned to placebo.[40] A phase 3 study (SAPHYR, ClinicalTrials.gov identifier: NCT03600818) compared sarilumab, a fully human anti-IL-6 receptor monoclonal antibody, plus 14 weeks of glucocorticoids with placebo plus 52 weeks of glucocorticoids. The study terminated early for reasons not related to efficacy or safety. Nevertheless, the analysis of the patients that completed treatment showed that patients randomized to sarilumab had better rates of sustained remission at 52 weeks (28% vs 10% placebo; $P = .02$), lower rate of relapse (17% vs 29%; $P = .02$), and improved health-related quality of life.[41] Based on the results of this study, the FDA recently approved sarilumab for the treatment of adult patients with polymyalgia rheumatica who have had an inadequate response to corticosteroids or who cannot tolerate corticosteroid taper.

Methotrexate

Methotrexate for Giant Cell Arteritis

The evidence supporting the use of methotrexate for GCA is conflicting. One single-center RCT of methotrexate (10 mg weekly) versus placebo[42] in combination with glucocorticoids observed a benefit with regard to relapse. Patients in the methotrexate arm received a lower cumulative dose of prednisone (4187 ± 1529 mg) than those in the placebo arm (5489.5 ± 1396 mg). Two other RCTs,[43,44] however, observed no significant improvements in relapse rate or cumulative prednisone dose. A meta-analysis of the three RCTs including 161 patients suggests that methotrexate may offer modest benefits in terms of remission maintenance and glucocorticoid-sparing with a number needed to treat to prevent a first and second relapse of 3.6 and 4.7 patients, respectively.[45] Notably, the methotrexate dose in these trials (7.5 m to 15 mg weekly) was lower than that typically used in rheumatoid arthritis, which could have limited the efficacy of this agent. Despite the mixed results, ACR/VF and EULAR both recommend the use of the methotrexate as an alternative to tocilizumab for those in need for glucocorticoid-sparing agents who have contraindication, intolerance, or limited access to tocilizumab.[23,24] A phase 3 head-to-head RCT comparing methotrexate to tocilizumab for patients with GCA is currently underway (METOGiA, ClinicalTrials.gov identifier: NCT03892785).

Methotrexate for Polymyalgia Rheumatica

Studies with varying designs (eg, different methotrexate dosing, treatment duration, and prednisone tapers) have evaluated the efficacy and safety of methotrexate for PMR with mixed results.[46–49] In two RCTs of methotrexate dosed at 10 mg weekly, higher rates of remission and decreased cumulative prednisone dose were observed.[46,48] Other studies found no benefit from adding methotrexate to conventional glucocorticoid regimens.[47,49] Practice guidelines conditionally recommend methotrexate for those patients who relapse or develop glucocorticoid-related adverse events or are at a high risk of glucocorticoid toxicity.[3,29]

NEW TARGETS FOR GIANT CELL ARTERITIS AND POLYMYALGIA RHEUMATICA

Even within these successful trials, relapses occurred in over 40% of patients, a figure that has been corroborated by recent meta-analyses.[50] Major relapses, defined by clinical features of ischemia or active aortic inflammation, occurred less frequently but still affected 1 in 30 patients with GCA.[51] Hence, there is a need for additional disease-modifying agents with glucocorticoid sparing effects for these patient populations. Following significant advances in the knowledge of the pathophysiology of GCA and PMR, numerous newer agents are under investigation and discussed below.

CD4+ T-Cell Costimulation Blockade

Abatacept is a fusion protein composed of the Fc region of the immunoglobulin IgG1 and the extracellular domain of cytotoxic T-lymphocyte-associated protein 4 (CTLA-4). The CTLA-4 domain binds to CD80 and CD86 expressed on dendritic cells and blocks the interaction between these costimulatory molecules and CD28 expressed by CD4+ T cells, an important step in the activation of autoreactive lymphocytes (**Fig. 1**). Abatacept was studied in a phase 2 treatment-withdrawal RCT.[52] In this study, 41 GCA patients in remission after receiving 4 doses of IV abatacept (10 mg/kg on days 1, 15, 29, and week 8) and a prednisone taper from 40 to 60 mg/d to 20 mg/d were randomized to receive monthly abatacept infusions or a placebo along with the continuation of the prednisone taper completed by week 28. Compared to placebo, patients receiving abatacept had a lower rate of relapse-free survival at 12 months (48% vs 31%, $P = .049$) and a longer median time of remission duration (9.9 months vs 3.9 months, $P = .023$). Abatacept was relatively well tolerated. In light of these findings, the ACR/VF recommends the use of abatacept as an alternative agent when tocilizumab would be indicated but cannot be used or is not effective.[23] EULAR noted the data at the moment are limited, precluding a specific recommendation.[24] Studies comparing abatacept and tocilizumab have been limited but include a prospective study involving 33 GCA patients,[53] which observed a better clinical response among those who received tocilizumab (100% vs 62%). Additional data are necessary, but no such head-to-head RCTs are currently registered. Abatacept is also currently being evaluated for use in PMR (ClinicalTrials.gov identifier: NCT03632187).

IL-12/IL-23 Signaling Inhibition

Ustekinumab is a human IgG1 kappa monoclonal antibody against the shared P40 subunit of IL-12 and IL-23 (see **Fig. 1**). These cytokines are secreted by dendritic cells and participate in the differentiation of Th1 (IL-12) and Th17 (IL-23) CD4+ cells. Two prospective, open-label, uncontrolled studies with different study designs evaluated ustekinumab in GCA and had mixed results.[54,55] One of these studies evaluated ustekinumab in refractory GCA patients who had relapsed while tapering glucocorticoids.[54] With ustekinumab, the median dose of prednisolone decreased to 5 mg at week 52 from 15 mg at baseline. No disease relapses were reported while patients were on ustekinumab. However, 75% of the patients were still receiving glucocorticoids by the time the efficacy outcomes were evaluated at week 52.[54] In contrast, a second study involving 13 new-onset or relapsing GCA patients was stopped prematurely after 7 of the initial 10 patients enrolled relapsed.[55] The mean time to relapse was 23 weeks, and the mean daily prednisone dose at relapse was 3 mg. Unlike in the prior ustekinumab study, in the second study, all patients followed a rigorous prednisone taper regimen aiming for prednisone discontinuation at 6 months. Therefore, it is possible that the better response seen in the first ustekinumab study[54] was due to the effects of glucocorticoids instead of ustekinumab. Adequately powered RCTs are necessary to properly evaluate the efficacy of ustekinumab in GCA. A phase 2 RCT of ustekinumab versus placebo is currently underway, but additional phase 3 studies may be needed (ClinicalTrials.gov identifier: NCT03711448). No studies to date have evaluated the role of IL-12/IL-23 inhibitors in PMR.

IL-17 Signaling Inhibition

Secukinumab is a fully human IgG1 kappa monoclonal antibody that selectively inhibits IL-17A (see **Fig. 1**). IL-17 A produced by Th17 CD4+ cells and CD8+ T cells acts on macrophages, endothelial cells, and vascular smooth muscle cells, leading to inflammation, vascular injury, and remodeling. IL-17 inhibition may offer a steroid-sparing opportunity as glucocorticoids primarily act on the Th17 pathway in GCA. A phase 2 study evaluated secukinumab in 52 new or relapsing GCA patients (TitAIN trial; ClinicalTrials.gov identifier: NCT03765788). Participants were randomized to receive secukinumab (300 mg weekly for 4 weeks, then every 4 weeks) or placebo.[56] All patients received a 26-week prednisone taper. Results showed that the

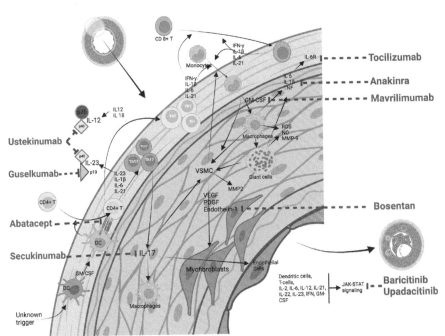

Fig. 1. GCA immuno-pathophysiology and sites of interventions of approved and investigational targeted biologic therapy. DC in the adventitia layer activated by unknown triggers secrete chemokines and cytokines that recruit and activate CD4+ T cells toward the Th1 or Th17 pathway. IL-12 and IL-18 lead to the Th1 pathway, and IL-23, IL-1β, IL-6, and IL-21 transform and maintain CD4+ T cells toward the Th17 pathway. In the next stage, chemokines and cytokines (IFN-γ, IL-1β, IL-6, IL-21) from Th1 cells help recruit monocytes and CD8+ T cells. These in turn activate VSMCs. VSMC and CD8+ T cells help amplify the monocytic recruitment and inflammation in GCA. Monocytes then transform into macrophages and merge to form multinucleated giant cells. IL-6, IL-1β, and TNF-α released by macrophages lead to the local inflammation and the systemic constitutional symptoms of GCA. In the final stage of the GCA pathogenesis, vascular injury and remodeling occur. VSMC produces MMP-2 and undergoes apoptosis. Macrophages and giant cells (in the media) produce additional mediators (ROS, NO, MMP-9) of vascular injury. In addition, macrophages and injured VSMC produce VEGF, PDGF that facilitates neoangiogenesis (in media and intima) and vascular remodeling, a process that includes myofibroblast differentiation of VSMC. These myofibroblasts then migrate to the intima and lead to intimal hyperplasia. The Th17 pathway (maintained by IL-23) secretes IL-17, which acts on cells including macrophages, endothelial cells, and VSMC, thus playing a vital role in further vascular remodeling and intimal proliferation of GCA. Additionally, GM-CSF plays a vital role in multiple crucial steps of GCA including DC activation, monocytic recruitment, and activation. Finally, various cells and cytokines implicated in the GCA pathogenesis use JAK-STAT signaling. DC, dendritic cells; GCA, giant cell arteritis; GM-CSF, granulocyte-macrophage colony-stimulating factor; IFN, interferon; IL, interleukin; JAK-STAT, Janus kinase–signal transduction and activator of transcription; MMP, metalloproteinase; NO, nitric oxide; PDGF, platelet-derived growth factor; ROS, reactive oxygen species; Th, T helper cells; VEGF, vascular endothelial growth factor; VSMC, vascular smooth muscle cells. (Created with BioRender.com.)

secukinumab treatment group had higher sustained remission rates at 28 weeks (70.1% vs 20.3%) and 52 weeks (59.3% vs 8.0%).[57] A phase 3 RCT is currently ongoing (ClinicalTrials.gov identifier: NCT04930094). No studies to date have evaluated the role of IL-17 inhibitors in PMR.

Granulocyte-Macrophage Colony-Stimulating Factor Signaling Inhibition

Granulocyte-macrophage colony-stimulating factor (GM-CSF), a multifunctional cytokine that modulates the biology of dendritic cells, CD4[+] T cells, and macrophages,[58] is implicated in the pathogenesis of GCA. GM-CSF, its receptor, and downstream signaling molecules are expressed by immune and endothelial cells in temporal arteries from patients, and GM-CSF receptor blockade in cultured arterial biopsies leads to decreased expression of dendritic cell, CD4[+] T cell, and macrophage markers along with downregulation in transcription of Th1- and Th17-related genes (eg, interferon [IFN]-γ and IL-6).[59] Furthermore, GM-CSF seems to be crucial for macrophage-induced tissue destruction and remodeling,[60,61] and the blockade of this pathway in animal models was associated with reduced arterial inflammation, neovascularization, and intimal hyperplasia.[62]

Mavrilimumab is a fully human immunoglobulin G4 monoclonal antibody that inhibits GM-CSF activity by binding to its receptor alpha subunit. A recent phase 2 RCT was successful in demonstrating the efficacy of blocking GM-CSF for maintaining disease remission in GCA. In this study, 42 patients were randomized (3:2) to receive either mavrilimumab 150 mg or placebo. Both groups received a 26-week prednisone taper. Mavrilimumab was associated with longer time to relapse (hazard ratio 0.38, 95% confidence interval 0.15–0.92), and significantly more patients receiving this agent were in remission by week 26 (83% vs 50% for placebo, $P = .004$).[63] No studies to date have evaluated the role of GM-CSF in PMR.

Janus Kinase Signaling Inhibition

Various immune cells (eg, dendritic cells, CD4[+] T cells) implicated in the pathogenesis of GCA respond to cytokines (eg, IL-2, IL-6, IL-12, IL-21, IL-22, IL-23, IFN-γ, GM-CSF) that signal through the Janus kinase–signal transduction and activator of transcription (JAK-STAT) pathway.[64] JAK inhibitors (JAKi) affect JAK-STAT signaling, potentially impacting the Th1 (IL-12, IFN-γ, GM-CSF) and Th17 pathways (IL-23, IL-6, GM-CSF) and dendritic cell activity (GM-CSF). Theoretically this strategy may overcome the limitations of other treatments, where vascular inflammation mediated by additional cytokines may go unchecked. Currently, baricitinib and upadacitinib are being studied in GCA. Baricitinib, which inhibits JAK1/JAK2, was investigated in an uncontrolled, open-label pilot study involving 15 relapsing GCA patients.[65] Patients received baricitinib (4 mg/d) and a glucocorticoid taper over 15 to 22 weeks. Overall, 13 patients were able to discontinue glucocorticoids and remained in clinical remission through week 52. These findings require confirmation in an RCT. Upadacitinib, which more selectively inhibits JAK1, is currently being studied in a phase 3 RCT (SELECT-GCA; ClinicalTrials.gov identifier: NCT03725202). The role of JAKi in PMR is currently being assessed in phase 2 studies using baricitinib (ClinicalTrials.gov identifier: NCT04027101) and tofacitinib (selective for JAK1/JAK3) (ClinicalTrials.gov identifier: NCT04799262).

It should be noted that ongoing and future studies of JAKi will require careful safety assessments in view of the recently published oral surveillance study. This large randomized FDA-mandated safety study of the JAKi tofacitinib identified an increased incidence of cardiovascular events and malignancy among patients with rheumatoid arthritis older than 50 years and with at least 1 cardiovascular risk factor.[66]

B-Cell-Depleting Therapies

Decreased number of circulating B cells has been noted in GCA and PMR,[67] and dysregulation of B-cell function has been observed in GCA.[68] Although B cells can modulate CD4$^+$ T-cell responses via the production of IL-6,[69] a clear role for B cells in the pathogenesis of GCA and PMR has not been established. In fact, biopsies of GCA patients do not exhibit significant amounts of B-cell infiltrates. That said, rituximab, an anti-CD20 B-cell-depleting monoclonal antibody, was tested in PMR.[70] In this RCT (BRIDGE-PMR), a single infusion of 1000 mg of rituximab was compared to placebo on a background of 17 weeks of glucocorticoids. Patients receiving rituximab had a higher rate of glucocorticoid-free remission at 21 weeks than those receiving placebo (48% vs 21%; $P = 0.049$). Further studies to clarify the role of rituximab in GCA and PMR are needed.

IL-23 Signaling Inhibition

Guselkumab is a monoclonal antibody that selectively inhibits IL-23 by binding to its P19 subunit (see Fig. 1). IL-23 is secreted by dendritic cells and promotes Th17 CD4$^+$ cell differentiation and survival.[64] A phase 2 RTC is currently underway to assess the safety and efficacy of IL-23 inhibition with guselkumab in GCA (ClinicalTrials.gov identifier: NCT04633447). No studies to date have evaluated the role of IL-23 inhibitors in PMR.

IL-1β Signaling Inhibition

Anakinra is a recombinant IL-1 receptor antagonist (IL-1ra). IL-1β is produced by macrophages and leads to inflammation by binding to IL-1 receptors. IL-1β is believed to contribute to GCA's systemic symptoms and stimulate the production of other cytokines, including IL-6 and TNF-α. Along with other cytokines (eg, IL-6 and IL-23), IL-1β may help maintain the Th-17 pathway.[64] Anakinra is currently under investigation in a phase 3 RCT in GCA (ClinicalTrials.gov identifier: NCT02902731). No studies to date have evaluated the role of IL-1ra in PMR.

Endothelin-1 Signaling Inhibition

Endothelin-1, a potent vasoconstrictor, may be implicated in the vascular remodeling occurring in GCA.[71] In GCA patients, tissue endothelin-1 levels do not decrease early on despite the use of glucocorticoids.[72] Bosentan, an endothelin-1 receptor antagonist, inhibits the action of endothelin-1 and might help prevent vision loss. The role of bosentan in preventing blindness is currently being studied in a phase 3 RCT for GCA (ClinicalTrials.gov identifier: NCT03841734).

Fig. 1 summarizes the pathogenesis of GCA including established and speculated therapeutic targets. Table 1 summarizes prior and ongoing pharmacologic studies including drug mechanism of action.

Glucocorticoid Tapers Lasting Less than 6 Months

In the wake of the GiACTA study, current and planned phase 3 clinical trials in GCA typically evaluate patients against a background of a 26-week steroid taper. While this represents a substantial reduction in glucocorticoid exposure as compared to previous tapering regimens, glucocorticoid-related adverse events may still occur, and additional lowering would be of benefit. The uncontrolled, open-label, proof-of-concept GUSTO (GCA treatment with ultra-short glucocorticoids and tocilizumab) study evaluated an ultra-short glucocorticoid regimen in combination with tocilizumab for new-onset GCA patients.[73] In this study, 18 patients received 500 mg of IV methylprednisolone for 3 days and 1 dose of IV tocilizumab (8 mg/kg body weight) followed by weekly subcutaneous tocilizumab injections (162 mg) until week 52. No additional glucocorticoids were provided unless patients experienced a relapse. The primary outcome of remission achieved by day 31 and maintained through week 24 was achieved only by 25% of the patients. In contrast, the secondary outcome of

Table 1
Therapeutic targets in GCA based on pathogenesis

Agent	Pathogenic Mechanism Targeted or Potentially Targeted	Stage of Development
Methotrexate	Several cell types are involved in the pathogenesis of GCA including CD4+ T cells, CD8+ T cells, and macrophages. Methotrexate is a nontargeted immunosuppressant that inhibits AICAR formyl transferase that ultimately leads to increase in adenosine. Increased adenosine in turn leads to increased intracellular cAMP that causes immunosuppression.[75]	Phase 2[42–44]
Abatacept	Abatacept interferes with the costimulation provided by DCs to CD4+ T cells, which prevents CD4+ T-cell activation.	Phase 2 (completed)[52]
Guselkumab	IL-23 is involved in the differentiation of CD4+ T cells toward the Th17 phenotype. Guselkumab inhibits the signaling of IL-23.	Phase 2 (ongoing) (ClinicalTrials.gov identifier: NCT04633447)
Secukinumab	IL-17 acts on macrophages, endothelial cells, and VSMC causing vascular injury and remodeling by affecting VSMC apoptosis and monocytic recruitment. Secukinumab inhibits IL-17A.	Phase 2 (completed) (TitAIN) trial (ClinicalTrials.gov identifier: NCT03765788) Phase 3 (ongoing) (ClinicalTrials.gov identifier: NCT04930094)
Tocilizumab, Sirukumab	IL-6 secreted by DC, Th17 cells, macrophages, and giant cells leads to local inflammation and systemic symptoms of GCA; it also affects Treg cells leading to Th17 pathway. Tocilizumab (an IL-6 receptor antagonist) and sirukumab (an IL-6 inhibitor) affect IL-6-mediated changes in GCA.	Tocilizumab: phase 3 (completed)[34], FDA approved Sirukumab: phase 3 (withdrawn) (ClinicalTrials.gov identifier: NCT02531633)[76]

Drug	Mechanism	Status
Mavrilimumab	GM-CSF is implicated in multiple steps in GCA including DC activation, monocytic recruitment, and activation. Mavrilimumab is a GM-CSF inhibitor	Phase 2 (completed)[63]
Ustekinumab	The Th1 pathway is maintained by IL-12, and the Th17 pathway by IL-23. IL-12 and IL-23 both have a common subunit P40. Ustekinumab binds to P40 and inhibits Th1 and Th17 pathways.	Open label (completed)[54] Phase 1 open label (terminated)[55] Phase 2 (ongoing) (ClinicalTrials.gov identifier: NCT03711448)
Adalimumab, etanercept, infliximab	Macrophage and giant cells secrete TNF along with IL-1β and IL-6, which leads to local inflammation and systemic symptoms of GCA. Adalimumab, etanercept, and infliximab are TNF inhibitors.	No benefit seen[77–79]
Baricitinib, upadacitinib	JAK-STAT signaling is integral to multiple cells (DC, T cells, monocytes) and various cytokines (IL-6, IL-12, IL-23, IL-2, IFN-γ) implicated in GCA pathogenesis. Baricitinib and upadacitinib are JAK inhibitors with varying selectivity to JAK subtypes.	Phase 2 open-label study[65] Phase 3 (ongoing) (SELECT-GCA, (ClinicalTrials.gov identifier: NCT03725202)
Anakinra	IL-1β secreted by DC, Th17 cells, macrophage, and giant cells leads to local inflammation and systemic symptoms of GCA. Anakinra, IL-1 receptor inhibitor, affects IL-1β-mediated changes in GCA.	Phase 3 (ClinicalTrials.gov identifier: NCT02902731)
Bosentan	Endothelin-1 causes vascular remodeling in GCA. Bosentan, an endothelin-1 receptor antagonist, blocks the effect of endothelin-1.	Phase 3 (ongoing) (ClinicalTrials.gov identifier: NCT03841734)

Abbreviations: AICAR, amino-imidazolecarboxamidoribonucleotide; cAMP, cyclic adenosine monophosphate; DC, dendritic cell; FDA, Food and Drug Administration; GCA, giant cell arteritis; GM-CSF, granulocyte-macrophage colony-stimulating factor; IL, interleukin; JAK-STAT, Janus kinase–signal transduction and activator of transcription; Th, T helper cells; TNF, tumor necrosis factor; VSMC, vascular smooth muscle cells.

relapse-free remission at week 52 was achieved by 72% of the participants. Of note, 1 patient developed AION on day 17.

A second uncontrolled, open-label, proof-of-concept study evaluated the efficacy of weekly tocilizumab injections in combination with 8 weeks of prednisone for new-onset and relapsing GCA patients.[74] The primary endpoint, sustained remission, was defined as the absence of relapse from induction of remission up to week 52 while adhering to the prednisone taper. The initial prednisone dose was 60 mg (n = 7), 50 mg (n = 1), 40 mg (n = 7), 30 mg (n = 6), and 20 mg (n = 9). All patients entered remission within 4 weeks of baseline. The primary endpoint was achieved by 23 (77%) patients. The mean (standard deviation) cumulative prednisone dose in these 23 responder patients was 1052 (390) mg. No cases of permanent vision loss occurred during the study. Confirmation of these findings in an RCT trial is required.

Nonimmunosuppressive Adjunctive Therapy

A number of nonimmunosuppressive measures are recommended for patients with GCA and PMR. These include agents to treat or prevent glucocorticoid-induced osteoporosis, vaccines according to age and the use of nonglucocorticoid immunosuppressive medications, and aspirin for certain type of patients. The ACR/VF guidelines currently recommend against the use of statins to treat GCA[23] while conditionally recommending aspirin in cases of hemodynamically significant extra-cranial vessel involvement.[23] The EULAR guidelines[24] recommend against such use of anti-platelet agents or anticoagulation unless indicated for other reasons. Both professional societies recommend surgical or endovascular revascularization in cases of clinically significant ischemia not responding to medical therapy.[23,24] However, high-quality studies to guide revascularization in GCA are lacking. In nonemergent cases, vascular interventions should be done when GCA is in remission.[23]

SUMMARY

After several decades with prolonged glucocorticoid tapers as the cornerstone for the treatment of GCA and primary PMR, the therapeutic landscape for these disorders is rapidly changing. IL-6 signaling blockade in combination with shorter glucocorticoid tapers has shown efficacy in terms of remission maintenance, glucocorticoid-sparing effects, and improvement of health-related quality of life in both GCA and PMR patients. Phase 2 RCTs with the GM-CSF antagonist mavrilimumab and the IL-17A inhibitor secukinumab recently met their respective primary efficacy outcomes in patients with GCA. Phase 2 and 3 RCTs with tocilizumab and sarilumab have also shown positive results in patients with primary PMR. Tocilizumab might facilitate even further reduction in glucocorticoid use for patients with GCA, but confirmatory RCTs are needed before shorter glucocorticoid tapers can be recommended. Lastly, several phase 2 and 3 RCTs are currently underway with medications including guselkumab, abatacept, upadacitinib, and secukinumab. In view of the robust research agenda in both GCA and primary PMR, the therapeutic armamentarium against these conditions will hopefully continue to expand in the coming years.

CLINICS CARE POINTS

- Early initiation of glucocorticoids remains a key aspect of GCA and PMR management. Glucocorticoid route, dose, duration and taper are affected by clinical presentations and co-morbid conditions.

- GCA and PMR patients are at risk of significant glucocorticoid-related toxicities. Initiating glucocorticoid-sparing agents should be considered to minimize toxicities when indicated.
- New options for GCA and PMR are under development and may be available in the coming years.

DISCLOSURE

M. Putman participates in clinical trials funded by Abbvie, United States (SELECT-GCA) and AstraZeneca (MANDARA) and receives consulting payments from Novartis. S. Unizony receives consulting payments from Kiniksa and Janssen and research support from Genentech, United States. D. Nepal has nothing to disclose.

FUNDING

Supported in part by a Scientist Development Grant from the Rheumatology Research Foundation, United States.

REFERENCES

1. Gonzalez-Gay MA, Vazquez-Rodriguez TR, Lopez-Diaz MJ, et al. Epidemiology of giant cell arteritis and polymyalgia rheumatica. Arthritis Rheum 2009;61(10): 1454–61.
2. Jennette JC, Falk RJ, Bacon PA, et al. 2012 revised International Chapel Hill Consensus Conference Nomenclature of Vasculitides. Arthritis Rheum 2013; 65(1):1–11.
3. Buttgereit F, Dejaco C, Matteson EL, et al. Polymyalgia Rheumatica and Giant Cell Arteritis: A Systematic Review. JAMA 2016;315(22):2442–58.
4. Dejaco C, Brouwer E, Mason JC, et al. Giant cell arteritis and polymyalgia rheumatica: current challenges and opportunities. Nat Rev Rheumatol 2017;13(10): 578–92.
5. Kermani TA, Warrington KJ. Polymyalgia rheumatica. Lancet 2013;381(9860): 63–72.
6. Salvarani C, Cantini F, Hunder GG. Polymyalgia rheumatica and giant-cell arteritis. Lancet 2008;372(9634):234–45.
7. Weyand CM, Goronzy JJ. Clinical practice. Giant-cell arteritis and polymyalgia rheumatica. N Engl J Med 2014;371(1):50–7.
8. Weyand CM, Goronzy JJ. Medium- and large-vessel vasculitis. N Engl J Med 2003;349(2):160–9.
9. Adriawan IR, Atschekzei F, Dittrich-Breiholz O, et al. Novel aspects of regulatory T cell dysfunction as a therapeutic target in giant cell arteritis. Ann Rheum Dis 2022;81(1):124–31.
10. Miyabe C, Miyabe Y, Strle K, et al. An expanded population of pathogenic regulatory T cells in giant cell arteritis is abrogated by IL-6 blockade therapy. Ann Rheum Dis 2017;76(5):898–905.
11. Samson M, Corbera-Bellalta M, Audia S, et al. Recent advances in our understanding of giant cell arteritis pathogenesis. Autoimmun Rev 2017;16(8):833–44.
12. Wen Z, Shen Y, Berry G, et al. The microvascular niche instructs T cells in large vessel vasculitis via the VEGF-Jagged1-Notch pathway. Sci Transl Med 2017; 9:399.
13. Weyand CM, Goronzy JJ. Immune mechanisms in medium and large-vessel vasculitis. Nat Rev Rheumatol 2013;9(12):731–40.

14. Weyand CM, Watanabe R, Zhang H, et al. Cytokines, growth factors and proteases in medium and large vessel vasculitis. Clin Immunol 2019;206:33–41.

15. Unizony S, Arias-Urdaneta L, Miloslavsky E, et al. Tocilizumab for the treatment of large-vessel vasculitis (giant cell arteritis, Takayasu arteritis) and polymyalgia rheumatica. Arthritis Care Res 2012;64(11):1720–9.

16. Deng J, Younge BR, Olshen RA, et al. Th17 and Th1 T-cell responses in giant cell arteritis. Circulation 2010;121(7):906–15.

17. Alba MA, Garcia-Martinez A, Prieto-Gonzalez S, et al. Relapses in patients with giant cell arteritis: prevalence, characteristics, and associated clinical findings in a longitudinally followed cohort of 106 patients. Medicine (Baltimore) 2014; 93(5):194–201.

18. Labarca C, Koster MJ, Crowson CS, et al. Predictors of relapse and treatment outcomes in biopsy-proven giant cell arteritis: a retrospective cohort study. Rheumatology 2016;55(2):347–56.

19. Muratore F, Boiardi L, Restuccia G, et al. Relapses and long-term remission in large vessel giant cell arteritis in northern Italy: Characteristics and predictors in a long-term follow-up study. Semin Arthritis Rheum 2020;50(4):549–58.

20. Gonzalez-Gay MA, Blanco R, Rodriguez-Valverde V, et al. Permanent visual loss and cerebrovascular accidents in giant cell arteritis: predictors and response to treatment. Arthritis Rheum 1998;41(8):1497–504.

21. Hayreh SS, Zimmerman B. Visual deterioration in giant cell arteritis patients while on high doses of corticosteroid therapy. Ophthalmology 2003;110(6):1204–15.

22. Hocevar A, Rotar Z, Jese R, et al. Do Early Diagnosis and Glucocorticoid Treatment Decrease the Risk of Permanent Visual Loss and Early Relapses in Giant Cell Arteritis: A Prospective Longitudinal Study. Medicine (Baltimore) 2016; 95(14):e3210.

23. Maz M, Chung SA, Abril A, et al. 2021 American College of Rheumatology/Vasculitis Foundation Guideline for the Management of Giant Cell Arteritis and Takayasu Arteritis. Arthritis Care Res 2021;73(8):1071–87.

24. Hellmich B, Agueda A, Monti S, et al. 2018 Update of the EULAR recommendations for the management of large vessel vasculitis. Ann Rheum Dis 2020;79(1): 19–30.

25. Stone JH, Tuckwell K, Dimonaco S, et al. Glucocorticoid Dosages and Acute-Phase Reactant Levels at Giant Cell Arteritis Flare in a Randomized Trial of Tocilizumab. Arthritis Rheumatol 2019;71(8):1329–38.

26. Hernandez-Rodriguez J, Cid MC, Lopez-Soto A, et al. Treatment of polymyalgia rheumatica: a systematic review. Arch Intern Med 2009;169(20):1839–50.

27. Dasgupta B, Dolan AL, Panayi GS, et al. An initially double-blind controlled 96 week trial of depot methylprednisolone against oral prednisolone in the treatment of polymyalgia rheumatica. Br J Rheumatol 1998;37(2):189–95.

28. Cimmino MA, Parodi M, Montecucco C, et al. The correct prednisone starting dose in polymyalgia rheumatica is related to body weight but not to disease severity. BMC Musculoskelet Disord 2011;12(1):94.

29. Dejaco C, Singh YP, Perel P, et al. 2015 Recommendations for the management of polymyalgia rheumatica: a European League Against Rheumatism/American College of Rheumatology collaborative initiative. Ann Rheum Dis 2015;74(10): 1799–807.

30. Matteson EL, Dejaco C. Polymyalgia Rheumatica. Ann Intern Med 2017;166(9): ITC65–80.

31. Proven A, Gabriel SE, Orces C, et al. Glucocorticoid therapy in giant cell arteritis: duration and adverse outcomes. Arthritis Rheum 2003;49(5):703–8.

32. Stone JH, McDowell PJ, Jayne DRW, et al. The glucocorticoid toxicity index: Measuring change in glucocorticoid toxicity over time. Semin Arthritis Rheum 2022;55:152010.

33. Miloslavsky EM, Naden RP, Bijlsma JW, et al. Development of a Glucocorticoid Toxicity Index (GTI) using multicriteria decision analysis. Ann Rheum Dis 2017; 76(3):543–6.

34. Stone JH, Tuckwell K, Dimonaco S, et al. Trial of Tocilizumab in Giant-Cell Arteritis. N Engl J Med 2017;377(4):317–28.

35. Strand V, Dimonaco S, Tuckwell K, et al. Health-related quality of life in patients with giant cell arteritis treated with tocilizumab in a phase 3 randomised controlled trial. Arthritis Res Ther 2019;21(1):64.

36. Stone JH, Han J, Aringer M, et al. Long-term effect of tocilizumab in patients with giant cell arteritis: open-label extension phase of the Giant Cell Arteritis Actemra (GiACTA) trial. Lancet Rheumatology 2021;3(5):e328–36.

37. Reichenbach S, Adler S, Bonel H, et al. Magnetic resonance angiography in giant cell arteritis: results of a randomized controlled trial of tocilizumab in giant cell arteritis. Rheumatology 2018;57(6):982–6.

38. Unizony S, McCulley TJ, Spiera R, et al. Clinical outcomes of patients with giant cell arteritis treated with tocilizumab in real-world clinical practice: decreased incidence of new visual manifestations. Arthritis Res Ther 2021;23(1):8.

39. Unizony SH, Bao M, Han J, et al. Treatment failure in giant cell arteritis. Ann Rheum Dis 2021;80(11):1467–74.

40. Bonelli M, Radner H, Kerschbaumer A, et al. Tocilizumab in patients with new onset polymyalgia rheumatica (PMR-SPARE): a phase 2/3 randomised controlled trial. Ann Rheum Dis 2022;81(6):838–44.

41. Dasgupta B, Unizony S, Warrington KJ, et al. LB0006 sarilumab in patients with relapsing polymyalgia rheumatica: a phase 3, multicenter, randomized, double blind, placebo controlled trial (SAPHYR). Ann Rheum Dis 2022;81:210–1.

42. Jover JA, Hernandez-Garcia C, Morado IC, et al. Combined treatment of giant-cell arteritis with methotrexate and prednisone. a randomized, double-blind, placebo-controlled trial. Ann Intern Med 2001;134(2):106–14.

43. Hoffman GS, Cid MC, Hellmann DB, et al. A multicenter, randomized, double-blind, placebo-controlled trial of adjuvant methotrexate treatment for giant cell arteritis. Arthritis Rheum 2002;46(5):1309–18.

44. Spiera RF, Mitnick HJ, Kupersmith M, et al. A prospective, double-blind, randomized, placebo controlled trial of methotrexate in the treatment of giant cell arteritis (GCA). Clin Exp Rheumatol 2001;19(5):495–501.

45. Mahr AD, Jover JA, Spiera RF, et al. Adjunctive methotrexate for treatment of giant cell arteritis: an individual patient data meta-analysis. Arthritis Rheum 2007; 56(8):2789–97.

46. Caporali R, Cimmino MA, Ferraccioli G, et al. Prednisone plus methotrexate for polymyalgia rheumatica: a randomized, double-blind, placebo-controlled trial. Ann Intern Med 2004;141(7):493–500.

47. Feinberg HL, Sherman JD, Schrepferman CG, et al. The use of methotrexate in polymyalgia rheumatica. J Rheumatol 1996;23(9):1550–2.

48. Ferraccioli G, Salaffi F, De Vita S, et al. Methotrexate in polymyalgia rheumatica: preliminary results of an open, randomized study. J Rheumatol 1996;23(4):624–8.

49. van der Veen MJ, Dinant HJ, van Booma-Frankfort C, et al. Can methotrexate be used as a steroid sparing agent in the treatment of polymyalgia rheumatica and giant cell arteritis? Ann Rheum Dis 1996;55(4):218–23.

50. Mainbourg S, Addario A, Samson M, et al. Prevalence of Giant Cell Arteritis Relapse in Patients Treated With Glucocorticoids: A Meta-Analysis. Arthritis Care Res 2020;72(6):838–49.

51. Aussedat M, Lobbes H, Samson M, et al. Epidemiology of major relapse in giant cell arteritis: A study-level meta-analysis. Autoimmun Rev 2022;21(1):102930.

52. Langford CA, Cuthbertson D, Ytterberg SR, et al. A Randomized, Double-Blind Trial of Abatacept (CTLA-4Ig) for the Treatment of Giant Cell Arteritis. Arthritis Rheumatol 2017;69(4):837–45.

53. Rossi D, Cecchi I, Sciascia S, et al. An agent-to-agent real life comparison study of tocilizumab versus abatacept in giant cell arteritis. Clin Exp Rheumatol 2021; 39(Suppl 129):125–8.

54. Conway R, O'Neill L, Gallagher P, et al. Ustekinumab for refractory giant cell arteritis: A prospective 52-week trial. Semin Arthritis Rheum 2018;48(3):523–8.

55. Matza MA, Fernandes AD, Stone JH, et al. Ustekinumab for the Treatment of Giant Cell Arteritis. Arthritis Care Res 2021;73(6):893–7.

56. Venhoff N, Schmidt WA, Lamprecht P, et al. Efficacy and safety of secukinumab in patients with giant cell arteritis: study protocol for a randomized, parallel group, double-blind, placebo-controlled phase II trial. Trials 2021;22(1):543.

57. Venhoff N, Schmidt W, Bergner R, et al. Secukinumab in giant cell arteritis: a randomized, parallel-group, double-blind, placebo-controlled, multicenter phase 2 trial Arthritis. Rheum 2021;73.

58. Wicks IP, Roberts AW. Targeting GM-CSF in inflammatory diseases. Nat Rev Rheumatol 2016;12(1):37–48.

59. Corbera-Bellalta M, Alba-Rovira R, Muralidharan S, et al. Blocking GM-CSF receptor alpha with mavrilimumab reduces infiltrating cells, pro-inflammatory markers and neoangiogenesis in ex vivo cultured arteries from patients with giant cell arteritis. Ann Rheum Dis 2022;81(4):524–36.

60. Jiemy WF, van Sleen Y, van der Geest KS, et al. Distinct macrophage phenotypes skewed by local granulocyte macrophage colony-stimulating factor (GM-CSF) and macrophage colony-stimulating factor (M-CSF) are associated with tissue destruction and intimal hyperplasia in giant cell arteritis. Clin Transl Immunology 2020;9(9):e1164.

61. van Sleen Y, Jiemy WF, Pringle S, et al. A Distinct Macrophage Subset Mediating Tissue Destruction and Neovascularization in Giant Cell Arteritis: Implication of the YKL-40/Interleukin-13 Receptor alpha2 Axis. Arthritis Rheumatol 2021; 73(12):2327–37.

62. Watanabe R, Zhang H, Maeda T. GM-CSF is a pro-inflammatory cytokine in experimental vasculitis of medium and large arteries [abstract 1766]. Arthritis Rheumatol 2019;71.

63. Cid MC, Unizony SH, Blockmans D, et al. Efficacy and safety of mavrilimumab in giant cell arteritis: a phase 2, randomised, double-blind, placebo-controlled trial. Ann Rheum Dis 2022. https://doi.org/10.1136/annrheumdis-2021-221865.

64. Koster MJ, Warrington KJ. Giant cell arteritis: pathogenic mechanisms and new potential therapeutic targets. BMC Rheumatol 2017;1:2.

65. Koster MJ, Crowson CS, Giblon RE, et al. Baricitinib for relapsing giant cell arteritis: a prospective open-label 52-week pilot study. Ann Rheum Dis 2022. https://doi.org/10.1136/annrheumdis-2021-221961.

66. Ytterberg SR, Bhatt DL, Mikuls TR, et al. Cardiovascular and Cancer Risk with Tofacitinib in Rheumatoid Arthritis. N Engl J Med 2022;386(4):316–26.

67. van der Geest KS, Abdulahad WH, Chalan P, et al. Disturbed B cell homeostasis in newly diagnosed giant cell arteritis and polymyalgia rheumatica. Arthritis Rheumatol 2014;66(7):1927–38.

68. Koster MJ, Matteson EL, Warrington KJ. Recent advances in the clinical management of giant cell arteritis and Takayasu arteritis. Curr Opin Rheumatol 2016; 28(3):211–7.

69. Barr TA, Shen P, Brown S, et al. B cell depletion therapy ameliorates autoimmune disease through ablation of IL-6-producing B cells. J Exp Med 2012;209(5): 1001–10.

70. Marsman DE, den Broeder N, van den Hoogen FH, et al. Efficacy of Rituximab in Patients with Polymyalgia Rheumatica: A Double-Blind, Randomised, Placebo-Controlled, Proof-of-Concept Trial The. Lancet Rheumatol 2021;3(11):e758-e766.

71. Planas-Rigol E, Terrades-Garcia N, Corbera-Bellalta M, et al. Endothelin-1 promotes vascular smooth muscle cell migration across the artery wall: a mechanism contributing to vascular remodelling and intimal hyperplasia in giant-cell arteritis. Ann Rheum Dis 2017;76(9):1624–34.

72. Lozano E, Segarra M, Corbera-Bellalta M, et al. Increased expression of the endothelin system in arterial lesions from patients with giant-cell arteritis: association between elevated plasma endothelin levels and the development of ischaemic events. Ann Rheum Dis 2010;69(2):434–42.

73. Christ L, Seitz L, Scholz G, et al. Tocilizumab monotherapy after ultra-short glucocorticoid administration in giant cell arteritis: a single-arm open-label, proof-of-concept study. Lancet Rheumatol 2021;3(9):E619–26.

74. Unizony S, Matza M, Jarvie A, et al. Tocilizumab in combination with 8 weeks of prednisone for giant cell arteritis. Ann Rheum Dis 2022;81:123.

75. Cutolo M, Sulli A, Pizzorni C, et al. Anti-inflammatory mechanisms of methotrexate in rheumatoid arthritis. Ann Rheum Dis 2001;60(8):729–35.

76. Schmidt WA, Dasgupta B, Luqmani R, et al. A Multicentre, Randomised, Double-Blind, Placebo-Controlled, Parallel-Group Study to Evaluate the Efficacy and Safety of Sirukumab in the Treatment of Giant Cell Arteritis. Rheumatol Ther 2020;7(4):793–810.

77. Seror R, Baron G, Hachulla E, et al. Adalimumab for steroid sparing in patients with giant-cell arteritis: results of a multicentre randomised controlled trial. Ann Rheum Dis 2014;73(12):2074–81.

78. Martinez-Taboada VM, Rodriguez-Valverde V, Carreno L, et al. A double-blind placebo controlled trial of etanercept in patients with giant cell arteritis and corticosteroid side effects. Ann Rheum Dis 2008;67(5):625–30.

79. Hoffman GS, Cid MC, Rendt-Zagar KE, et al. Infliximab for maintenance of glucocorticosteroid-induced remission of giant cell arteritis: a randomized trial. Ann Intern Med 2007;146(9):621–30.

Isolated Aortitis
Workup and Management

Tanaz A. Kermani, MD, MS[a],*, Kevin Byram, MD[b]

KEYWORDS

- Isolated aortitis • Idiopathic aortitis • Aortitis • Noninfectious aortitis
- Large-vessel vasculitis • Treatment • Prognosis

KEY POINTS

- Aortitis noted on surgical pathologic condition should prompt evaluation for rheumatologic conditions, especially systemic vasculitis, although the majority is clinically isolated aortitis (CIA).
- Imaging of the entire aorta and branches is recommended in patients with isolated aortitis, and a large proportion of patients have disease outside of the surgically treated area.
- The role of immunosuppressive therapies such as glucocorticoids for aortitis incidentally found on histopathology without systemic vasculitis is uncertain.
- Patients with CIA need to be monitored longitudinally with imaging and regular clinical examination to evaluate for recurrence and need for further intervention.

INTRODUCTION

Aortitis, or inflammatory vasculopathy involving the aorta, can be detected either histologically at the time of surgical intervention of an aortic aneurysm or radiographically with luminal and/or vessel wall imaging. Aortitis has been associated with infectious causes such as syphilis and mycobacterial disease as well as systemic vasculitis like giant cell arteritis (GCA) and Takayasu arteritis (TAK).[1] In cases where no cause is found and patients do not meet established criteria for GCA or TAK, a diagnosis of clinically isolated aortitis (CIA) is made.[2,3] During the last several decades, large cohorts of patients with CIA have been published.[4–13] Controversy exists as to whether CIA represents a forme fruste of a systemic vasculitis such as GCA or TAK or a distinct entity. No specific global definition of CIA exists. The Chapel Hill Consensus Conference includes CIA as a type of "single organ vasculitis."[3]

[a] Division of Rheumatology, University of California Los Angeles, 2020 Santa Monica Boulevard, Suite 540, Santa Monica, CA 90404, USA; [b] Division of Rheumatology and Immunology, Vanderbilt University Medical Center, 1161 21st Avenue South, T3113, MCN, Nashville, TN 37232, USA
* Corresponding author.
E-mail address: TKermani@mednet.ucla.edu

Rheum Dis Clin N Am 49 (2023) 523–543
https://doi.org/10.1016/j.rdc.2023.03.013
0889-857X/23/© 2023 Elsevier Inc. All rights reserved.

rheumatic.theclinics.com

Although 30% to 50% of patients with aortitis may be asymptomatic, some may present with nonspecific symptoms such as chest or abdominal pain, palpitations, malaise, fevers, or weight loss.[7,14] Ischemic manifestations such as limb claudication or even stroke can occur as well if stenotic lesions develop in branches of the aorta. In some cases, aortitis may be incidentally noted on cross-sectional imaging such as computed tomography (CT), MRI, or PET with findings of thickening, ectasia, aneurysms, or dissections.[1] However, many cases of CIA in the medical literature are incidentally identified at the time of surgical intervention of an aortic aneurysm repair.[4-13] This review summarizes our current knowledge on the epidemiology, diagnostic evaluation, and therapeutic approach to CIA.

EPIDEMIOLOGY
Prevalence of Aortitis on Surgical Specimens of the Thoracic Aorta

The true prevalence of CIA is difficult to estimate because CIA is a diagnosis of exclusion and is often incidentally noted on surgical specimens. Large surgical cohorts of patients undergoing thoracic aortic aneurysm repair report prevalence of aortitis on surgical specimens from 2% to 12%, in which many are further classified as having CIA.[4,5,12,14-16]

Prevalence of Clinically Isolated Aortitis

The diagnosis and evaluation of aortitis requires exclusion of several systemic rheumatologic conditions. The prevalence of CIA, where no other cause is found, differs in surgical versus clinical series with higher prevalence noted in surgical series. In series with surgical specimens, CIA accounts for 47% to 81% of cases (**Table 1**).[4-13] In contrast, in a large study that included 353 patients with aortitis either on imaging (77%) or histopathology (23%), CIA accounted for only 21% of the cases of aortitis with the majority of the cases occurring in patients with large-vessel vasculitis (LVV).[17] Similarly, in a smaller study evaluating 32 patients with aortitis based on imaging, majority of the cases were in patients with GCA (41%) with CIA accounting for only 2 cases (6%).[18]

Risk Factors

Overwhelmingly, CIA affects the ascending aortic arch more than other portions of the aorta, although most of the data are from thoracic surgical cohorts.[4,5,14] In one study, the presence of aortic branch involvement by definition, ruled out a diagnosis of CIA, favoring other diagnoses such as TAK or GCA,[12] whereas in other cohorts, frequency of aortic branch involvement up to 72% has been reported.[7,9,11,19]

In most cohorts, 50% to 78% of patients with CIA are women with average age in the seventh decade.[7,9,11-14,19-23] Potential risk factors for CIA have been identified (**Table 2**). Many patients with CIA have typical cardiovascular risk factors such as hypertension, coronary artery disease, or tobacco use.[9,11,13,14,19-23]

Two studies have compared patients with findings of aortitis on surgical resection to patients without aortitis. In a case-control study of 43 patients with aortitis without preexisting autoimmune disease, Quimson and colleagues found higher incidence of female sex, presence of hypertension, and older age in patients compared with 219 nonaortitis controls.[14] Interestingly, absence of coronary artery disease was also associated with aortitis in this study.[14] Similarly, in the study by Caterson and colleagues older age, female sex and hypertension were associated with aortitis compared with patients without aortitis, although fewer patients in that study had CIA.[21]

Other studies have compared patients with CIA to patients with aortitis from other inflammatory conditions. In a small series of 9 patients with CIA and 7 patients with

Table 1
Surgical series of thoracic aortitis with prevalence of clinically isolated aortitis, or other systemic conditions

Study	Total Number with Aortitis	Clinically Isolated Aortitis	Giant Cell arteritis/ Polymyalgia Rheumatica	Takayasu Arteritis	Other	Other Diagnoses
Rojo-Leyva F et al,[4] 2000[a]	52	36 (70%)	4 (8%)	2 (4%)	8 (15%)	2 SLE, 1 SS, 2 RPF, 1 PAN, 1 IBD, 1 GPA
Miller DV et al,[5] 2006	45	21 (47%)	14 (31%)	6 (13%)	4 (9%)	2 RA, 2 unclassified
Liang KP et al,[7] 2009	64	52 (81%)	10 (16%)	0	2 (3%)	1 inflammatory arthritis, 1 CD
Schmidt J et al,[8] 2011[a]	37	27 (78%)	5 (14%)	0	3 (8%)	1 RA, 1 CD, 1 SLE
Wang H et al,[9] 2012[a]	42	24 (57%)	0	8 (19%)	6 (14%)	2 BD, 1 Kawasaki, 3 unclassified
Ryan C et al,[10] 2015	71	34 (48%)	5 (7%)	1 (1%)	7 (10%)	1 SLE, 1 Cogan, 1 relapsing polychondritis, 1 ulcerative colitis, 2 unclassified, 1 elevated rheumatoid factor without diagnosis
Murzin DL et al,[11] 2017[a]	47	32 (68%)	7 (13%)	1 (2%)	1 (2%)	1 RA
Clifford AH et al,[12] 2019	196	129 (66%)	42 (63%)	14 (7%)	11 (5.6%)	1 RA, 2 sarcoidosis, 1 IgG4-related disease, 1 undifferentiated systemic disease, 1 RPF
De Martino A et al,[13] 2019	26	19 (73%)	5 (19%)	0	0	N/A

Abbreviations: CD, Crohn disease; GPA, granulomatosis with polyangiitis; IBD, inflammatory bowel disease; PAN, polyarteritis nodosa; RA, rheumatoid arthritis; RPF, retroperitoneal fibrosis; SLE, systemic lupus erythematosus; SS, Sjogren syndrome
[a] Percentages do not add up to 100 because infectious, malignant or genetic causes also included in the study.

Table 2
Demographics and potential risk factors of patients with clinically isolated aortitis from various surgical cohorts

Study	Clinical Setting	Number of Aortitis Cases	Percent CIA	Age, Mean (years)	Female (%)	Hypertension (%)	CAD (%)	Tobacco Use (%)	Aortic Branch Involvement at Presentation (%)
Zehr KJ et al,[23] 2005	United States	37[a]	92%	69.6	78	73	29.7	67.6	–
Liang KP et al,[7] 2009	United States	64	52 (81%)	69.1	50	–	–	–	42
Wang H et al,[9] 2012	Chinese Cohort	24	24 (100%)	46.3[b]	50	54	–	33	8
Murzin DL et al,[11] 2017	Canada	32	32 (100%)	66.0	56	62	44	69	71
Espitia O et al,[22] 2016	France	44	44 (100%)	65.0[g]	64	45	–	43[f]	–
De Martino A et al,[13] 2019	Italy	26	19 (73%)	69	54	81	–	–	–
Clifford AH et al,[12] 2019	United States	196	129 (65.8%)	65.6	67	–	–	–	–
Goldhar HA et al,[19] 2019	Canada	16	9 (56%)	72.9	78	67	22	100[d]	56
Quimson L et al,[14] 2020	United States	43	43 (100%)	70.0[c]	65[c]	88[c]	21[e]	–	–
Aghayev A et al,[20] 2021	United States	23	23 (100%)	67.5	65	65[g]	35	57	–
Caterson HC et al,[21] 2022	Australia	41	27 (66%)	69.7[c]	54[c]	83[c]	–	48	–

[a] Up to 25% likely had GCA/PMR.
[b] Significantly older than TAK comparator group.
[c] Significantly more than nonaortitis comparator group.
[d] Significantly more than in secondary aortitis comparator group.
[e] Significantly less compared with nonaortitis controls.
[f] Significantly more than in GCA comparator group.
[g] Significantly less than in GCA comparator group.

secondary aortitis, patients with CIA had significantly more tobacco use.[19] In another study of 73 patients with GCA and 44 patients with CIA, Espitia and colleagues, found that patients with CIA were younger with a higher frequency of tobacco use.[22] Finally, Wang and colleagues, compared 24 patients with CIA to 8 patients with TAK and found older age (46 years in CIA vs 34 years for TAK), similar sex distribution, and lower frequency of hypertension in CIA.[9]

Potential Causes and Their Frequencies in Thoracic Aortitis

The rheumatologic conditions most commonly associated with aortitis also vary depending on the nature of the series (surgical vs radiographic).[4–8,11–13,17,18] In surgical series of thoracic aortitis, among cases where an underlying systemic rheumatologic condition was identified, not surprisingly, GCA was common accounting for 36% to 63% of these cases (see **Table 1**).[4–13] Other rheumatologic conditions associated with aortitis included TAK, polymyalgia rheumatica (PMR), Behcet disease, relapsing polychondritis, Cogan syndrome, IgG4-related disease (IgG4-RD), granulomatosis with polyangiitis (GPA), polyarteritis nodosa, sarcoidosis, retroperitoneal fibrosis, systemic lupus erythematosus (SLE), Sjogren syndrome, rheumatoid arthritis (RA), ankylosing spondylitis, psoriatic arthritis, inflammatory bowel disease (IBD; see **Table 1**).[4–8,11–13] Among 353 patients with radiographic or histopathologic findings of aortitis, of the 280 cases due to a systemic rheumatologic condition, the most common diagnoses were GCA (48%), TAK (34%), Behcet disease (6%), relapsing polychondritis (4%), IgG4-RD (3%), Cogan syndrome (0.7%), ankylosing spondylitis (0.7%), and sarcoidosis (0.3%).[17]

DIAGNOSTIC APPROACH

The diagnostic approach to aortitis noted on surgical pathology includes the evaluation for systemic rheumatologic conditions. Once these have been carefully ruled out, the diagnosis of CIA is likely. Histopathologic findings may provide some clues as to the cause of the aortitis, although majority of the cases of CIA have granulomatous inflammation that is indistinguishable from that found in GCA, so called "giant cell aortitis."[2] Imaging of the entire aorta to evaluate for lesions in other territories is also an important part of the diagnostic evaluation given the high prevalence of abnormalities in other vascular beds.[7,9,11,19]

Systemic Conditions that Cause Aortitis

There are several systemic rheumatologic diseases that can cause aortitis (**Table 3**). A careful history is essential in the evaluation of patients with CIA to identify any potential causes, especially in patients who have no earlier history of a rheumatic disease. This section provides an overview of these conditions and clinical aspects that may suggest their presence.

Constitutional symptoms such as fevers, night sweats, appetite changes, weight loss may indicate a systemic inflammatory condition (assuming infection has been ruled out). Involvement of the aorta and its branches are known manifestations of GCA and TAK. In prospective studies using computed tomography angiography (CTA) and PET, the prevalence of aortitis in newly diagnosed GCA ranges from 45% to 65% of patients.[24–28] Furthermore, as noted above, a large proportion of cases of aortitis identified on surgical specimens where a secondary cause is identified are in patients with GCA.[4–13] In patients aged older than 50 years, with aortitis found on imaging or at surgery, history should focus on the presence of any cranial manifestations such as headaches, jaw claudication, scalp tenderness, vision changes. It is

Table 3
Systemic conditions that can cause aortitis and the patterns noted on histopathology of the aorta

Condition	Histopathology of Aorta	Predominant Vessel Size Affected	Distinguishing Clinical Features	Diagnostic Testing
Clinically isolated aortitis	Granulomatous inflammation and/or lymphoplasmacytic inflammation	Large vessels	Often incidentally noted on surgical pathology of the ascending aorta, absence of other autoimmune diseases or features to suggest a systemic inflammatory condition	Large-vessel imaging, exclusion of other causes of aortitis
Giant cell arteritis	Granulomatous inflammation, occasional giant cells, lymphoplasmacytic infiltrate	Large vessels	Age >50 y, cranial symptoms, constitutional symptoms, vascular ischemia	Temporal artery biopsy, temporal artery imaging, large-vessel imaging
Polymyalgia rheumatica	Granulomatous inflammation	Large vessels	Age >50 y, proximal myalgias, constitutional symptoms	Clinical diagnosis made on history, exclusion of other conditions including inflammatory arthritis, elevated acute phase reactants
Takayasu arteritis	Granulomatous inflammation	Large vessels (aorta and branches)	Age <50 y, constitutional symptoms, carotidynia, limb claudication, renovascular hypertension, peripheral pulse loss/asymmetry, vascular bruits	Large-vessel imaging
Sarcoidosis	Granulomatous inflammation, noncaseating with	Any vessel size	Pulmonary involvement, mediastinal or hilar lymphadenopathy,	Imaging, biopsy of affected tissue, laboratory testing may include elevated

Disease	Histopathology	Vessel size	Clinical manifestations	Diagnosis
	accompanying lymphoplasmacytic infiltrate		erythema nodosum, inflammatory eye disease (uveitis, dacryoadenitis), cardiac manifestations	angiotensin converting enzyme, elevated 1,25-dihydroxyvitamin D
Antineutrophil cytoplasmic antibody-associated vasculitis	Granulomatous inflammation, necrotizing	Small vessels but rare involvement of the aorta	Upper airway involvement with sinus disease, otitis media, sensorineural hearing loss, tracheal stenosis, pulmonary nodulosis, alveolar hemorrhage, rapidly progressive glomerulonephritis, mononeuropathy multiplex, cranial neuropathies, ocular manifestations (scleritis, inflammatory orbital tumors), palpable purpura	ANCA positivity, biopsy of affected tissue
Rheumatoid arthritis	Granulomatous inflammation with possible presence of rheumatoid nodules characterized by necrosis and palisading histiocytes/macrophages	Small to medium vessels but aorta can be affected	Inflammatory arthritis, extra-articular manifestations including cutaneous nodulosis, scleritis, cutaneous ulcerations, cutaneous vasculitis, vasculitic neuropathy, pericarditis	Inflammatory arthritis on exam, erosions on imaging, positive rheumatoid factor, positive cyclic citrullinated peptide antibodies
Inflammatory bowel disease	Granulomatous inflammation, noncaseating	Any vessel size	Involvement of the small intestine and/or colon, erythema nodosum, inflammatory arthritis,	Enterography, endoscopic evaluation with biopsies

(continued on next page)

Table 3
(continued)

Condition	Histopathology of Aorta	Predominant Vessel Size Affected	Distinguishing Clinical Features	Diagnostic Testing
			uveitis, hepatic involvement	
Relapsing polychondritis	Mixed inflammatory pattern	Any vessel size	Nasal and/or auricular chondritis, inflammatory eye disease, tracheal/bronchial abnormalities	Clinical diagnosis, imaging to evaluate the trachea and upper airways
Cogan syndrome	Mixed inflammatory pattern	Any vessel size	Interstitial keratitis, uveitis, episcleritis/scleritis, vestibular dysfunction, sensorineural hearing loss, vasculitis	Clinical diagnosis
Behcet syndrome	Mixed inflammatory pattern	Any vessel size	Recurrent oral and/or genital ulcerations, cutaneous lesions including erythema nodosum, pustules, uveitis, gastrointestinal manifestations, venous and arterial disease	Clinical diagnosis, pathergy test
IgG4-related disease	Lymphoplasmacytic inflammation, presence of IgG4-positive plasma cells, fibrosis	Large vessels	Lacrimal gland inflammation, sialadenitis, lymphadenopathy, autoimmune pancreatitis, periaortitis	Elevated plasma IgG4 but this is a histopathologic diagnosis with affected tissue with characteristic histologic features and positive IgG4 staining plasma cells

Systemic lupus erythematosus	Lymphoplasmacytic inflammation	Any vessel size	Rashes, photosensitivity, oral ulcerations, arthralgia, renal manifestations with glomerulonephritis, serositis, cytopenias, central nervous system manifestations	Positive antinuclear antibody, positive extractable nuclear antigen, positive antiphospholipid antibodies, hypocomplementemia, renal biopsy
Ankylosing spondylitis	Lymphoplasmacytic inflammation	Large vessel	Inflammatory back pain, sacroiliitis, enthesitis, inflammatory arthritis, extra-articular manifestations including uveitis, enteritis	Positive HLA B27, imaging findings of sacroiliitis or ankylosis of the spine

mportant to recognize that approximately 12% of patients with GCA may present with isolated large-vessel manifestations and are less likely to present with cranial symptoms and more likely to present with symptoms of vascular insufficiency such as limb claudication.[29] There is also a close and well-recognized association between PMR, characterized by proximal myalgias, and GCA. In imaging studies, up to 30% of individuals with PMR have subclinical GCA.[30] Patients with TAK tend to be younger at disease onset (<50 years) and often present with symptoms of vascular insufficiency including carotidynia, limb claudication, arterial events including strokes, and renovascular hypertension.[31]

Other systemic vasculitides that can rarely affect the aorta and cause aortitis include relapsing polychondritis, GPA, or other forms of antineutrophil cytoplasmic antibody (ANCA)-associated vasculitis, Behcet disease, and Cogan syndrome. Clinical features of relapsing polychondritis include nasal chondritis, auricular chondritis, involvement of the airways including the trachea and bronchi, and ocular inflammation.[32] Aortitis in addition to the involvement of the branches (predominantly supra-aortic vessels) has been associated with this condition.[33] GPA is a systemic, necrotizing small-vessel vasculitis characterized by the presence of ANCA.[3,34] Although any organ can be involved, the sinuses, lungs, kidneys with glomerulonephritis, and nervous system are the most commonly and severely affected.[34] Large-vessel manifestations including the involvement of the aorta has been rarely reported in GPA.[35] Behcet disease is a rare systemic vasculitis characterized by recurrent oral ulcerations, genital ulcerations, cutaneous lesions, ocular manifestations, gastrointestinal involvement, venous and arterial involvement (all vessel sizes).[3,36] Finally, Cogan syndrome is a rare autoimmune condition characterized by interstitial keratitis, vestibule-auditory involvement, and manifestations including large-vessel vasculitis.[3,37]

Other multisystem diseases such as IBD and sarcoidosis, which are characterized by granulomatous inflammation, should also be on the differential for a patient with aortitis. Manifestations of sarcoidosis include involvement of the lungs, lymphatic system, skin, and eyes.[38] It can also cause vasculitis including the involvement of the large vessels/aorta.[39–41] In the case of IBD, extraintestinal manifestations include aortitis in rare cases.[42] However, there are also reports of association with GCA and TAK in patients with IBD at a higher frequency than would be expected by chance alone, which may account for findings of aortitis.[43–46]

IgG4-RD is a multisystem disease characterized by infiltration of the organs by lymphoplasmacytic inflammation with IgG4-positive plasma cells and fibrosis.[47] In a large cohort, 4 different phenotypic groups of IgG4-RD were identified, with aortitis being most commonly observed in the group with retroperitoneal and aortic disease followed by the group with Mikulicz disease and systemic disease.[48] The presence of lymphoplasmacytic inflammation on aortic specimens should raise concern for this entity and prompt additional staining for IgG4.[2]

Finally, other systemic rheumatologic conditions including RA, ankylosing spondylitis and connective tissue diseases such as SLE, Sjogren syndrome have also been rarely associated with aortitis.[49–51]

Laboratory Testing

Data are scarce regarding the utility of elevated acute phase reactants such as erythrocyte sedimentation rate (ESR) and c-reactive protein (CRP) in aortitis. Limitations again include the retrospective nature of most series. Furthermore, baseline values were not uniformly tested. In a large cohort of 129 patients with CIA, baseline markers of inflammation were available in only 20 patients (15%).[12] The mean ESR and CRP were normal. Additionally, there were no differences when compared with patients with GCA and TAK with surgical evidence of aortitis.[12] Similarly, in another series of 64 patients with aortitis, the preoperative ESR was available in 20 patients (31%) and was elevated (>25 mm/h) in only 2 patients.[7] Finally, in another surgical series with markers of inflammation measured in 13 of 32 patients (41%), elevated ESR and/or CRP was noted in 77% but there are no details about when these were tested making interpretation challenging.[11] In a study evaluating radiographic aortitis, mean ESR and CRP were elevated in patients with CIA and GCA with aortitis with no differences between the groups.[22] Based on these data, the clinical utility of acute phase reactants in ruling out other systemic inflammatory conditions in patients with thoracic aortitis noted either on histopathology or on imaging is unclear. Other serologic studies including rheumatoid factor, cyclic citrullinated peptide, antinuclear antibody with extractable nuclear antigens, ANCA, IgG subclasses and other testing including complement levels, angiotensin converting enzyme may be considered depending on the clinical history and suspicion for an alternate cause (see **Table 3**).

Histopathology

The pathologic findings of aortitis are classified into 4 patterns of inflammation: granulomatous/giant cell, lymphoplasmacytic, suppurative, and mixed pattern.[2,52] Although certain systemic diseases have been associated with the different patterns of inflammation, the histopathologic findings by themselves are insufficient to distinguish CIA from other causes of aortitis and clinical correlation is crucial.

The granulomatous/giant cell pattern (**Fig. 1**) is the most commonly observed pattern in CIA, accounting for about 66% cases.[2] This is characterized by the presence of large epithelioid macrophages with or without giant cells with significant overlap with the pattern observed in GCA. An accompanying lymphoplasmacytic pattern is often present. The granulomatous/giant cell pattern has been observed in other systemic conditions that cause aortitis including GCA, TAK, RA, sarcoidosis, GPA, and IBD. Infections such as mycobacterial and fungal infections should also be considered with this pattern.[2,52] Some studies have found the presence of necrotizing inflammation with medial laminar necrosis may distinguish CIA from other systemic causes but this is controversial.[10] In a study comparing patients with CIA to TAK, the presence of intimal medial thickness, was more commonly observed in TAK.[9] Patients with CIA had more active features of aortitis including giant cell aortitis, inflammatory necrosis or plasma cell infiltration but this may have been due to differences in treatment with 50% TAK patients being on corticosteroid therapy compared with 20% with CIA.[9]

The next most frequently observed pattern in CIA is the lymphoplasmacytic pattern characterized by lymphocytes and plasma cells without granulomatous inflammation.[2,52] It is important to recognize that under sampling can also cause this pattern by missing an area with the granulomatous pattern. This pattern should prompt evaluation of IgG4-RD but this pattern is also observed in other conditions including SLE, ankylosing spondylitis, and syphilis.[2,52]

The mixed pattern is characterized by a mixture of inflammatory cells including lymphocytes, plasma cells, macrophages, neutrophils, mast cells, and eosinophils. This is an uncommon pattern and has been reported in aortitis in Cogan syndrome, Behcet disease, and relapsing polychondritis.[2,52]

Finally, the suppurative pattern, characterized by marked neutrophilic infiltrates with extensive necrosis should raise concern for a bacterial infectious process.[2,52]

A recent study of surgical tissue from 49 patients with inflammatory and noninflammatory aneurysms (12 CIA, 14 GCA, 23 noninflammatory) found that the aortic tissue is not sterile and contains a microbiome.[53] Patients with inflammatory aneurysms had evidence of reduced phylogenic diversity and increased prevalence of pathogens that

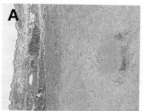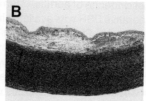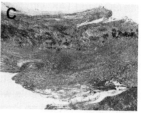

Fig. 1. Histopathology from the ascending aorta of a 29-year-old female patient with clinically isolated aortitis. Hematoxylin and eosin stain of the ascending aorta at medium power with medial necrosis with focal giant cell formation consistent with necrotizing granulomatous inflammation, plasma cell-rich and lymphocyte-rich infiltrates of the vasa vasorum (Panel *A*). Elastin stain at low power of uninvolved aortic tissue in the same patient with CIA with dense, organized fibers of the elastic lamellar units of the aortic media (Panel *B*) and elastin stain at low power of involved aortic tissue with disorganized and disjointed fibers of the elastic lamellar units of the aortic media in the setting of inflammatory aortitis (Panel *C*).

can cause a proinflammatory environment compared with patients with noninflammatory aneurysms but the microbiomes between patients with GCA and CIA were not different.[53] Another study evaluating transcriptomic profile in patients with inflammatory (8 GCA with or without PMR, 17 CIA) and noninflammatory aneurysms (25 patients) found similar signatures in patients with GCA and CIA.[54] Patients with inflammatory aneurysms had upregulated genes enriched in immune-related functions and downregulated genes enriched in neuronal processes.[54] These studies not surprisingly, suggest differences in the causes and mechanism of inflammatory and noninflammatory aneurysms but also raise the question about whether CIA is a limited presentation of GCA.[53,54]

Imaging Abnormalities

Imaging findings in patients characterized as clinically isolated aortitis
Imaging of the entire aorta and its branches is important in all patients with aortitis. CTA or magnetic resonance angiography (MRA) are usually preferred because they can visualize the vessel wall and the lumen. Findings suggestive of vasculitis include vessel wall thickening, vessel wall enhancement, ectasia, aneurysms, stenosis (especially smooth, tapered stenosis), occlusions (**Fig. 2**). Frequency of involvement of the other vascular beds including aortic lesions or branch lesions is variable by the series, although in all cases, abnormalities beyond the surgically resected area are noted in a significant proportion of patients.[7,11,12] It is important to keep several limitations in mind when interpreting the currently available data. First, all the series are retrospective, and imaging studies are not uniformly available. There are no standardized protocols for which imaging studies are used (usually CTA, MRA). Finally, not all vascular beds may have been imaged, which may underestimate the findings.

In the series of 64 patients with thoracic aortitis on surgical resection from the Mayo Clinic, 89% patients with CIA and other rheumatologic causes of aortitis had vascular imaging studies with abnormalities of other vascular beds noted in 72%.[7] This included stenosis/ectasia of the aortic branches (42%), descending thoracic aortic aneurysms (32%), descending thoracic and abdominal aortic aneurysms (21%), and abdominal aortic aneurysms (7%).[7] In the study from the Cleveland Clinic of 129 patients with CIA, 64 patients (50%) had imaging of the chest and abdomen, which demonstrated isolated thoracic disease in 52% and involvement of the thoracic and abdominal aorta in the remainder.[12] In this series, no branch vessel disease was

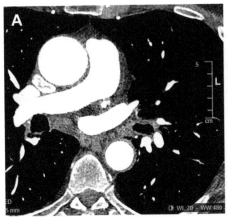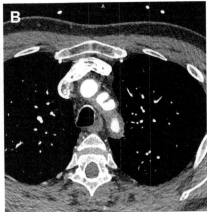

Fig. 2. Computed tomography angiography from a 75-year-old man with clinically isolated aortitis showing ascending aortic aneurysm with thickening of the wall of the descending thoracic aorta (Panel A) and branch vessels (Panel B). Findings were incidentally noted on computed tomography of the coronary arteries.

present in patients with CIA at baseline by definition.[12] In the study from Canada, 21 of the 32 patients (66%) with CIA had imaging of the aorta and branch vessels at baseline with branch lesions in 71% and additional aortic lesions in 14%.[11]

Comparison of imaging findings in clinically isolated aortitis to other LVV

Several studies comparing radiographic findings in CIA to other LVV have been published.[12,17,22,55] In a study that included patients with either radiographic or histopathologic evidence of aortitis, only data on the aortic distribution of the lesions was reported.[17] In 73 patients with CIA, abnormalities on baseline imaging was noted in the descending aorta (73%), aortic arch (69%), ascending aorta (64%), and abdominal aorta (63%) with similar frequencies also reported in 136 patients with GCA and 96 patients with TAK.[17] Another series of radiographic aortitis, 44 patients with CIA were compared with 73 patients with GCA and aortic involvement found suprarenal abdominal aorta (but not other aortic regions) were more frequent in patients with GCA (63%) compared with CIA (46%), p value .06.[22] Aneurysms were more frequent in the CIA group (39%) compared with the GCA group (21%), p value .03, and patients with CIA also had a higher mean aortic wall thickening (4.6 mm) compared with patients with GCA (3.9 mm), p value .08.[22] Again, data for nonaortic involvement were not reported. In another cohort of radiographic aortitis using PET, comparing 11 patients with CIA to 7 patients with GCA with aortitis, thoracic aorta and abdominal aorta were more frequently observed in CIA (91% and 82%, respectively) compared with GCA (14% each) and aortic branches were involved in 29% with GCA but no patient with CIA.[55] In a study from the Cleveland Clinic, dilatation of the distal aorta was more frequently observed in patients with GCA (71%) compared with CIA (52%) or TAK (57%), $P < .05$, and none of the patients with CIA had branch vessel disease at baseline (by definition) compared with 36% with TAK and 24% with GCA ($P < .001$).[12]

THERAPEUTIC APPROACH

CIA is a challenging disease state for clinicians. The prognosis and relapse rate of patients with CIA are difficult to predict, and role of immunosuppressive therapy is unclear. This leads to much uncertainty regarding how to approach the patient with aortitis on histopathology but without signs and symptoms of systemic vasculitis. Patients with CIA benefit from being evaluated longitudinally by a multidisciplinary team composed of rheumatologists, vascular specialists, cardiologists, and radiologists. Longitudinal assessment relies on careful history taking, physical examination, and serial imaging to evaluate for new or worsening areas of vascular involvement or development of features that suggest a more specific underlying diagnosis. Patients with a more specific diagnosis such as GCA or TAK should be treated according to established guidelines, and their management is beyond the scope of this article.[56,57]

Medical Therapy

The role of systemic immunosuppression in patients with CIA is unclear. No randomized controlled studies exist specific to CIA to inform the clinician of the optimal approach to therapy. Many cohorts of patients with CIA have a proportion of patients that were ultimately treated with immunosuppressive therapy but the number of patients is too small to conclude definitive benefit or risk. Although glucocorticoids are a mainstay of therapy in patients with established GCA or TAK, the role of glucocorticoids is unclear in patients with CIA. In series, 9% to 48% of patients with CIA are treated postoperatively with immunosuppressive therapy, mainly glucocorticoids (**Table 4**).[7,9,11–13,19–21,23,58] Regimens vary per institution, although high-to-moderate doses of prednisone (0.5–1.0 mg/kg/d) are used and tapered over weeks to months.[11,12,23]

The potential benefit of immunosuppressive therapy has not been reliably demonstrated in all cohorts. Interestingly, in the large Cleveland Clinic cohort of patients with CIA, patients treated with immunosuppression had lower incidence of relapse compared with those that did not receive immunosuppressive therapy (18% vs 50%, $P = .09$), although the number of treated patients were small (only 9%).[12] Similarly, in the Mayo Clinic series, lower rate of new or worsening vascular events (38% vs 46%) were seen in treated patients compared with the whole aortitis cohort.[23] All 3 patients in that series that had fatal complication of aortic aneurysm had not received glucocorticoids. However, the number of patients treated is small (n = 13, 35%).[23] A subsequent cohort study from the same institution reported one death in the 22 patients (4.5%) treated with glucocorticoids compared with 5 deaths in 42 patients (11.9%) that did not receive treatment.[7]

In other studies, no differences in outcomes were noted in patients treated with immunosuppressive therapy compared with untreated patients.[11,21] Murzin and colleagues showed no difference in new vascular involvement when considering treatment status.[11] Similarly, Caterson and colleagues showed no significant difference in 30-day mortality, morbidity, or resource utilization in those treated with glucocorticoids.[21] Some studies even suggest a potential harm in treated patients. In a smaller study, where about half the patients received glucocorticoid therapy, Aghayev and colleagues reported higher rate of descending aortic dilation (0.23 cm/y vs 0.06 cm/y) in patients that received glucocorticoids, although the result was not statistically significant.[20] Additionally, impaired wound healing and infectious risks are important considerations that frequently outweigh the unknown benefit of glucocorticoids, especially in patients without a systemic vasculitis.

Disease modifying agents such as methotrexate, azathioprine, mycophenolate mofetil, and infliximab have been used in some cases of aortitis determined to be refractory to monotherapy with glucocorticoids.[11,12,19,23] Transcriptomics represents an exciting field which may help tailor therapy in these challenging cases of aortitis of unclear cause.[54] Nonimmunosuppressive pharmacologic management includes blood pressure management, particularly in those patients with aneurysmal disease.[59,60]

Although the role of antiplatelet agents and statins have not been specifically established in the management of CIA, they might be considered on a case-by-case basis should the patient be at high risk for cardiovascular disease otherwise.[59,60]

Surgery

Large or enlarging aortic aneurysms should be evaluated by a vascular surgeon to explore whether intervention is indicated. The diameter criterion for intervention of known inflammatory thoracic aortic aneurysm is the same as for noninflammatory aneurysms.[59,60] Open repair is the current standard of intervention but there might be a role in some cases for an endovascular approach.[61] There is debate about whether in cases of CIA, surgical resection of the affected aorta itself is considered therapeutic, especially if the diseased tissue has been fully excised. It is for this reason that many patients with IA do not receive immunosuppressive treatment but rather are monitored longitudinally. On follow-up though, distal aortic dilatation or evolution of aneurysm is reported in some patients with CIA or giant cell aortitis without systemic vasculitis.[20,23,58] Because cases of CIA specifically were not included for consideration in the development of treatment guidelines for GCA and TAK, application of similar guiding principles with respect to surgical intervention and preop immunosuppressive agents in patients known to have CIA has an unclear role.[57] Ultimately, the decision to pursue medical treatment or rely on surgical intervention is challenging and should be made in the context of close consultation with an experienced pathologist, surgical team, radiologist, and rheumatologist.

Monitoring and Prognosis including Data on New Abnormalities or Need for Surgery

Follow-up duration varies per series but long-term survival of patients with CIA is 69% to 92%.[7,9,12,13,20,21,23] Various series report 25% to 56% of patients with CIA will develop new or worsening vascular involvement on follow-up (see **Table 4**).[11–13,19,20,23,58] Future dissection is rare but reported as well in a minority of cases.[19,20] Up to 40% of patients with CIA will require further surgical intervention for new aneurysm, dissection, or other vascular involvement (see **Table 4**).[11,12,19,23] It is also important to note that patients with CIA may later be diagnosed with a systemic inflammatory condition. In a study from the Cleveland Clinic, of the 196 patients with aortitis on surgical specimens from the thoracic aorta, during follow-up, 11 of the 73 patients (15%) initially classified as CIA were reclassified as having a systemic disease including GCA (63%), TAK (18%), spondyloarthritis (9%), undifferentiated systemic disease with migratory polyarthritis, and elevated markers of inflammation (9%).[12] For these reasons, regardless of the decision to treat or not with systemic immunosuppression, patients should be monitored serially with large-vessel cross-sectional imaging. Expertise in each imaging modality will vary by center and choice of modality should be made in consultation with the local radiologist.

SUMMARY

CIA is a rare and challenging disease often noted incidentally on surgical resection of the thoracic aorta. The diagnosis of CIA requires consideration for, and careful exclusion of, systemic rheumatologic conditions, which can cause aortitis. It remains unclear whether this represents an aortic limited form of LVV. Patients with CIA often have abnormalities in other vascular beds. They are at increased risk of recurrence and need to be monitored longitudinally for new vascular involvement, with a multidisciplinary team including vascular specialists, radiologists, and rheumatologists. The

Table 4
Outcomes of patients with clinically isolated aortitis from various surgical cohorts

Study	Number of CIA Cases	Duration of Follow up of Study (Mean)	Treated with Immunosuppression	New or Worsening Vascular Involvement	New Surgeries	CIA Revised to Systemic Disease	Death
Zehr KJ et al,[23] 2005[b]	34	2.8 ± 2.3 y	13 (35%)	17 (46%) – all	5 (13.5%)	–	8 (21.6%)
Liang KP et al,[7] 2009	52	15.4 mo (median)	22 (34%)	–	–	–	6 (9.4%)
Wang H et al,[9] 2012	24	45 mo (median)	5 (20%)	–	–	–	2 (8%)
Murzin DL et al,[11] 2017	32	47.5 mo	12 (38%)	5/12 [a](42%)	3 (9%)	6%	–
De Martino A et al,[13] 2019	19	30.5 mo	–	5/20 (25%)	–	–	6 (31%)
Clifford AH et al,[12] 2019	129	56.2 mo	12 (9%)	45%	29 (40%)	15%	9 (12%)
Goldhar HA et al,[19] 2019	9	3.6 y	2 (22%)	5 (56%)	3 (33%)	0%	–
Aghayev A et al,[20] 2021	23	8.8 y	11 (48%)	3 (12%)[c]	1 (4%)	–	5 (22%)
Caterson HC et al,[21] 2022	27	30 d	0	–	–	–	1 (3.7%)
Wang H et al,[58] 2012	15	58 mo	3 (20%)	7 (47)	5 (33%)	13%	–

Where possible, the percentages represent proportion of patients in that study with CIA.
a Only 12 patients had longitudinal imaging. Development of longitudinal lesions did not differ significantly by treatment status.
b Only 20 patients had follow-up imaging.
c All in patients that did not receive initial surgical management. A higher rate of descending aortic dilation (0.23 cm/y vs 0.06 cm/y) occurred in patients that received glucocorticoid therapy (P = ns).

decision to treat or intervene surgically should be made in the context of this multidisciplinary team. Glucocorticoids, immunosuppressive, and biologic therapy have all been described as potential treatment modalities in the patient with CIA but their role and benefit are uncertain. Next-generation transcriptomics represents a promising new technology to further understanding and potential therapies for this challenging disease entity.

CLINICS CARE POINTS

- CIA accounts for 47% to 81% of incidentally noted aortitis from surgical resection of the aorta, typically the ascending aorta.
- Several rheumatologic conditions, especially GCA can cause aortitis and evaluation of CIA requires a broad differential.
- The different patterns of inflammation noted on histopathology may provide clues as to the cause of aortitis.
- Imaging of the large-vessels with CTA or MRA should be performed in all patients with aortitis noted on surgical resection because 48% to 72% have abnormalities in other vascular beds.
- Treatment of CIA, especially when the affected aorta has been surgically resected, is controversial with much uncertainty about whether immunosuppressive therapy alters the natural course of the disease.
- Longitudinal multidisciplinary teams including vascular surgeons, radiologists, and rheumatologists are important in the monitoring of these patients, and 25% to 56% may be developing new vascular abnormalities over follow-up.

DISCLOSURE

The authors have nothing to disclose.

REFERENCES

1. Pugh D, Grayson P, Basu N, et al. Aortitis: recent advances, current concepts and future possibilities. Heart 2021;107:1620–9.
2. Cinar I, Wang H, Stone JR. Clinically isolated aortitis: pitfalls, progress, and possibilities. Cardiovasc Pathol 2017;29:23–32.
3. Jennette JC, Falk RJ, Bacon PA, et al. 2012 revised International Chapel Hill Consensus Conference Nomenclature of Vasculitides. Arthritis Rheum 2013; 65:1–11.
4. Rojo-Leyva F, Ratliff NB, Cosgrove DM 3rd, et al. Study of 52 patients with idiopathic aortitis from a cohort of 1,204 surgical cases. Arthritis Rheum 2000;43: 901–7.
5. Miller DV, Isotalo PA, Weyand CM, et al. Surgical pathology of noninfectious ascending aortitis: a study of 45 cases with emphasis on an isolated variant. Am J Surg Pathol 2006;30:1150–8.
6. Mennander AA, Miller DV, Liang KP, et al. Surgical management of ascending aortic aneurysm due to non-infectious aortitis. Scand Cardiovasc J 2008;42: 417–24.
7. Liang KP, Chowdhary VR, Michet CJ, et al. Noninfectious ascending aortitis: a case series of 64 patients. J Rheumatol 2009;36:2290–7.

8. Schmidt J, Sunesen K, Kornum JB, et al. Predictors for pathologically confirmed aortitis after resection of the ascending aorta: a 12-year Danish nationwide population-based cross-sectional study. Arthritis Res Ther 2011;13:R87.

9. Wang H, Li L, Wang L, et al. Comparison of clinical and pathological characteristics of isolated aortitis and Takayasu arteritis with ascending aorta involvement. J Clin Pathol 2012;65:362–6.

10. Ryan C, Barbour A, Burke L, et al. Non-infectious aortitis of the ascending aorta: a histological and clinical correlation of 71 cases including overlap with medial degeneration and atheroma–a challenge for the pathologist. J Clin Pathol 2015; 68:898–904.

11. Murzin DL, Belanger EC, Veinot JP, et al. A case series of surgically diagnosed idiopathic aortitis in a Canadian centre: a retrospective study. CMAJ Open 2017;5:E483–7.

12. Clifford AH, Arafat A, Idrees JJ, et al. Outcomes Among 196 Patients With Noninfectious Proximal Aortitis. Arthritis Rheumatol 2019;71:2112–20.

13. De Martino A, Ballestracci P, Faggioni L, et al. Incidence of Aortitis in Surgical Specimens of the Ascending Aorta Clinical Implications at Follow-Up. Semin Thorac Cardiovasc Surg 2019;31:751–60.

14. Quimson L, Mayer A, Capponi S, et al. Comparison of Aortitis Versus Noninflammatory Aortic Aneurysms Among Patients Who Undergo Open Aortic Aneurysm Repair. Arthritis Rheumatol 2020;72:1154–9.

15. Pacini D, Leone O, Turci S, et al. Incidence, etiology, histologic findings, and course of thoracic inflammatory aortopathies. Ann Thorac Surg 2008;86:1518–23.

16. Svensson LG, Arafat A, Roselli EE, et al. Inflammatory disease of the aorta: patterns and classification of giant cell aortitis, Takayasu arteritis, and nonsyndromic aortitis. J Thorac Cardiovasc Surg 2015;149:S170–5.

17. Ferfar Y, Morinet S, Espitia O, et al. Spectrum and Outcome of Noninfectious Aortitis. J Rheumatol 2021;48:1583–8.

18. Loricera J, Blanco R, Hernandez JL, et al. Non-infectious aortitis: a report of 32 cases from a single tertiary centre in a 4-year period and literature review. Clin Exp Rheumatol 2015;33:19–31.

19. Goldhar HA, Walker KM, Abdelrazek M, et al. Characteristics and outcomes in a prospective cohort of patients with histologically diagnosed aortitis. Rheumatol Adv Pract 2019;3:rky051.

20. Aghayev A, Bay CP, Tedeschi S, et al. Clinically isolated aortitis: imaging features and clinical outcomes: comparison with giant cell arteritis and giant cell aortitis. Int J Cardiovasc Imaging 2021;37:1433–43.

21. Caterson HC, Li A, March L, et al. Post-operative outcomes of inflammatory thoracic aortitis: a study of 41 patients from a cohort of 1119 surgical cases. Clin Rheumatol 2022;41:1219–26.

22. Espitia O, Samson M, Le Gallou T, et al. Comparison of idiopathic (isolated) aortitis and giant cell arteritis-related aortitis. A French retrospective multicenter study of 117 patients. Autoimmun Rev 2016;15:571–6.

23. Zehr KJ, Mathur A, Orszulak TA, et al. Surgical treatment of ascending aortic aneurysms in patients with giant cell aortitis. Ann Thorac Surg 2005;79:1512–7.

24. Agard C, Barrier JH, Dupas B, et al. Aortic involvement in recent-onset giant cell (temporal) arteritis: a case-control prospective study using helical aortic computed tomodensitometric scan. Arthritis Rheum 2008;59:670–6.

25. Hommada M, Mekinian A, Brillet PY, et al. Aortitis in giant cell arteritis: diagnosis with FDG PET/CT and agreement with CT angiography. Autoimmun Rev 2017;16: 1131–7.

26. Blockmans D, Coudyzer W, Vanderschueren S, et al. Relationship between fluorodeoxyglucose uptake in the large vessels and late aortic diameter in giant cell arteritis. Rheumatology 2008;47:1179–84.

27. de Boysson H, Liozon E, Lambert M, et al. 18F-fluorodeoxyglucose positron emission tomography and the risk of subsequent aortic complications in giant-cell arteritis: A multicenter cohort of 130 patients. Medicine (Baltim) 2016;95:e3851.

28. Prieto-Gonzalez S, Arguis P, Garcia-Martinez A, et al. Large vessel involvement in biopsy-proven giant cell arteritis: prospective study in 40 newly diagnosed patients using CT angiography. Ann Rheum Dis 2012;71:1170–6.

29. Gribbons KB, Ponte C, Craven A, et al. Diagnostic Assessment Strategies and Disease Subsets in Giant Cell Arteritis: Data From an International Observational Cohort. Arthritis Rheumatol 2020;72:667–76.

30. Hemmig AK, Gozzoli D, Werlen L, et al. Subclinical giant cell arteritis in new onset polymyalgia rheumatica A systematic review and meta-analysis of individual patient data. Semin Arthritis Rheum 2022;55:152017.

31. Pugh D, Karabayas M, Basu N, et al. Large-vessel vasculitis. Nat Rev Dis Primers 2022;7:93.

32. Kingdon J, Roscamp J, Sangle S, et al. Relapsing polychondritis: a clinical review for rheumatologists. Rheumatology 2018;57:1525–32.

33. Tomelleri A, Campochiaro C, Sartorelli S, et al. Large-vessel Vasculitis Affecting the Aorta and its Branches in Relapsing Polychondritis: Case Series and Systematic Review of the Literature. J Rheumatol 2020;47:1780–4.

34. Kitching AR, Anders HJ, Basu N, et al. ANCA-associated vasculitis. Nat Rev Dis Primers 2020;6:71.

35. Skeik N, Hari G, Nasr R. Aortitis caused by antineutrophil cytoplasmic antibodies (ANCA)-associated vasculitis: a case-based review. Rheumatol Int 2019;39:1983–8.

36. Greco A, De Virgilio A, Ralli M, et al. Behcet's disease: New insights into pathophysiology, clinical features and treatment options. Autoimmun Rev 2018;17:567–75.

37. Durtette C, Hachulla E, Resche-Rigon M, et al. Cogan syndrome: Characteristics, outcome and treatment in a French nationwide retrospective study and literature review. Autoimmun Rev 2017;16:1219–23.

38. Drent M, Crouser ED, Grunewald J. Challenges of Sarcoidosis and Its Management. N Engl J Med 2021;385:1018–32.

39. Fernandes SR, Singsen BH, Hoffman GS. Sarcoidosis and systemic vasculitis. Semin Arthritis Rheum 2000;30:33–46.

40. Weiler V, Redtenbacher S, Bancher C, et al. Concurrence of sarcoidosis and aortitis: case report and review of the literature. Ann Rheum Dis 2000;59:850–3.

41. Kimbrough BA, Warrington KJ, Langenfeld HE, et al. Vasculitis in Patients With Sarcoidosis: A Single-Institution Case Series of 17 Patients. J Clin Rheumatol 2022;28:217–22.

42. Bunu DM, Timofte CE, Ciocoiu M, et al. Cardiovascular Manifestations of Inflammatory Bowel Disease: Pathogenesis, Diagnosis, and Preventive Strategies. Gastroenterol Res Pract 2019;2019:3012509.

43. Bekele DI, Warrington KJ, Koster MJ. Giant cell arteritis associated with inflammatory bowel disease: a case-series and review of the literature. Rheumatol Int 2021;41:487–92.

44. Sy A, Khalidi N, Dehghan N, et al. Vasculitis in patients with inflammatory bowel diseases: A study of 32 patients and systematic review of the literature. Semin Arthritis Rheum 2016;45:475–82.

45. de Almeida Martins C, Caon AER, Facanali CBG, et al. Coexistence of Takayasu's Arteritis in Patients with Inflammatory Bowel Diseases. Gastroenterol Res Pract 2021;2021:8831867.

46. Gudbrandsson B, Molberg O, Garen T, et al. Prevalence, Incidence, and Disease Characteristics of Takayasu Arteritis by Ethnic Background: Data From a Large, Population-Based Cohort Resident in Southern Norway. Arthritis Care Res 2017;69:278–85.

47. Perugino CA, Stone JH. IgG4-related disease: an update on pathophysiology and implications for clinical care. Nat Rev Rheumatol 2020;16:702–14.

48. Wallace ZS, Zhang Y, Perugino CA, et al. Clinical phenotypes of IgG4-related disease: an analysis of two international cross-sectional cohorts. Ann Rheum Dis 2019;78:406–12.

49. Kaneko S, Yamashita H, Sugimori Y, et al. Rheumatoid arthritis-associated aortitis: a case report and literature review. SpringerPlus 2014;3:509.

50. Palazzi C, Salvarani C, D'Angelo S, et al. Aortitis and periaortitis in ankylosing spondylitis. Joint Bone Spine 2011;78:451–5.

51. Akebo H, Sada R, Matsushita S, et al. Lupus Aortitis Successfully Treated with Moderate-dose Glucocorticoids: A Case Report and Review of the Literature. Intern Med 2020;59:2789–95.

52. Stone JR, Bruneval P, Angelini A, et al. Consensus statement on surgical pathology of the aorta from the Society for Cardiovascular Pathology and the Association for European Cardiovascular Pathology: I. Inflammatory diseases. Cardiovasc Pathol 2015;24:267–78.

53. Getz TM, Hoffman GS, Padmanabhan R, et al. Microbiomes of Inflammatory Thoracic Aortic Aneurysms Due to Giant Cell Arteritis and Clinically Isolated Aortitis Differ From Those of Non-Inflammatory Aneurysms. Pathog Immun 2019;4: 105–23.

54. Hur B, Koster MJ, Jang JS, et al. Global Transcriptomic Profiling Identifies Differential Gene Expression Signatures Between Inflammatory and Noninflammatory Aortic Aneurysms. Arthritis Rheumatol 2022;74:1376–86.

55. Talarico R, Boiardi L, Pipitone N, et al. Isolated aortitis versus giant cell arteritis: are they really two sides of the same coin? Clin Exp Rheumatol 2014;32:S55–8.

56. Hellmich B, Agueda A, Monti S, et al. 2018 Update of the EULAR recommendations for the management of large vessel vasculitis. Ann Rheum Dis 2020;79: 19–30.

57. Maz M, Chung SA, Abril A, et al. 2021 American College of Rheumatology/Vasculitis Foundation Guideline for the Management of Giant Cell Arteritis and Takayasu Arteritis. Arthritis Rheumatol 2021;73:1349–65.

58. Wang H, Smith RN, Spooner AE, et al. Giant cell aortitis of the ascending aorta without signs or symptoms of systemic vasculitis is associated with elevated risk of distal aortic events. Arthritis Rheum 2012;64:317–9.

59. Hiratzka LF, Bakris GL, Beckman JA, et al. 2010 ACCF/AHA/AATS/ACR/ASA/ SCA/SCAI/SIR/STS/SVM guidelines for the diagnosis and management of patients with Thoracic Aortic Disease: a report of the American College of Cardiology Foundation/American Heart Association Task Force on Practice Guidelines, American Association for Thoracic Surgery, American College of Radiology, American Stroke Association, Society of Cardiovascular Anesthesiologists, Society for Cardiovascular Angiography and Interventions, Society of Interventional Radiology, Society of Thoracic Surgeons, and Society for Vascular Medicine. Circulation 2010;121:e266–369.

60. Accf/Aha/Aats/Acr/Asa/Sca/Scai/Sir/Sts/Svm Guidelines For The Diagnosis, Management Of Patients With Thoracic Aortic Disease Representative Members, Hiratzka LF, et al. Surgery for Aortic Dilatation in Patients With Bicuspid Aortic Valves: A Statement of Clarification From the American College of Cardiology/ American Heart Association Task Force on Clinical Practice Guidelines. Circulation 2016;133:680–6.
61. Oishi K, Mizuno T, Fujiwara T, et al. Surgical strategy for inflammatory thoracic aortic aneurysms in the endovascular surgery era. J Vasc Surg 2022;75: 74–80 e72.

Treatment Approaches to Granulomatosis with Polyangiitis and Microscopic Polyangiitis

Check for updates

Alvise Berti, MD, PhD[a], Divi Cornec, MD, PhD[b],*, Anisha B. Dua, MD, MPH[c]

KEYWORDS

- ANCA vasculitis ● Granulomatosis with polyangiitis ● Microscopic polyangiitis
- Treatment

Continued

BACKGROUND/INTRODUCTION

Granulomatosis with polyangiitis (GPA) and microscopic polyangiitis (MPA) are antineutrophilic cytoplasmic antibody (ANCA)-associated vasculitides (AAV) that cause inflammation and necrosis of the small blood vessels, leading to downstream ischemia and organ damage. GPA is associated with the presence of granulomas on pathology, serine proteinase-3 (PR3) positivity, higher frequency of ENT and upper airway involvement, and a higher risk of relapses compared with MPA, which pathologically demonstrates inflammation and necrosis without granulomas, and with myeloperoxidase (MPO) positivity. Despite differences in pathology and clinical manifestations, both of these entities have been included together in most randomized controlled trials evaluating induction and maintenance of remission regimens in patients with AAV.

We have made significant strides in our ability to effectively induce and maintain remission in our patients with GPA and MPA, but challenges still remain. The use of glucocorticoids (GC), cyclophosphamide, and rituximab has changed the face of AAV from an almost uniformly fatal disease to one where remission is achieved in 80% to 90% of patients. However, mortality at 5 years is still 10% to 20%, with 50% of deaths in the first year being attributed to infection, and relapses occur in

[a] Center for Medical Sciences (CISMed), Department of Cellular, Computational and Integrative Biology (CIBIO), University of Trento, and Division of Rheumatology, Santa Chiara Hospital, APSS Trento, Italy; [b] Rheumatology Department, INSERM UMR1227 LBAI, Lymphocytes B, Autoimmunité et Immunothérapies, University of Brest, National Reference Center for Rare Systemic Autoimmune Diseases CERAINO, CHRU Brest, Brest, France; [c] Division of Rheumatology, Northwestern University Feinberg School of Medicine, 675 North Saint Clair Street, Suite 14-100, Chicago, IL 60611, USA
* Corresponding author. INSERM U1227 "B cell, Autoimmunity and Immunotherapies", Brest University Hospital, Bd Tanguy Prigent, Brest Cedex 29609, France.
E-mail address: divi.cornec@chu-brest.fr

Rheum Dis Clin N Am 49 (2023) 545–561
https://doi.org/10.1016/j.rdc.2023.03.004
0889-857X/23/

Continued

KEY POINTS

- Glucocorticoids are a mainstay of induction therapy in patients with granulomatosis with polyangiitis (GPA) and microscopic polyangiitis (MPA), although recent trials and guidelines have demonstrated that we can successfully induce remission with significantly lower doses.
- Both cyclophosphamide and rituximab are effective for inducing remission in GPA/MPA, and patient- as well as disease-specific factors must be considered in choosing a therapeutic agent.
- Plasmapheresis should not be used routinely for induction in patients with GPA/MPA.
- Rituximab has demonstrated efficacy in maintaining remission for patients with GPA/MPA although the length of therapy and the role of long-term low-dose glucocorticoid treatment remain unclear.
- Unmet needs in GPA/MPA include disease refractory to our current induction regimens, persistent low-grade disease activity, relapses, and side effects from the medications used to treat the underlying disease. Active research is underway to try and address many of these concerns.

up to 20% of patients within 18 months.[1] Side effects and toxicities of the medications used to control disease activity remain significant issues in the management of our patients.[2] Many ongoing trials are evaluating new or repurposed drugs for the management of AAV. In this review, we discuss various classes of medication that have been evaluated in the management of AAV including GC, cyclophosphamide, disease-modifying antirheumatic drugs, B-cell–targeted therapies, complement inhibition, and plasmapheresis. We additionally discuss some of the variations in treatment strategies between the American College of Rheumatology/Vasculitis Foundation (ACR/VF) and the European Alliance of Associations for Rheumatology (EULAR) guidelines in the management of GPA and MPA and highlight ongoing therapeutic trials that are underway.

PATIENT ASSESSMENT

After AAV is diagnosed, individual patient assessment should govern the choice of induction remission therapy. The disease activity and the damage, quantified respectively with the Birmingham vasculitis Activity Score (BVAS)[3] and the Vasculitis Damage Index (VDI),[4] the clinical phenotype (GPA versus MPA) and antibody profile (PR3-ANCA, MPO-ANCA, ANCA–negative),[5] the patient age and body mass index, the prognosis, and quality of life should be considered in this choice (**Table 1**).

For instance, clinical diagnosis, ANCA subtype, and new versus relapsing disease are 3 nonindependent risk factors for relapse. Disease activity, prognosis, age, and comorbidities may help to guide the choice of immunosuppression, for example, older age and renal dysfunction for reducing the dose of cyclophosphamide for disease induction. Weight is important in determining the initial GC dose. A high degree of chronicity in kidney biopsy and disease damage may influence the intensity of immunosuppression initiated. Fertility and quality of life may also influence therapy choice (eg, avoiding cyclophosphamide in younger patients and so forth).[6–8]

Before starting immunosuppressive therapy, a risk assessment for comorbidities (eg, cardiovascular disease, diabetes mellitus, and psychiatric disorders that increase the risk of associated adverse events to corticosteroids) or any concomitant infections (eg, chronic carrier of hepatitis B infection that requires prophylaxis) or susceptibility to

Table 1
Patient factors to be evaluated before starting or changing immunosuppressive therapy

Clinical diagnosis	GPA versus MPA
ANCA serology	PR3-ANCA, MPO-ANCA ANCA—negative
Previous disease course	New vs relapsing disease
Disease activity	Birmingham Vasculitis Activity Score (BVAS)[3]
Disease prognosis projection	Eg, Five-Factor Score[62]
BMI/weight	—
Age	—
Chronicity on kidney biopsy[a]	Berden Score,[6] Mayo Clinic Chronicity Score,[7] and so forth
Prior disease damage	Vasculitis Damage Index (VDI)[4]
Comorbidities	Eg, cardiovascular disease, diabetes mellitus, osteoporosis, and psychiatric disorders
Immune status and infection	Risk assessment for any concomitant infections or latent infection, possible immunodeficiencies, and so forth
Fertility	—
HRQoL	Eg, AAV—patient-reported outcome[8]

Abbreviation: HRQoL, health-related quality of life.
[a] When kidney biopsy is performed in patients with glomerulonephritis due to AAV.

infections (ie, hypogammaglobulinemia after prolonged GC, potentially affecting the choice of rituximab therapy) should be performed.[9]

Treatment should not be delayed, particularly with severe pulmonary and/or renal disease. GC can be started in the absence of a definite diagnosis with high clinical suspicion for AAV (ie, awaiting biopsy) to avoid diagnostic delays and worse prognosis.[10]

GLUCOCORTICOIDS
Induction of Remission

GC are recommended as part of the induction of remission strategy for GPA/MPA. GC therapy should be started immediately at diagnosis or when a diagnosis of AAV is likely. Different regimens have been used in prospective trials (**Table 2**) over the years, with a progressive reduction of the cumulative dose. For more severe disease, intravenous pulses of methylprednisolone at a dose of 500 to 1000 mg per day for 3 days (1000–3000 mg) are common practice in many institutions, with no head-to-head comparisons.[11] Alternatively, oral GC at a dose of 1 mg/kg per day of prednisone (or equivalent) with a relatively prolonged taper were used in previous trials (see **Table 2**).[12–17] Importantly, observational studies have reported increased rates of infections with the use of higher initial doses GC (including pulses).

However, we have been moving toward GC-sparing regimens. The PEXIVAS and LOVAS trials showed that reduced GC regimens are equally effective in inducing remission in AAV.[15,17] In addition, the concept of tailoring GC based on the patients' weight has clearly emerged from recent trials. The PEXIVAS trial compared 2 regimens of GC in severe patients (with life-/organ-threatening disease) initially treated with methylprednisolone pulses. The "reduced" GC regimen (faster taper than the standard regimen) decreases prednisone to 20 mg per day within 7 weeks and 5 mg per day within 19 weeks. This reduced GC regimen is associated with a lower risk of serious

Table 2
Main corticosteroid (per day)-tapering schemes for induction of remission according to different randomized controlled trials

Weeks[a]	EUVAS/ CYCLOPS	WEGENT	CORTAGE	RAVE	PEXIVAS (Reduced Dose Arm <50 kg)	PEXIVAS (Reduced Dose Arm 50–75 kg)	PEXIVAS (Reduced Dose Arm >75 kg)	ADVOCATE (Control Arm ≥ 55 kg)	ADVOCATE (Control Arm < 55 kg)	LOVAS (0.5 mg/ kg/day Arm)
GC Pulse	Yes	Yes	Yes	Yes	Yes	Yes	Yes	No	No	No
0	1 mg/kg	1 mg/kg	60 mg	1 mg/kg	50 mg	60 mg	75 mg	60 mg	45 mg	0.5 mg/kg
1	0.75 mg/kg	1 mg/kg	60 mg	—	50 mg	60 mg	75 mg	60 mg	45 mg	0.5 mg/kg
2	0.5 mg/kg	1 mg/kg	60 mg	—	25 mg	30 mg	40 mg	45 mg	45 mg	0.5 mg/kg
4	0.4 mg/kg	0.75 mg/kg	50 mg	40 mg	20 mg	25 mg	30 mg	30 mg	30 mg	0.25 mg/kg
6	0.33 mg/kg	0.5 mg/kg	40 mg	30 mg	15 mg	20 mg	25 mg	25 mg	25 mg	7.5 mg
8	0.28 mg/kg	0.4 mg/kg	30 mg	20 mg	12.5 mg	15 mg	20 mg	20 mg	20 mg	5 mg
10	0.25 mg/kg	0.33 mg/kg	27.5 mg	15 mg	10 mg	12.5 mg	15 mg	15 mg	15 mg	4 mg
12	0.25 mg/kg	0.33 mg/kg	22.5 mg	10 mg	7.5 mg	10 mg	12.5 mg	10 mg	10 mg	3 mg
20	10 mg	—	—	0 mg	5 mg	5 mg	5 mg	5 mg	5 mg	1 mg
24	10/7.5 mg	12.5 mg	7 mg	0 mg	5 mg	5 mg	5 mg	0 mg	0 mg	0 mg

Footnotes: all trials (excluding LOVAS and ADVOCATE) allowed 1 to 3 g of methylprednisolone pulses before starting oral prednisolone. In ADVOCATE trial patients were excluded if they had received more than 3 g of intravenous GC within 4 weeks or more than 10 mg per day of oral prednisone (or equivalent) for more than 6 weeks continuously; in LOVAS trial, except for the protocolized dose of prednisolone, systemic administration of GC, including intravenous methylprednisolone pulse therapy, was not allowed in either treatment group.

a According to RAVE protocol, the use of glucocorticoids followed a strict protocol. Patients received 1 to 3 (1000 mg) pulses of methylprednisolone at enrollment, followed by prednisone 1 mg/kg/day (maximum 80 mg/day). The dose was tapered such that by month 5 all patients who achieved remission without flaring had completely discontinued glucocorticoids. The prednisone dose was reduced to 40 mg/day no later than by the completion of week 4 and maintained for 2 weeks. Stepwise dose reductions then continued every 2 weeks: 30 mg, 20 mg, 15 mg, 10 mg, 7.5 mg, 5 mg, 2.5 mg, and 0 mg/day. Within these parameters, the protocol allowed for investigator discretion about the oral prednisone dose between randomization and completion of week 4.

infection at 1 year while being equally effective at induction of remission when compared with the standard regimen.[15] More recently, the LOVAS trial demonstrated that a "reduced" regimen, starting with lower dose of 0.5 mg/kg/day of GC may be enough to induce remission in newly diagnosed, less severe AAV (without life-/severe organ-threatening disease).[17] Unfortunately, different inclusion criteria (eg, more severe patients enrolled in PEXIVAS), patients characteristics (eg, new diagnosis only in LOVAS, different ethnicities in PEXIVAS whereas only Japanese in LOVAS, and so forth), and treatment protocols (eg, GC pulses in PEXIVAS, no pulses in LOVAS) have impaired a more direct comparison of the 2 protocols (**Fig. 1**). In addition, the RITAZAREM trial, a prospective study of rituximab in relapsing patients with AAV, allowed a reduced GC dose for induction (0.5 mg/kg/day vs 1 mg/kg/day, based on clinical judgment) and demonstrated that the incidence of hypogammaglobulinemia (IgG <5 g/L) during follow-up of the patients receiving lower dose induction GCs was half that of the standard dose group.[18] In addition, the ADVOCATE trial control arm used relatively low GC doses, reflecting the current practice to keep GC at minimum.[16]

Maintenance of Remission

After remission-induction it is common practice to reduce the GC dose possibly until discontinuation.[5] No robust data exist to guide this decision, with different trials showing different approaches, but with a propensity to discontinue GCs if possible within the first year after diagnosis. This approach of clinical practice was initially proposed in the RAVE trial, and more recently has been used in the ADVOCATE and CLEAR control arms.[16,19] In clinical practice, GC treatment has to be individualized for each patient.

A meta-analysis in 2010 showed that longer courses of GC after remission-induction was associated with fewer relapses, with a proportion of relapse of 14% (95% confidence interval [CI] 10%–19%) in those studies that continue GCs and 43% (95% CI 33%–52%) in those studies that discontinued GCs during follow-up. Notably, these trials with GC continuation (regardless of the dose) enrolled only newly diagnosed patients, whereas the trials that discontinued GC enrolled both newly diagnosed and relapsing patients, possibly influencing the final results.[20]

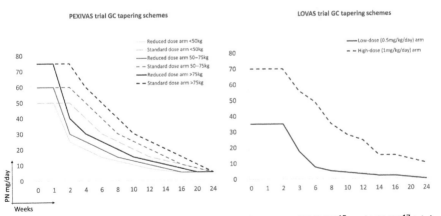

Fig. 1. Glucocorticoids (GC)-tapering schemes from the recent PEXIVAS[15] and LOVAS[17] trials, aiming to use lower dose of GC to induce remission. To ensure some degree of comparability between the 2 schemes, the LOVAS scheme was calculated for a subject of 70 kg.

Considering these uncertainties in defining the optimal dosing and duration of GC for remission maintenance in AAV, in recent trials (ie, PEXIVAS), the decision to stop or continue low-dose GC in the long term was left to the physician/investigator.[15]

CYCLOPHOSPHAMIDE, AZATHIOPRINE, METHOTREXATE, MYCOPHENOLATE MOFETIL

Major steps in the development of effective therapies for AAV have been first the use of GC in the 60s and then the introduction of immunosuppressive regimens using cyclophosphamide (CYC) after the experience of Anthony Fauci at the National Institutes of Health in the early 70s.[21] However, it was soon described that long-term use of CYC leads to frequent and severe cancerous, hematological and infectious side effects. Several strategies were therefore evaluated to limit the use of CYC. The concept of a 2-phase treatment strategy using first CYC + GC to induce remission followed by azathioprine to prevent relapses was evaluated and validated in a seminal study published in 2003.[22] This strategy became the standard of care for severe AAV for 2 decades until the publication of the first rituximab studies in 2010 (see next section).

Cyclophosphamide can be administered as intermittent intravenous boluses or oral daily doses, with intravenous (IV) protocols leading to a 50% lower cumulative dose compared with oral administration with similar efficacy to induce remission (CYCLOPS trial)[12] but potentially higher rates of subsequent relapses.[23] IV CYC doses can be safely further reduced in older patients and in those with renal insufficiency, leading to a similar efficacy and a lower rate of adverse events.[14]

Other immunosuppressive drugs have been evaluated to induce or maintain remission in patients with AAV. Methotrexate has been shown to induce remission in patients with nonsevere forms of GPA with similar rates compared with CYC in the NORAM study,[24] but it is associated with an increased long-term risk of relapses.[25] Methotrexate (MTX) has also been evaluated for remission maintenance after CYC and showed a similar efficacy compared with azathioprine.[13] Mycophenolate mofetil (MMF) has been compared with CYC to induce remission in the MYCYC trial and showed similar rates of remission, but an increased relapse rate was observed in patients treated with MMF, particularly in PR3-ANCA–positive patients.[26] The noninferiority of MMF compared with cyclophosphamide to induce remission has been suggested by a recent meta-analysis of phase II and III trials,[27] but it is currently used only as a second-line agent in selected patients with MPA/GPA.

B-Cell–Targeting Therapies: Rituximab, Obinutuzumab, Belimumab

Because ANCAs have been shown to be pathogenic and induce vasculitis by direct transfer in mouse models,[28] the idea of targeting and depleting B cells, the precursors of ANCA-secreting cells, using anti-CD20 antibodies to treat AAV arose soon after rituximab was commercialized for the treatment of B-cell lymphomas.[29] After an initial positive experience in a few refractory patients,[30] 2 randomized controlled studies were published in 2010. Both the RAVE[31] and the RITUXVAS[32] studies demonstrated that, in addition to high-dose GC, treatment with rituximab (4 weekly 375 mg/m² infusions with no maintenance infusions) was noninferior to CYC followed by azathioprine, with similar rates of remission off GC at 6 months (around 70% of the patients) and similar relapse rates at 18 months (around 40% of the patients who had first reached remission in the RAVE study).[5] Furthermore, rituximab was shown to be superior to CYC in the subsets of patients with relapsing disease and PR3-AAV.[33] Soon after, the MAINRITSAN study demonstrated that semestrial infusions of rituximab for 2 years (500 mg every 6 months) was superior to azathioprine to maintain remission after induction using CYC.[34] The MAINRITSAN 2 study then demonstrated that fixed semestrial dosing of rituximab had a similar efficacy compared with a tailored regimen (based on ANCA titers and CD20 B-cell recurrence),[35] but long-term outcomes of the 2 regimens have yet to be studied. The RITAZAREM study, completed more recently and using higher doses of rituximab (1 g infusions every 4 months for 2 years) in patients in remission after induction using rituximab, led to similar conclusions but is not yet published. Therefore, rituximab is currently considered the gold standard for maintenance of remission in patients with AAV. The optimal duration of maintenance treatment is yet ill-defined, with longer durations of treatments leading to less frequent relapses, but we are still lacking actionable predictive factors to personalize the treatment according to an individual risk of relapse.[36]

However, some patients are refractory to rituximab or develop anaphylaxis to the drug, so other B-cell–depleting agents have been evaluated in open-label studies. A case series reported good tolerance and efficacy of ofatumumab,[37] and another of obinutuzumab,[38] more recently developed humanized anti-CD20 antibodies. Although promising, these observations need to be confirmed in prospective controlled trials.

Finally, B-cell activating factor of the tumor necrosis factor family (BAFF), a cytokine involved in the activation of B cells and suspected to provide survival signal to autoreactive B cells, can be targeted by belimumab, a drug currently labeled for the treatment of systemic lupus erythematosus. Belimumab has been evaluated as a remission maintenance treatment in association with azathioprine in patients with AAV in the BREVAS study. However, because of difficulties in enrollment after the publication of the MAINRITSAN study that showed the superiority of rituximab over azathioprine, the BREVAS study was terminated after only 105 patients were treated, and no efficacy signal emerged from these incomplete data.[39]

New B-cell–depleting strategies are currently being evaluated in other autoimmune diseases, such as anti-BAFF receptor monoclonal antibodies in patients with Sjögren disease[40] or CD19-CAR T cells in patients with refractory systemic lupus erythematosus.[41,42] These treatments may be able to lead to a more profound B-cell depletion in the inflamed tissues and a better control of the autoimmune processes, but they have not been tested yet in patients with AAV.

COMPLEMENT INHIBITION
The Role of the Alternative Complement Pathway

Although hypocomplementemia is relatively uncommon in AAV and biopsies of tissue show scarce complement deposition or a "pauci-immune" pattern, multiple studies have demonstrated the importance of the complement pathway in mediating tissue injury in AAV.[43,44] Neutrophil activation is a key component in the pathogenesis of AAV, resulting in increased expression of PR3 and MPO on the surface of the neutrophil, thus allowing ANCAs to bind, with downstream respiratory burst, degranulation, vascular inflammation and damage.

Studies have shown that when MPO ANCA is injected into mice, they develop a necrotizing glomerulonephritis resembling human AAV and that when the alternative complement pathway, specifically the interaction between C5a and its receptor (C5aR), is blocked, these mice are protected from developing glomerulonephritis.[28,45,46] Results of human in-vitro experiments also revealed that C5a acts as a primer of neutrophils, increasing their expression of ANCA targets and enhancing their response to ANCA, and that ANCA activated neutrophils release factors that activate complement and generate further C5a.[47] This establishes an amplification loop that sustains ANCA-induced vascular inflammation. A meta-analysis revealed higher levels of circulating C5a, membrane attack complex, and factor B in patients with active AAV compared with those in remission or healthy controls.[48] These insights into the role of the alternative complement pathway has translated into a new target for the therapeutic management of AAV, specifically by blocking the interaction between C5a and its receptor.

Clinical Implications

Avacopan, an orally administered inhibitor of C5aR, prevents the binding of C5a and was approved by the Food and Drug Administration in October 2021 in combination with standard therapy for induction in GPA and MPA. Avacopan was initially studied in the phase II trials CLEAR and CLASSIC, which demonstrated the safety and efficacy of avacopan, 30 mg, twice a day.[19,49,50] The phase III ADVOCATE trial included 331 MPO- or PR3-positive patients with new or relapsing AAV.[16] All participants were induced with cyclophosphamide (oral or IV) for 12 weeks or rituximab weekly for 4 weeks, and those treated with cyclophosphamide were given maintenance therapy with azathioprine. The participants were randomized to receive avacopan, 30 mg, BID or prednisone, 60 mg, daily tapered to 0 by week 20.

Study results demonstrated that avacopan was noninferior to GC in inducing remission at 26 weeks (72.3% avacopan vs 70.1% prednisone, p < 0.001) and was superior at achieving sustained remission at 1 year (65.7% avacopan vs 54.9% prednisone p = 0.007). There was a 54% relative risk reduction in relapses in the avacopan arm (10.1% avacopan vs 21% prednisone). Improvements in estimated glomerular filtration rate (eGFR) were numerically higher in the avacopan arm at 26 weeks (5.8 vs 2.8 mL/min/1.73 m^2, p = 0.04) and 1 year (7.3 vs 4.0 mL/min/1.73 m^2, p = 0.02), but this did not reach statistical significance for superiority compared with GC. It is important to note that participants in both arms who were induced with rituximab did not get a maintenance dose of rituximab or other maintenance agent at 26 weeks, which may have influenced the trial results. Importantly, the GC toxicity index and health related quality of life measures were superior in the avacopan treated patients, and serious adverse events and serious infections were comparable in both arms. Avacopan was significantly GC sparing (mean dose of 1349 mg vs 3655 mg, median dose 400 mg vs 2939 mg in the avacopan vs GC arms, respectively). Because the critical role of C5a in the pathogenesis of MPA/GPA has been elucidated, we now have a new drug approved that can significantly reduce steroid burden in patients with AAV.

Also targeting the interaction of C5a and its receptor, vilobelimab, an anti-C5a antibody, has demonstrated positive phase II results in both the United States (US IXPLORE, NCT03712345) and Europe (IXCHANGE–NCT03895801). Vilobelimab (in addition to cyclophosphamide or rituximab), dosed at 800 mg IV every 2 weeks for 16 weeks (after loading doses at 1, 4, and 8 days), was shown to be comparable to standard of care with high-dose corticosteroids in clinical response and Vasculitis Damage Index (VDI), with lower GC toxicities and adverse events in the vilobelimab arm. These positive findings have yet to be evaluated in a phase III trial.

Targeting the alternative complement pathway (along with cyclophosphamide or rituximab) has enabled significantly less GC exposure during induction of remission in patients with AAV. Questions regarding the efficacy of avacopan in advanced renal failure, its effect on other extrarenal disease manifestations, the optimal length of treatment, long-term outcomes beyond one year, and cost-effectiveness still remain.

PLASMA EXCHANGE

The PEXIVAS trial, which included 704 patients, indicates that the routine use of plasma exchange (7 plasma exchanges within 14 days after randomization) for severe GPA and MPA with glomerulonephritis (eGFR <50 mL/min/1.73 m^2) or alveolar hemorrhage has no benefit.[15] Reported death from any cause or end-stage kidney disease at 12 months from randomization was 28.4% in the plasma exchange group versus 31% in the control group (hazard ratio [HR] 0.86; 95% confidence interval [CI] 0.65 to 1.13). Several subgroup analyses were conducted to evaluate if plasma exchange was beneficial, including stratifying the patients by age (≥60 years old), serum creatinine level (≥500 μmol), ANCA type (PR3-ANCA versus MPO-ANCA), presence of alveolar hemorrhage (<85% O2 saturation in ambient air), and type of induction therapy (CYC iv/CYC oral/RTX), but no subgroup was found to significantly benefit from plasma exchange.

The previous MEPEX trial, including 137 patients, showed that plasma exchange increased the rate of renal recovery in severe AAV presenting with renal failure when compared with intravenous methylprednisolone alone.[51] There are several reasons that may explain the conflicting results of MEPEX and PEXIVAS; first, all participants in the MEPEX trial had severe (serum creatinine >5.8 mg/dL) glomerulonephritis, whereas the criteria to establish severity was less stringent (eGFR <50 mL/min/1.73 m^2 or diffuse pulmonary hemorrhage) in PEXIVAS (**Table 3**). Second, all the patients in MEPEX had a biopsy-proven glomerulonephritis, whereas only a minority of PEXIVAS participants were biopsy-confirmed. In addition, in MEPEX,

Table 3
Comparison between MEPEX and PEIXVAS trial

MEPEX[51]	PEXIVAS[15]
137 patients (European)	704 patients (International)
Inclusion criteria: serum creatinine >5.8 mg/dL, biopsy-proven glomerulonephritis	Inclusion criteria: eGFR <50 mL/min/1.73 m^2 and/or diffuse pulmonary hemorrhage; biopsy not required for inclusion
Design: PLEX vs IV methylprednisolone	Design: PLEX vs No PLEX; Reduced vs standard GC dose
5 to 7 sessions of PLEX Albumin as plasma substitute	5 to 7 sessions of PLEX Albumin as plasma substitute
Immunosuppressive treatment: Oral CYC (100%)	Immunosuppressive treatment: CYC (85%) or rituximab (15%) + IV methylprednisolone for 1–3 days (1–3 g)
Serology: PR3-ANCA 43% MPO-ANCA 52%	Serology: PR3-ANCA 41% MPO-ANCA 59%
Disease activity: BVAS.v3: 21	Disease activity: BVAS.v3: 9
Creatinine (μmol/L; median [range]): 735 (498 to 1669)	Creatinine (μmol/L; median [IQR]: 327 (206–491) for PLEX, 336 (209–495) for No PLEX)
Dialysis: PLEX (67%) vs methylprednisolone (71%)	Dialysis: PLEX (19%) vs NO PLEX (21%)
Primary endpoint: 3 months Secondary endpoint: 12 months	Primary endpoint: 12 months Secondary endpoint: 12 months
ESRD: HR 0.47 (95% CI: 0.24–0.91)	ESRD: HR 0.81 (95% CI: 0.57–1.13)
Deaths and AEs at 1 year: no difference	Deaths and AEs at 1 year: no difference

Abbreviations: AEs, adverse events; BVAS.v3, Birmingham Vasculitis Activity Score version 3; CYC, cyclophosphamide; ESRD, end-stage renal disease; GC, glucocorticoids; HR, hazard ratio; PLEX, plasma exchange.

baseline disease activity was higher than those enrolled in PEXIVAS, as demonstrated by a higher BVAS.

A recent meta-analysis of the published trials suggested a possible benefit of plasma exchange on renal outcome at 12 months in patients with severe renal disease, with a 4.6% reduction of the EKSD risk at 12 months for creatinine greater than 300 μmol/L and a 16% reduction of the EKSD risk at 12 months for creatinine greater than 500 μmol/L. However, the use of plasma exchange significantly increased the risk of serious infection at 12 months (HR 1.27, 95% CI 1.08–1.49).[52] Consequently, the use of plasma exchange remains highly controversial and should not be used routinely and rather be reserved for patients with severe renal disease in select situations, while balancing the risk of severe infection.

DIFFERENCES AND SIMILARITIES BETWEEN SELECTED INTERNATIONAL CLINICAL GUIDELINES IN ANTIBODY-ASSOCIATED VASCULITIDES

The main international guidelines have slightly different positions about the management of GPA/MPA (**Table 4**),[9,10] depending on the specific recommendation. We compared the Kidney Disease Improving Global Outcomes (KDIGO) 2021, focusing on glomerulonephritis, that were written by nephrologists, the American College of Rheumatology/Vasculitis Foundation (ACR/VF) 2021 written by rheumatologists, and European Alliance of Association for Rheumatology (EULAR) 2022 (recommendations not yet published but presented at the EULAR meeting 2022 in Copenhagen) that are the effort of a mixed panel mainly composed of nephrologists and rheumatologists.

For instance, for induction treatment, KDIGO 2021 and EULAR 2022 recognized similar efficacy of CYC and RTX to induce remission in severe active disease, whereas ACR/VF conditionally recommends RTX over CYC. This statement for ACR/VF was based on the fact that RTX is considered less toxic than CYC and therefore should be preferred. On the other hand, all the guidelines agree on the use of RTX in relapsing disease (as shown by RAVE and, more recently, by RITA-ZAREM),[5,18] whereas only in KDIGO 2021 there is an explicit alert for severe kidney disease (creatinine >4 mg/dL), because these patients were not included in the RAVE trial, and therefore, CYC is still considered the preferred agent for induction of remission.

The international guidelines have quite different positions about plasma exchange in AAV. KDIGO 2021 considers plasma exchange in patients requiring dialysis or with rapidly increasing creatinine greater than 500 μmol/L (>5.8 mg/dL). However, if AAV overlaps with antiglomerular basement membrane antibody glomerulonephritis, plasma exchange should be used.[53] ACR/VF 2021 guidelines recommend against the routine use of plasma exchange in both active AAV glomerulonephritis and alveolar hemorrhage. Finally, EULAR 2022 recommendations are that plasma exchange can be considered in patients with rapidly increasing creatinine greater than 300 μmol/L, with no evidence for its routine use in alveolar hemorrhage.

The reduced GC PEXIVAS regimen is recommended by all the guidelines over the standard dose, preceded by IV pulse of methylprednisolone in cases of severe disease. Similarly, RTX for maintenance became the standard of care for maintenance of remission, regardless of the induction of remission treatment used, although in KDIGO 2021 the option to use azathioprine after induction of CYC remains equivalent to RTX, whereas RTX should be preferred after RTX induction. Only EULAR 2022 has a specific recommendation on the new complement inhibitor avacopan (that may be used as part of induction therapy), likely because the phase III trial was not published

Table 4
Differences and similarities in the main published guidelines on granulomatosis with polyangiitis and microscopic polyangiitis

		KDIGO 2021[10]	ACR/VF 2021[9]	EULAR 2022[a]
Biopsy		If clinical presentation compatible and positive MPO or PR3-ANCA serology, waiting for a kidney biopsy to be performed or reported should not delay starting immunosuppressive therapy	—	Recommended to assist in establishing a new diagnosis of AAV and for further evaluation of patients suspected of having relapsing vasculitis
Induction therapy	Active severe	RTX = CYC RTX preferred in relapsing disease In severe (creatinine >4 mg/dL [>354 mmol/L]) kidney disease, limited data for induction therapy with RTX are available. Combination of RTX + CYC can also be considered	RTX over CYC RTX preferred in relapsing active severe disease (that received other induction treatments)	RTX = CYC RTX preferred in relapsing disease
	Active nonsevere	MMF might be an alternative to CYC for nonlife-threatening MPO-ANCA subgroup	MTX over RTX or CYC or AZA or MMF	RTX over or CYC or MTX or MMF
Glucocorticoids		Reduced GC *PEXIVAS* regimen recommended (+ IV pulses in severe disease) For CYC: *achieve 5 mg/d by 6 months;* *for RTX can be withdrawn by 6 mo*	Reduced GC *PEXIVAS* regimen recommended Either IV pulse GC or high-dose oral GC may be prescribed as part of initial therapy	Reduced GC *PEXIVAS* regimen recommended (+ IV pulses in severe disease)
Plasma exchange		*Consider* PLEX for patients with creatinine >500 mmol/L requiring dialysis or with rapidly increasing creatinine *Consider* PLEX for patients with diffuse alveolar hemorrhage who has hypoxemia	*Against* routine PLEX for active GN *Against* routine PLEX for alveolar hemorrhage	PLEX *may be considered* for GN with creatinine >300 µmol/L Routine PLEX for alveolar hemorrhage not recommended

(continued on next page)

Table 4
(continued)

	KDIGO 2021[10]	ACR/VF 2021[9]	EULAR 2022[a]
Maintenance therapy	Following CYC induction, either AZA (+GC) or RTX (without GC) Following RTX induction, maintenance immunosuppressive therapy should be given (with RTX) MMF and MTX (if eGFR > 60) are alternatives	RTX over AZA/MTX (regardless of induction with CYC or RTX) AZA/MTX over MMF or LEF	RTX over AZA/MTX (regardless of induction with CYC or RTX)
Duration	Between 18 mo and 4 y for AZA (+GC); ≥18 months for RTX	For ≥18 months	For 24 to 48 months
Avacopan	—	—	Avacopan may be considered for induction of remission
Renal Tx	Delay transplantation until patients are in complete clinical remission for ≥6 mo Persistence of ANCA should not delay transplantation	For patients with GPA/MPA in remission and stage 5 CKD, we conditionally recommend evaluation for renal transplantation	

Abbreviations: ACR/VF, American College of Rheumatology/Vasculitis Foundation; AZA, Azathioprine; CKD, chronic kidney disease; CYC, cyclophosphamide; EULAR, European Alliance of Associations for Rheumatology; GC, glucocorticoids; GN, glomerulonephritis; KDIGO, Kidney Disease—Improving Global Outcomes; LEF, leflunomide; MTX, methotrexate; PLEX, plasma exchange; RTX, rituximab; SVV, small-vessel vasculitis; —, no specific recommendation.
[a] EULAR recommendations are not yet published but have been presented at the EULAR meeting 2022 in Copenhagen.

until 2021.[16] The diagnostic role of biopsy and indication for kidney transplant are not discussed by all the guidelines. In conclusion, there are differences and similarities between the 3 main sets of international guidelines that may reflect the varying expertise and sensibilities from different expert panels. Knowing these aspects may be crucial for clinicians to help them to navigate among these different guidelines/ recommendations.

ONGOING TRIALS AND NEW THERAPEUTICS ON THE HORIZON
Induction

We have previously discussed the role of B-cell depletion in AAV, and trials are currently evaluating this target to see if we can minimize GC exposure and improve the clinical response to induction therapy. The COMBIVAS trial (NCT03967925) includes severe active PR3-positive patients, evaluating belimumab (200 mg subcutaneously weekly for 1 year) in combination with rituximab 1 g (day 0 and 14) compared with placebo with rituximab. The starting dose of prednisone is 20 mg daily tapered over 3 months, and participants will be followed for 2 years. The primary outcome of this trial is time to PR3 negativity, which is associated with a lower risk of relapse.[54] It is hypothesized that the addition of belimumab will potentiate the effect of rituximab on B-cell depletion and prevent the return of autoreactive cells,[55] or suppress a broader repertoire of B cells (including those not expressing CD20) than can be achieved with rituximab alone, thus inducing more rapid and sustained remission.[56] Obinutuzumab is a newer generation anti-CD20 antibody that causes more direct cell death and increased antibody-dependent cellular cytotoxicity and phagocytosis than rituximab.[57] It has been used effectively in patients with anaphylaxis to rituximab or refractory disease,[38] and a phase II clinical trial is being planned comparing obinutuzumab with rituximab to evaluate the antibody response and ability to achieve remission in patients with PR3+ GPA and MPA (NCT05376319).

Refractory Disease

Current ACR/VF recommendations in refractory disease are to switch from rituximab to cyclophosphamide or visa versa,[9] and the SATELITE trial (NCT04871191) will look at the group of patients who did not respond to both of these therapies or have a contraindication to cyclophosphamide. There is increasing evidence supporting the role of interleukin-6 (IL-6) in the pathogenesis of AAV.[58-60] The 3 arms of an ongoing study will assess the combination of rituximab and methotrexate (or azathioprine or mycophenolate mofetil) compared with tocilizumab (an antibody against IL-6) compared with abatacept in this refractory population of patients.

Nonsevere Relapses and Maintenance Regimens

Another area of unmet need in AAV is persistent low-grade disease activity or nonsevere relapses. Abatacept, which works by blocking costimulatory signals required for T-cell activation, is being studied in the ABROGATE study, which includes relapsing patients with nonsevere GPA (NCT02108860) to see if the addition of abatacept can allow for GC-free sustained remission. In an open-label study of 20 patients, the addition of abatacept resulted in 80% remission rates and greater than 70% were able to wean GC.[61] Hydroxychloroquine, used frequently in the management of rheumatoid arthritis and various connective tissue diseases, is being evaluated in addition to background treatments in patients with low-level disease activity to see if there is improvement in disease activity and quality of life in patients with AAV (NCT04316494). Long-term GC use in maintaining remission is being evaluated in 2 parallel studies in France (NCT03290456) and the United States/Canada (NCT01940094) and will hopefully provide insight into the risks and benefits of GC tapering, as well as the phenotypes that would benefit most from the use of long-term prednisone.

CLINICS CARE POINTS

- The choice of therapy used for management of GPA/MPA must be individualized with consideration of prognosis, serologic profile, disease severity/activity, comorbidities, and other patient-specific factors.
- Understanding of the pathogenesis of GPA/MPA has led to therapeutic regimens that are better able to induce and maintain remission in our patients.
- Although there are nuanced differences between international guidelines for induction and maintenance therapy, there has been significant headway in limiting the use of GCs as evidenced by trials as well as guideline recommendations
- Recent insights into the role of plasmapheresis and complement inhibition are changing the landscape for management of AAV, and multiple other targeted therapeutic trials are underway.

DISCLOSURE

A.B. Dua is on advisory boards/consults for Chemocentryx, Novartis, Abbvie, and Sanofi.

REFERENCES

1. He P, Hu JP, Tian XJ, et al. Prevalence and risk factors of relapse in patients with ANCA-associated vasculitis receiving cyclophosphamide induction: a systematic review and meta-analysis of large observational studies. Rheumatol Oxf Engl 2021;60(3):1067–79.
2. Flossmann O, Berden A, Groot K de, et al. Long-term patient survival in ANCA-associated vasculitis. Ann Rheum Dis 2011;70(3):488–94.
3. Mukhtyar C, Lee R, Brown D, et al. Modification and validation of the Birmingham Vasculitis Activity Score (version 3). Ann Rheum Dis 2009;68(12):1827–32.
4. Exley AR, Bacon PA, Luqmani RA, et al. Development and initial validation of the vasculitis damage index for the standardized clinical assessment of damage in the systemic vasculitides. Arthritis Rheum 1997;40(2):371–80.
5. Specks U, Merkel PA, Seo P, et al. Efficacy of remission-induction regimens for ANCA-associated vasculitis. N Engl J Med 2013;369(5):417–27.
6. Berden AE, Ferrario F, Hagen EC, et al. Histopathologic classification of ANCA-associated glomerulonephritis. J Am Soc Nephrol 2010;21(10):1628–36.
7. Sethi S, D'Agati VD, Nast CC, et al. A proposal for standardized grading of chronic changes in native kidney biopsy specimens. Kidney Int 2017;91(4):787–9.
8. Robson JC, Dawson J, Doll H, et al. Validation of the ANCA-associated vasculitis patient-reported outcomes (AAV-PRO) questionnaire. Ann Rheum Dis 2018;77(8):1157–64.
9. Chung SA, Langford CA, Maz M, et al. 2021 American college of rheumatology/vasculitis foundation guideline for the management of antineutrophil cytoplasmic antibody-associated vasculitis. Arthritis Care Res 2021;73(8):1088–105.

10. Kidney Disease: Improving Global Outcomes (KDIGO) Glomerular Diseases Work Group. KDIGO 2021 clinical practice guideline for the management of glomerular diseases. Kidney Int 2021;100(4S):S1-276.

11. Chanouzas D, McGregor JAG, Nightingale P, et al. Intravenous pulse methylprednisolone for induction of remission in severe ANCA associated Vasculitis: a multi-center retrospective cohort study. BMC Nephrol 2019;20(1):58.

12. de Groot K, Harper L, Jayne DRW, et al. Pulse versus daily oral cyclophosphamide for induction of remission in antineutrophil cytoplasmic antibody—associated vasculitisa randomized trial. Ann Intern Med 2009;150(10):670–80.

13. Pagnoux C, Mahr A, Hamidou MA, et al. Azathioprine or methotrexate maintenance for ANCA-associated vasculitis. N Engl J Med 2008;359(26):2790–803.

14. Pagnoux C, Quéméneur T, Ninet J, et al. Treatment of systemic necrotizing vasculitides in patients aged sixty-five years or older: results of a multicenter, open-label, randomized controlled trial of corticosteroid and cyclophosphamide-based induction therapy. Arthritis Rheumatol Hoboken NJ 2015;67(4):1117–27.

15. Walsh M, Merkel PA, Peh CA, et al. Plasma exchange and glucocorticoids in severe ANCA-associated vasculitis. N Engl J Med 2020;382(7):622–31.

16. Jayne DRW, Merkel PA, Schall TJ, et al, ADVOCATE Study Group. Avacopan for the treatment of ANCA-associated vasculitis. N Engl J Med 2021;384(7):599–609.

17. Furuta S, Nakagomi D, Kobayashi Y, et al. Effect of reduced-dose vs high-dose glucocorticoids added to rituximab on remission induction in ANCA-associated vasculitis: a randomized clinical trial. JAMA 2021;325(21):2178–87.

18. Smith RM, Jones RB, Specks U, et al. Rituximab as therapy to induce remission after relapse in ANCA-associated vasculitis. Ann Rheum Dis 2020;79(9):1243–9.

19. Jayne DRW, Bruchfeld AN, Harper L, et al. Randomized trial of C5a receptor inhibitor avacopan in ANCA-associated vasculitis. J Am Soc Nephrol JASN 2017; 28(9):2756–67.

20. Walsh M, Merkel PA, Mahr A, et al. Effects of duration of glucocorticoid therapy on relapse rate in antineutrophil cytoplasmic antibody-associated vasculitis: a meta-analysis. Arthritis Care Res 2010;62(8):1166–73.

21. Fauci AS, Wolff SM, Johnson JS. Effect of cyclophosphamide upon the immune response in Wegener's granulomatosis. N Engl J Med 1971;285(27):1493–6.

22. Jayne D, Rasmussen N, Andrassy K, et al. A randomized trial of maintenance therapy for vasculitis associated with antineutrophil cytoplasmic autoantibodies. N Engl J Med 2003;349(1):36–44.

23. Harper L, Morgan MD, Walsh M, et al. Pulse versus daily oral cyclophosphamide for induction of remission in ANCA-associated vasculitis: long-term follow-up. Ann Rheum Dis 2012;71(6):955–60.

24. De Groot K, Rasmussen N, Bacon PA, et al. Randomized trial of cyclophosphamide versus methotrexate for induction of remission in early systemic antineutrophil cytoplasmic antibody–associated vasculitis. Arthritis Rheum 2005;52(8):2461–9.

25. Faurschou M, Westman K, Rasmussen N, et al. Brief Report: long-term outcome of a randomized clinical trial comparing methotrexate to cyclophosphamide for remission induction in early systemic antineutrophil cytoplasmic antibody-associated vasculitis. Arthritis Rheum 2012;64(10):3472–7.

26. Jones RB, Hiemstra TF, Ballarin J, et al. Mycophenolate mofetil versus cyclophosphamide for remission induction in ANCA-associated vasculitis: a randomised, non-inferiority trial. Ann Rheum Dis 2019;78(3):399–405.

27. Berti A, Alsawas M, Jawaid T, et al. Induction and maintenance of remission with mycophenolate mofetil in ANCA-associated vasculitis: a systematic review and meta-analysis. Nephrol Dial Transplant 2022;37(11):2190–200.

28. Xiao H, Heeringa P, Hu P, et al. Antineutrophil cytoplasmic autoantibodies specific for myeloperoxidase cause glomerulonephritis and vasculitis in mice. J Clin Invest 2002;110(7):955–63.

29. Specks U, Fervenza FC, McDonald TJ, et al. Response of Wegener's granulomatosis to anti-CD20 chimeric monoclonal antibody therapy. Arthritis Rheum 2001; 44(12):2836–40.

30. Keogh KA, Wylam ME, Stone JH, et al. Induction of remission by B lymphocyte depletion in eleven patients with refractory antineutrophil cytoplasmic antibody-associated vasculitis. Arthritis Rheum 2005;52(1):262–8.

31. Stone JH, Merkel PA, Spiera R, et al. Rituximab versus cyclophosphamide for ANCA-associated vasculitis. N Engl J Med 2010;363(3):221–32.

32. Jones RB, Cohen Tervaert JW, Hauser T, et al. Rituximab versus cyclophosphamide in ANCA-associated renal vasculitis. N Engl J Med 2010;363(3):211–20.

33. Unizony S, Villarreal M, Miloslavsky EM, et al. Clinical outcomes of treatment of anti-neutrophil cytoplasmic antibody (ANCA)-associated vasculitis based on ANCA type. Ann Rheum Dis 2016;75(6):1166–9.

34. Guillevin L, Pagnoux C, Karras A, et al. Rituximab versus Azathioprine for Maintenance in ANCA-Associated Vasculitis. N Engl J Med 2014;371(19):1771–80.

35. Charles P, Terrier B, Perrodeau É, et al. Comparison of individually tailored versus fixed-schedule rituximab regimen to maintain ANCA-associated vasculitis remission: results of a multicentre, randomised controlled, phase III trial (MAINRITSAN2). Ann Rheum Dis 2018;77(8):1143–9.

36. Charles P, Perrodeau É, Samson M, et al. Long-term rituximab use to maintain remission of antineutrophil cytoplasmic antibody-associated vasculitis: a randomized trial. Ann Intern Med 2020;173(3):179–87.

37. McAdoo SP, Bedi R, Tarzi R, et al. Ofatumumab for B cell depletion therapy in ANCA-associated vasculitis: a single-centre case series. Rheumatol Oxf Engl 2016;55(8):1437–42.

38. Amudala NA, Boukhlal S, Sheridan B, et al. Obinutuzumab as treatment for ANCA-associated vasculitis. Rheumatol Oxf Engl 2022;61(9):3814–7.

39. Jayne D, Blockmans D, Luqmani R, et al. Efficacy and safety of belimumab and azathioprine for maintenance of remission in antineutrophil cytoplasmic antibody-associated vasculitis: a randomized controlled study. Arthritis Rheumatol Hoboken NJ 2019;71(6):952–63.

40. Bowman SJ, Fox R, Dörner T, et al. Safety and efficacy of subcutaneous ianalumab (VAY736) in patients with primary Sjögren's syndrome: a randomised, double-blind, placebo-controlled, phase 2b dose-finding trial. Lancet Lond Engl 2022;399(10320):161–71.

41. Mougiakakos D, Krönke G, Völkl S, et al. CD19-Targeted CAR T cells in refractory systemic lupus erythematosus. N Engl J Med 2021;385(6):567–9.

42. Mackensen A, Müller F, Mougiakakos D, et al. Anti-CD19 CAR T cell therapy for refractory systemic lupus erythematosus. Nat Med 2022;28(10):2124–32.

43. Jennette JC, Wilkman AS, Falk RJ. Anti-neutrophil cytoplasmic autoantibody-associated glomerulonephritis and vasculitis. Am J Pathol 1989;135(5):921–30.

44. Kettritz R. With complements from ANCA mice. J Am Soc Nephrol JASN 2014; 25(2):207–9.

45. Xiao H, Schreiber A, Heeringa P, et al. Alternative complement pathway in the pathogenesis of disease mediated by anti-neutrophil cytoplasmic autoantibodies. Am J Pathol 2007;170(1):52–64.

46. Schreiber A, Xiao H, Jennette JC, et al. C5a receptor mediates neutrophil activation and ANCA-induced glomerulonephritis. J Am Soc Nephrol JASN 2009;20(2): 289–98.

47. Trivioli G, Vaglio A. The rise of complement in ANCA-associated vasculitis: from marginal player to target of modern therapy. Clin Exp Immunol 2020;202(3): 403–6.

48. Moiseev S, Lee JM, Zykova A, et al. The alternative complement pathway in ANCA-associated vasculitis: further evidence and a meta-analysis. Clin Exp Immunol 2020;202(3):394–402.

49. Merkel PA, Niles J, Jimenez R, et al. Adjunctive treatment with avacopan, an oral C5a receptor inhibitor, in patients with antineutrophil cytoplasmic antibody-associated vasculitis. ACR Open Rheumatol 2020;2(11):662–71.

50. Jayne D. Complement inhibition in ANCA vasculitis. Nephrol Ther 2019;15(6): 409–12.

51. Jayne DRW, Gaskin G, Rasmussen N, et al. Randomized trial of plasma exchange or high-dosage methylprednisolone as adjunctive therapy for severe renal vasculitis. J Am Soc Nephrol JASN 2007;18(7):2180–8.

52. Walsh M, Collister D, Zeng L, et al. The effects of plasma exchange in patients with ANCA-associated vasculitis: an updated systematic review and meta-analysis. BMJ 2022;376:e064604.

53. McAdoo SP, Tanna A, Hrušková Z, et al. Patients double-seropositive for ANCA and anti-GBM antibodies have varied renal survival, frequency of relapse, and outcomes compared to single-seropositive patients. Kidney Int 2017;92(3): 693–702.

54. Morgan MD, Szeto M, Walsh M, et al. Negative anti-neutrophil cytoplasm antibody at switch to maintenance therapy is associated with a reduced risk of relapse. Arthritis Res Ther 2017;19(1):129.

55. Berti A, Hillion S, Hummel AM, et al. Circulating autoreactive proteinase 3+ B cells and tolerance checkpoints in ANCA-associated vasculitis. JCI Insight 2021;6(22):e150999.

56. Prendecki M, McAdoo SP. New therapeutic targets in antineutrophil cytoplasm antibody-associated vasculitis. Arthritis Rheumatol Hoboken NJ 2021;73(3):361–70.

57. Freeman CL, Sehn LH. A tale of two antibodies: obinutuzumab versus rituximab. Br J Haematol 2018;182(1):29–45.

58. Berti A, Cavalli G, Campochiaro C, et al. Interleukin-6 in ANCA-associated vasculitis: Rationale for successful treatment with tocilizumab. Semin Arthritis Rheum 2015;45(1):48–54.

59. Berti A, Warner R, Johnson K, et al. The association of serum interleukin-6 levels with clinical outcomes in antineutrophil cytoplasmic antibody-associated vasculitis. J Autoimmun 2019;105:102302.

60. Sakai R, Kondo T, Kurasawa T, et al. Current clinical evidence of tocilizumab for the treatment of ANCA-associated vasculitis: a prospective case series for microscopic polyangiitis in a combination with corticosteroids and literature review. Clin Rheumatol 2017;36(10):2383–92.

61. Langford CA, Monach PA, Specks U, et al. An open-label trial of abatacept (CTLA4-IG) in non-severe relapsing granulomatosis with polyangiitis (Wegener's). Ann Rheum Dis 2014;73(7):1376–9.

62. Guillevin L, Lhote F, Gayraud M, et al. Prognostic factors in polyarteritis nodosa and Churg-Strauss syndrome. A prospective study in 342 patients. Medicine (Baltim) 1996;75(1):17–28.

Therapeutic Advances in Eosinophilic Granulomatosis with Polyangiitis

Check for updates

Jessica L. Bloom, MD, MSCS[a], Carol A. Langford, MD, MHS[b],
Michael E. Wechsler, MD, MMSc[c],*

KEYWORDS

- EGPA • Churg-Strauss • Eosinophilia • Anti-IL-5 • ANCA-associated vasculitis
- Therapeutics • Mepolizumab

KEY POINTS

- Eosinophilic granulomatosis with polyangiitis (EGPA) is an eosinophilic vasculitis that affects a variety of organ systems.
- Because of its complexity, EGPA often requires a multi-disciplinary approach for both diagnosis and management and many specialties are called on to evaluate these patients at the time of diagnosis, during the course of disease, and/or to address clinical management questions.
- Historically, glucocorticoids and a variety of other immunosuppressants were used to abrogate the inflammation and tissue injury associated with EGPA.
- The goals of EGPA treatment are to induce remission, limit disease-related damage, prevent relapse, and ensure survival while minimizing treatment-related morbidity.
- The management of EGPA has evolved greatly during the last decade with the development of novel targeted therapeutics that have resulted in significantly improved outcomes for these patients including therapies that target B cells or modulate eosinophils; many more novel targeted therapies are emerging.

BACKGROUND

Eosinophilic granulomatosis with polyangiitis (EGPA) is an eosinophilic vasculitis that affects a variety of organ systems. Classically, EGPA histopathology is characterized by necrotizing vasculitis (most often of small vessels), extravascular granulomas, and infiltrative eosinophils (**Fig. 1**).[1] Although presentations may vary, the 2012 Chapel Hill

[a] Section of Rheumatology, Department of Pediatrics, University of Colorado School of Medicine, 13123 East 16th Avenue B-311, Aurora, CO 80045, USA; [b] Department of Rheumatic and Immunologic Diseases, Cleveland Clinic, 9500 Euclid Avenue A50, Cleveland, OH 44195, USA; [c] Division of Pulmonary, Critical Care, and Sleep Medicine, Department of Medicine, National Jewish Health, J215, 1400 Jackson Street, Denver, CO 80206, USA
* Corresponding author.
E-mail address: WechslerM@NJHealth.org

Rheum Dis Clin N Am 49 (2023) 563–584
https://doi.org/10.1016/j.rdc.2023.03.006
0889-857X/23/© 2023 Elsevier Inc. All rights reserved.

Consensus Conference distinguished EGPA from other vasculitides by the presence of eosinophilic and granulomatous inflammation involving the respiratory tract accompanied by necrotizing vasculitis and by the association with asthma and eosinophilia.[2] Although EGPA is considered one of the antineutrophil cytoplasmic antibody (ANCA)-associated vasculitides (AAV), only 30% to 40% of patients have a positive ANCA, most often with antimyeloperoxidase (MPO) antibodies.[3–5] Because of its complexity, EGPA often requires a multi-disciplinary approach for both diagnosis and management and many specialties are called on to evaluate these patients at the time of diagnosis, during the course of disease, and/or to address clinical management questions. Historically, glucocorticoids and a variety of other immunosuppressants were used to abrogate the inflammation and tissue injury associated with EGPA; however, the management of EGPA has evolved greatly during the last decade with the development of novel targeted therapeutics that have resulted in significantly improved outcomes for these patients.[6,7] This review gives an overview of the presentation of EGPA and the novel approaches toward treatments that have emerged in recent years.

EPIDEMIOLOGY

EGPA has an estimated incidence of 1 to 3 cases per million per year and a prevalence of 14 cases per million per year.[8] Thus, much of what we know about EGPA comes from diverse international cohorts. EGPA is the rarest form of AAV, and is likely underdiagnosed given its variegated clinical presentation, improvement with glucocorticoids, and similarities to severe asthma. There is no male or female predominance in adults with EGPA.[4,5] Although the average age of diagnosis is in the late 40s or early 50s, it often takes years to come to a formal diagnosis.[9] EGPA is quite rare in children but does occur in this age group and is often misdiagnosed, warranting thorough investigation of any child who presents with eosinophilia.

CAUSE

The cause of EGPA is unknown; however, it is suspected that both environmental and genetic factors play a role. Possible environmental triggers include allergens, infections, medications, and silica inhalation.[10–12] Some epidemiologic studies also suggest increased frequency at higher latitudes and more rural areas. An association between the development of EGPA and a variety of asthma therapies has long been

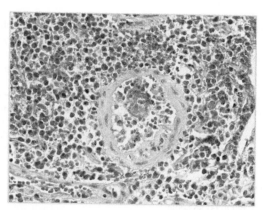

Fig. 1. Typical pathologic features of eosinophil tissue infiltration at the blood vessel wall with granulomata and evidence of eosinophilic vasculitis.

appreciated with cases reported in those taking inhaled glucocorticoids, leukotriene modifiers, and biologics including omalizumab and dupilumab.[13–16] Nonetheless, no causal link has been established and EGPA cases associated with these therapies have generally fallen into 2 categories—forme fruste EGPA, resulting from the withdrawal of systemic glucocorticoids that was masking the underlying eosinophilic vasculitis and coincidental cases of what was perceived to be worsening asthma treated with biologics or other therapies in lieu of administration of glucocorticoids for what was actually incipient EGPA. Genome wide association studies are currently ongoing but earlier genetic studies have implicated HLA-DRB1*07 and HLA-DRB4 as being associated with the development of EGPA.[17,18] ANCA negative subtypes have been associated with IL-10 polymorphisms.[19]

PATHOGENESIS

The pathophysiology of EGPA is complex, resulting in a significant immune dysregulation.[20] There is involvement of both T helper (Th)-1 and Th-2 cells, leading to the granulomatous pulmonary inflammation and the allergic and eosinophilic features, respectively. Additionally, decreased IL-10 levels in EGPA indicate reduced regulatory T-cells, whereas elevated immunoglobulin levels indicate dysregulated humoral immunity.[21–23] The hypereosinophilia in EGPA is most likely due to Th-2 cell or innate lymphoid cell (ILC2)-mediated upregulation of IL-5 predominantly, but also of IL-4 and IL-13.[24] Decreased eosinophil apoptosis can also play a role. Eosinophils are thought to be pathogenic by the release of toxic granular proteins locally in the tissue, including eosinophilic cationic protein, eosinophil derived neurotoxin (EDN), eosinophil peroxidase and major basic protein.[25–28] Deposition of these proteins can lead to local inflammation and damage to the blood vessel wall, resulting in vasculitis, hypercoagulability, and tissue damage, and to many of the features of asthma and chronic sinusitis that are seen in these patients. As IL-5 is involved in the maturation, proliferation, and activation of eosinophils, it has become a major target in EGPA management (see later discussion).[24] IL-4 is also implicated in EGPA pathophysiology because it is involved in B-cell mediated production of antibodies including ANCA, IgE and IgG4, all of which can be elevated in these patients.[29] ANCA is thought to bind to antigens present on the neutrophil, which then adheres to the blood vessel endothelium and migrates through the blood vessel wall, where they recruit other inflammatory cells to the site, causing local damage.[5]

A variety of biomarkers is under investigation for their potential role in disease monitoring and/or medication development. Possible markers of vasculitic activity include urinary-MCP-1 (correlates with renal disease activity and therapy response), urinary soluble-CD163 (correlates with necrotizing crescentic glomerulonephritis), serum and urinary soluble CD25, serum markers of the alternative complement pathway (correlates with disease activity in MPO-ANCA positive renal vasculitis), and markers of B-cell activation/repopulation.[30] Although potential markers of eosinophilic activity include IgG4, CCL26/Eotaxin-3, CL17/TARC, ECP, urinary EDN, and periostin, none has been shown to be more useful than absolute eosinophils in terms of predicting disease or response to the therapies.[30,31]

CLINICAL PRESENTATION

Patients typically develop EGPA during the course of many years and through 3 stages: prodromal, eosinophilic, and vasculitic.[32] The prodromal phase consists of allergic rhinitis, nasal polyposis, atopic disease, and asthma. Most often, this occurs in the second or third decades of life. During stage 2, or the eosinophilic phase, patients develop peripheral blood eosinophilia and infiltration of eosinophils into organs such as the lung, heart, and gastrointestinal tract. Finally, the vasculitic phase includes necrotizing vasculitis of small- sized to medium-sized vessels and granulomatous inflammation that can affect multiple organ systems such as the lungs, nerves, heart, intestines, skin, and kidneys. Constitutional symptoms occur more frequently in this stage, including weight loss, fever, malaise, and fatigue. Although classically in succession, phases may overlap or occur in any order.[9,33–35]

Although EGPA is typically a multisystem disease, pulmonary manifestations are the most common clinical feature. More than 90% of patients have asthma that is often severe and poorly controlled on inhaled glucocorticoids. Less commonly, some patients may have pleural effusions, pulmonary nodules, or, rarely, diffuse alveolar hemorrhage. Skin disease, such as urticaria, palpable purpura, tender subcutaneous nodules, or hemorrhagic vasculitic lesions, are among the most common presenting findings leading to a diagnosis. Up to three-quarters of patients experience peripheral sensory or motor neuropathy, most often due to mononeuritis multiplex, which can be debilitating for patients, resulting in permanent nerve damage. The most life-threatening manifestation of EGPA is cardiac involvement, which may present as eosinophilic myocarditis, heart failure, pericarditis, valvulitis, coronary vasculitis, and/or rhythm abnormalities. Although it can be asymptomatic, cardiac disease often presents early and is more prevalent in patients who are ANCA-negative and have high eosinophil counts at diagnosis.[36] Eosinophilic gastroenteritis is also common and may present with abdominal pain, diarrhea, gastrointestinal bleeding, or colitis. As with other AAV, venous thromboembolism can be prevalent and a cause of significant morbidity. Additional features seen commonly in EGPA include upper airway, sinus, and ear disease; ophthalmologic complications; hypertension; renal disease; lymphadenopathy; myalgias/myositis; and arthralgias/arthritis (**Table 1**).[9,20,35,37] ANCA-positive patients experience more glomerulonephritis, diffuse alveolar hemorrhage, ENT manifestations, palpable purpura, peripheral nerve pathologic condition, and are more likely to have vasculitis present on biopsy.[4,5,9]

EVALUATION OF SUSPECTED EOSINOPHILIC GRANULOMATOSIS WITH POLYANGIITIS

Evaluation of EGPA requires a thorough history and physical examination accompanied by laboratory and imaging tests. There is no single test to diagnose EGPA, although histopathology from a tissue sample is most specific.[9,38] Common laboratory findings include peripheral eosinophilia, elevated immunoglobulin E, positive rheumatoid factor, low-positive antinuclear antigen antibody, positive-anti-MPO antibody, and elevated C-reactive protein and erythrocyte sedimentation rates. Although peripheral eosinophilia is generally defined as greater than the upper limit of normal cells (roughly 500 cells/μL) or greater than 10% of the total leukocyte count, eosinophil counts greater or equal to 1500 cells/μL should raise suspicion for a hypereosinophilic syndrome such as EGPA. It is important to note that eosinophils respond rapidly to glucocorticoids and thus could be falsely diminished if checked after treatment. In this case, eosinophils may still be present in tissue. As discussed, ANCA are present in roughly 40% of patients with EGPA, almost all against MPO.

Imaging should be directed by the presenting signs and symptoms, although additional screening is often warranted once the diagnosis is confirmed. Patients typically undergo chest radiography followed by high-resolution chest computed tomography (CT), which often demonstrates ground glass opacities and nodular densities or fleeting pulmonary infiltrates.[39] When pulmonary infiltrates are present, bronchoalveolar lavage may be performed, which can be useful in demonstrating elevated

Table 1
Clinical manifestations of eosinophilic granulomatosis with polyangiitis[9,20,35,37,99,100]

Cardiovascular	Musculoskeletal
• Heart failure (41%)	• Arthralgia/arthritis (30%–40%)
• Eosinophilic myocarditis (16%)	• Myalgia/myositis (26%–39%)
• Cardiomyopathy (16%)	
• Pericarditis (10%–15%)	
• Valvulitis	
• Coronary vasculitis	
• Rhythm abnormalities	

Constitutional	Neurologic
• Fatigue (72%)	• Neuropathy (55%–72%)
• Weight loss (30%–50%)	○ Sensory neuropathy (51%)
• Fever (39%)	○ Mononeuritis multiplex (33%–46%)
• Lymphadenopathy (30%–40%)	• Cranial nerve palsies (3%)
	• Stroke (1%)

Mucocutaneous	Ocular (7%)
• Palpable purpura (23%–25%)	• Ischemic optic neuropathy
• Urticaria (10%)	• Central retinal artery or vein occlusion
• Tender subcutaneous nodules (7%–10%)	• Conjunctival nodules
• Ulcerations (4%)	• Orbital myositis
• Gangrene (1%–4%)	• Scleritis/episcleritis
• Hemorrhagic vasculitic lesions	
• Nasal or oral ulcers	

Ear, nose, and throat	Pulmonary
• Recurrent sinusitis (77%)	• Asthma, often severe (93%)
• Nasal polyposis (50%)	• Pulmonary infiltrates (39%–58%)
• Allergic rhinitis (17%)	• Pleural effusion (9%–10%)
• Sensorineural hearing loss	• Pulmonary nodules (5%–12%)
• Serous otitis media	• Diffuse alveolar hemorrhage (4%–6%)

Gastrointestinal	Renal
• Abdominal pain (59%)	• Hypertension (10%–30%)
• Eosinophilic gastroenteritis (4%)	• Proteinuria (6%–13%)
• Ischemic bowel (2%)	• Glomerulonephritis (8%)
Hematologic	• Hematuria (8%)
• Hypereosinophilia (all[a])	• Elevated creatinine (4%–5%)
• Venous thromboembolism (8%)	

[a] Hypereosinophilia may not be present if pretreated with glucocorticoids

eosinophil levels, to look for alveolar hemorrhage, and to rule out infection. Spirometry will likely show airflow obstruction. Sinus CT may demonstrate mucosal thickening and/or evidence of nasal or sinus polyps.

All patients suspected of having EGPA should receive an electrocardiogram and undergo echocardiography. Patients who have a reduced ejection fraction should undergo cardiac MRI assessing for valvular or mural thrombi and wall motion abnormalities.[40–44] Additional cardiac testing may include N-terminal-pro B-type natriuretic peptide, and troponin measurement. Cardiac fluorodeoxyglucose-positron emission tomography may be considered to assess for fibrosis versus inflammation.

Although a diagnosis of EGPA can often be made based on clinical history and supportive laboratory findings, ultimately, a tissue biopsy may be required for diagnosis. The most easily accessible affected tissue is often the best choice (skin, kidney, and so forth) although lung and endomyocardial biopsies may be necessary.

Nerve conduction studies and electromyograms can help characterize neuropathy due to EGPA.

CLASSIFICATION AND DIAGNOSIS

A variety of classification criteria exist for EGPA including the 1984 Lanham Diagnostic Criteria, 1990 American College of Rheumatology (ACR) Classification Criteria, 2012 revised International Chapel Hill Consensus Conference Nomenclature of Vasculitides definition, 2015 European Respiratory Society's EGPA Consensus Task Force Criteria, and 2022 ACR/European Alliance Of Associations For Rheumatology Classification Criteria (**Box 1**).[2,3,32,45,46] Although these criteria help distinguish different vasculitides or facilitate inclusion of patients into clinical trials, diagnostic criteria are limited. Although it is generally not difficult to distinguish EGPA from other vasculitides such as granulomatosis with polyangiitis (GPA) or microscopic polyangiitis (MPA) because of the presence of eosinophilia and asthma in EGPA and by the relative absence of ANCA in EGPA, it can be challenging to distinguish EGPA from the idiopathic hypereosinophilic syndrome (HES) and chronic eosinophilic pneumonia. Like EGPA, HES is characterized by high blood/tissue eosinophils, and can present with pulmonary infiltrates and multisystem involvement. One way to distinguish EGPA from HES is by the greater likelihood of asthma and the presence of ANCA or vasculitic disease features in EGPA or by the identification of specific myeloproliferative or lymphoproliferative features in HES. Although chronic eosinophilic pneumonia is also associated with asthma, eosinophilia, sinusitis and pulmonary infiltrates, it generally lacks the extrapulmonary manifestations seen in EGPA, and is not associated with ANCA or vasculitis.[47–49]

In any patient with eosinophilia, it is critical to take a good history. Drug reactions are among the most common causes of eosinophilia in North America and need to be excluded. Worldwide, parasites are the most common cause of hypereosinophilia so testing for ova and parasites should be considered in patients with a suggestive history or those coming from Africa, South America, or South East Asia. Strongyloides in particular should be excluded because treatment with glucocorticoids in these patients can result in systemic strongyloidiasis, which can be fatal.[50] Malignancies, especially leukemia and lymphoma, should also be excluded as should solid tumors that can also present with eosinophilia and systemic manifestations. Other diagnoses to consider include aspirin-exacerbated respiratory disease and allergic bronchopulmonary aspergillosis.

MANAGEMENT

Because of the rarity of EGPA, there have been very few randomized trials with most published experience being based on small open-label prospective studies, retrospective cohort studies and case series. The lack of randomized trials has led to the use of a wide range of different treatment approaches for EGPA. Some of the treatments used were derived from studies in other vasculitides or trials evaluating asthma. In Duobelt and colleagues' study of 354 adult patients with EGPA from 2003 to 2019, 42% received cyclophosphamide (CYC), 52% received azathioprine (AZA), 9% received mycophenolate mofetil (MMF), 9% received mepolizumab, and 10.5% received rituximab at some point during their disease course, highlighting the diversity of treatments that have been used in EGPA. Glucocorticoid dosing lasted a median of 12 months (interquartile range = 9) with only 12.6% able to discontinue systemic glucocorticoids and immunosuppressive agents for more than 2 years and 40.8% able to discontinue glucocorticoid therapy alone for more than 2 years. The length of time between diagnosis and the last follow-up visit in this study was 7.0 (±6.2) years.[37]

Box 1
Criteria and nomenclature for eosinophilic granulomatosis with polyangiitis[2,3,32,45,46]

1984 Lanham Diagnostic Criteria
  All 3 of the following:
  - Asthma
  - Peripheral eosinophilia greater than 1.5×10^6/cc
  - Systemic vasculitis involving 2 or more extrapulmonary organs

1990 American College of Rheumatology Classification Criteria
  At least 4 of the following:
  - Asthma
  - Eosinophilia greater than 10%
  - Neuropathy, mono or poly
  - Pulmonary infiltrates, nonfixed
  - Paranasal sinus abnormality
  - Extravascular eosinophils

2012 Revised International Chapel Hill Consensus Conference Definition
  - Eosinophil-rich and necrotizing granulomatous inflammation often involving the respiratory tract, and necrotizing vasculitis predominantly affecting small to medium vessels, and associated with asthma and eosinophilia. ANCA is more frequent in EGPA when glomerulonephritis is present.

2015 European Respiratory Task Force Diagnostic Criteria
  History or presence of asthma plus eosinophilia ($>1.0 \times 10^9$/L and/or > 10% of leukocytes)
  And 2 of the following:
  - A biopsy showing histopathological evidence of eosinophilic vasculitis
  - Perivascular eosinophilic infiltration, or eosinophil-rich granulomatous inflammation
  - Neuropathy, mono or poly (motor deficit or nerve conduction abnormality) Pulmonary infiltrates, non-fixed
  - Sino-nasal abnormality
  - Cardiomyopathy (established by echocardiography or MRI)
  - Glomerulonephritis (hematuria, red cell casts, proteinuria)
  - Alveolar hemorrhage (by bronchoalveolar lavage)
  - Palpable purpura
  - Positive test for ANCA (anti-MPO or anti-PR3)

2022 American College of Rheumatology/European Alliance of Associations for Rheumatology Classification Criteria
  - Only applies if the patient has already been diagnosed with small-vessel or medium-vessel vasculitis and alternative diagnoses mimicking vasculitis have been excluded.
  Total Score $\geq$ 6
    Clinical Criteria
    - Obstructive airway disease (+3 points)
    - Nasal polyps (+3 points)
    - Mononeuritis multiplex (+1 points)
    Laboratory and Biopsy Criteria
    - Blood eosinophil count >/ = 1×10^9/L (+5 points)
    - Extravascular eosinophilic-predominant inflammation on biopsy (+2 points)
    - Positive test for cytoplasmic antineutrophil cytoplasmic antibodies or anti-PR3 (−3 points)
    - Hematuria (−1 points)

Abbreviations: ANCA, antineutrophil cytoplasmic antibody; PR3, proteinase 3; MPO, myeloperoxidase.

Although EGPA treatment guidelines have been published by several groups and are useful in framing management approaches based on the published literature, they need to be viewed within the context of the individual patient.[46,51] Nonetheless, it is well established that the goals of treatment of EGPA are to induce remission, limit disease-related damage, prevent relapse, and ensure survival while minimizing treatment-related morbidity. Treatment is considered to have 2 phases: induction (when active disease is put into remission) and maintenance.

Remission Induction

The goal of induction of remission is to get active disease under control, whether at the time of diagnosis or recurrence of active disease, and to prevent organ damage from occurring. The approach to remission induction is based on whether the patient has mild-to-moderate disease or organ-threatening or life-threatening manifestations. The 1996 Five-Factor Score (FFS) may be used to assess disease severity and consists of 5 items: myocardial involvement, gastrointestinal disease (bleeding, perforation, infarction, or pancreatitis), renal insufficiency (plasma creatinine concentration greater than 1.6 mg/dL [141 μmol/L]), proteinuria (>1 g/d), and central nervous system involvement. All items are associated with a poor prognosis and are worth 1 point.[52] A revised FFS published in 2011 replaced proteinuria and central nervous system involvement with age greater than 65 years and the absence of ENT manifestations. Additionally, renal insufficiency was altered to signify a stabilized peak creatinine of 1.7 mg/dL (150 μmol/L). Still, prognostic studies based on FFS used the 1996 version.[53]

Organ-threatening or life-threatening disease

Patients who have organ or life-threatening disease should be treated with high dose glucocorticoids (500–1000 mg IV methylprednisolone daily for 3–5 days) and either CYC or rituximab. In addition to the factors within the FFS, diffuse alveolar hemorrhage, glomerulonephritis, cerebral vasculitis, vision threatening ocular disease, and significant mononeuritis multiplex also warrant more aggressive agents.

CYC is an alkylating neoplastic agent. Efficacy for CYC use in EGPA was explored in a 2001 meta-analysis by Gayraud and colleagues of patients with EGPA, MPA, and polyarteritis nodosa, in which 215 patients received glucocorticoids alone or glucocorticoids plus CYC. Although survival was similar between groups overall and for those with FFS scores of 0 and 1, the patients with an FFS score of 2 or greater experienced significantly greater survival with the combination of glucocorticoids plus CYC compared with those who received glucocorticoids alone ($P = .04$).[54] An earlier study in 1996, demonstrated a lower mortality rate in patients with EGPA and an FFS of 1 with the addition of CYC. Dosing for CYC is based off of treatment of GPA and includes daily dosing (1.5–2 mg/kg daily oral CYC for 3–6 months) and intermittent dosing (15 mg/kg given intravenously CYC every 2 weeks for 3 doses followed by every 3 weeks for at least 3 doses). The duration of therapy is typically 3 to 6 months followed by treatment with a conventional immunosuppressive agent such as AZA, methotrexate (MTX), or MMF based on GPA studies. Although CYC is often preferred in patients with cardiomyopathy, it can cause significant toxicity including increased risk of infections, cytopenias, malignancy, infertility, and hemorrhagic cystitis.

Rituximab, an anti-CD20 monoclonal antibody against B cells, is also used in severe EGPA based on compelling case series and rigorous studies in GPA and MPA.[55,56] A 2021 systematic review of 368 patients with EGPA demonstrated more than 80% of patients reached complete or partial remission with rituximab therapy.[57] Similar results were seen in a 2014 international study of 41 patients with EGPA demonstrating the ability to achieve remission or a partial response to therapy (83% by 6 months, 88% by 12 months) and taper glucocorticoids with rituximab therapy. Notably, those with a positive ANCA had a higher rate of remission at 12 months.[58] A 2020 retrospective analysis also demonstrated improved asthma control in EGPA and decreased glucocorticoid use.[59] A study by Wang and colleagues showed reduced eosinophils and improved cardiac dysfunction in patients with ANCA-negative EGPA-related myocarditis who received rituximab.[60] Finally, Teixeria and colleagues found that asthma and ear, nose, and throat relapse rates remained high despite decreased glucocorticoid use in EGPA patients who received rituximab due to refractory disease or contraindicated CYC use. Those with ANCA-positivity reached remission more quickly and experienced a longer relapse-free survival.[61] Further studies on rituximab use in EGPA are currently underway.

Dosing in adults with EGPA is 375 mg/m^2 IV rituximab every week for 4 weeks or 1000 mg IV for 2 doses given 2 weeks apart. Rituximab may be more useful in cases with a positive ANCA, active glomerulonephritis, or if there are concerns about CYC side effects. Possible side effects of rituximab include increased risk of infection, infusion reactions, lack of response to vaccines, hypogammaglobulinemia, progressive multifocal leukoencephalopathy, delayed onset neutropenia, and refractory B cell depletion.

Mild-to-moderate disease

For selected patients with mild-to-moderate disease, initial treatment with systemic glucocorticoids alone may be sufficient for patients with an FFS score of 0 or 1. This is based on results of randomized trial results showing high remission and high 5-year survival rates (93% and 97%, respectively) on glucocorticoids alone in patients with an FFS of 0. The relative treatment failures, relapse rate, or glucocorticoids use when on glucocorticoids alone did not change with the addition of AZA.[62,63] Still, although glucocorticoids remain extremely effective in reducing eosinophilia, they can cause significant side effects, even in the short term. Side effects may include infection, cataracts, glaucoma, osteoporosis, avascular necrosis, hypertension, cardiovascular disease, metabolic disease, and depression. It is important to taper glucocorticoids as able while recognizing that disease often recurs with lower doses. For this reason, additional glucocorticoid-sparing agents are often added alongside glucocorticoids from the start even in mild-to-moderate disease. Initial doses of oral prednisone range from 0.5 to 1 mg/kg/d (max 80 mg/d).

Refractory disease

Although glucocorticoids and CYC or rituximab are generally effective in terms of achieving disease control, some patients continue to have refractory disease despite these treatments. Refractory vasculitic disease is uncommon and should prompt a careful examination for whether what is being considered refractory disease is actually disease-related damage or from other causes such as infection or medication side effects. True refractory disease is most often due to persistent asthma and sinus disease. For these patients, adding an additional conventional immunosuppressive agent alongside glucocorticoids should be considered, with a goal of achieving remission and/or lessening glucocorticoid exposure. Historically, refractory disease has been treated with the addition of MTX, AZA, MMF, interferon alpha, intravenous immunoglobulin, imatinib, and plasma exchange without lot of data and with variable success.[64,65] More recently, anti-IL-5 therapies such as mepolizumab have been noted to be effective in predominantly eosinophilic patients with EGPA. Many of these medications are described in more detail below.

Remission Maintenance

The goals of remission maintenance are to prevent relapses and to facilitate the withdrawal of glucocorticoids and other toxic immunomodulators. In one series observed between 2003 and 2019, 50% of patients were reported to have at least 1 relapse, which was characterized by active asthma only (17%), ear/nose/throat (ENT) only

(21%), active asthma and ENT (18%), other lung disease (14%), cardiac (9%), skin manifestations (8%), and/or neuropathy (18%).[37] Relapses, which often manifest as asthma exacerbations or bouts of sinusitis with or without eosinophilia, typically require additional systemic glucocorticoids and additional therapies to optimize control (such as bronchodilators, inhaled glucocorticoids, and nasal glucocorticoids). However, vasculitic flares can also occur and be life-threatening. Vasculitic relapses should be managed with a remission-induction regimen based on disease severity as previously discussed.

Although many providers attempt to taper off of glucocorticoids first before initiating additional therapies in nonsevere EGPA, the approach to maintaining remission depends on a patient's disease severity at presentation and their induction therapy regimen. If CYC was used for induction, patients may receive AZA or other antimetabolites afterward. In GPA and MPA, rituximab has been used for remission maintenance after CYC but there has been less experience with this approach in EGPA. Newer practices may involve initiation of anti-IL-5 therapies in this scenario as well. Additionally, if used to induce remission, anti-IL-5 therapies are continued for maintenance. If rituximab is used for induction therapy, it may be continued every 6 months as maintenance therapy (500–1000 mg IV for adults).

Antimetabolites

Although a mainstay of treatment in the past, antimetabolites such as AZA, MTX, and MMF are used less often now as first-line therapies in EGPA.

AZA is a purine analog that disrupts RNA and DNA synthesis by interfering with purine synthesis. It is the most common antimetabolite used for management of EGPA in both remission induction and maintenance. In trials in GPA and MPA, there was no difference in relapse rates between AZA and oral daily CYC when used for remission maintenance and AZA reduced relapse rates and improved renal survival when continued beyond 18 to 24 months to 48 months.[66,67] However, a trial in GPA and MPA comparing AZA to rituximab for remission maintenance showed that rituximab was superior to AZA in preventing major relapses at 28 months.[68] In EGPA, AZA-induced remission in half of patients with an FFS of 0 and treatment failure or relapse while the addition of AZA to glucocorticoids in a double-blind 2017 trial study did not reduce treatment failures, relapse rate, or glucocorticoids use at 24 months.[62,63] Testing for thiopurine methyltransferase (TPMT) enzyme activity via both genotype and phenotype testing will assist in determining the most appropriate dose for individual patients with AZA being contraindicated in patients who have complete deficiency of TPMT or a homozygous TPMT mutation pattern. AZA is typically initiated at 50 mg/d while awaiting TPMT testing with a goal dose of 2 mg/kg/d (max 200 mg/d) if TPMT enzyme activity is normal. Potential side effects of AZA include increased infections, cytopenias, gastrointestinal upset, hepatotoxicity, and hypersensitivity.

MTX is an antimetabolite that inhibits dihydrofolate reductase and therefore inhibits DNA, RNA, thymidylate, and protein synthesis. It may be given orally or via subcutaneous injection. A 2004 open-label study found that 12 out of 23 patients with non–life-threatening EGPA maintained remission on MTX and glucocorticoids alone and allowed for a 53% reduction in glucocorticoids; however, relapses were frequent.[69] A trial in GPA and MPA comparing MTX to AZA for remission maintenance showed similar adverse event rates and relapse rates.[70] Typical dosing begins at 15 mg/wk by mouth or as a subcutaneous injection, with gradual increases up to 20 or 25 mg/wk if tolerated. Possible adverse effects of MTX include increased infections, nausea/vomiting, cytopenias, liver toxicity, teratogenicity, and MTX pneumonitis.

Targeting Eosinophils in EGPA

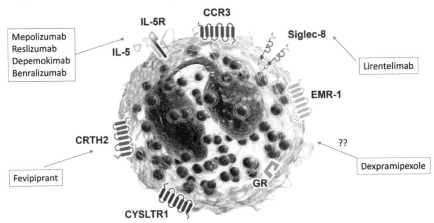

Fig. 2. There are many potential targets in EGPA but given the role of eosinophils in EGPA pathophysiology, targeting the eosinophil is a rational approach. Mepolizumab binds IL-5 and is the first therapy approved for EGPA management. Other therapies that target IL5 or its receptor include reslizumab, depemokimab, and benralizumab. Lirentelimab binds siglec 8 and fevipiprant binds the prostaglandin D2 receptor CRTH2; both can potentially block eosinophil activity. Dexpramipexole blocks eosinophil activity through an unknown mechanism. Upstream targeting of eosinophil production may be achieved by blocking TSLP with tezepelumab or IL-33 with itepekimab and eosinophil trafficking may be impeded by blocking IL-4/IL-13 with dupilumab. (*Adapted from* Wechsler ME, Fulkerson PC, Bochner BS, et al. Novel targeted therapies for eosinophilic disorders. J Allergy Clin Immunol. 2012;130(3):563-571.)

MMF is an antimetabolite that, once taken orally and converted to inosine-5'-monophosphate dehydrogenase, inhibits purine synthesis and therefore DNA replication in B cells and T cells. There are limited data on the use of MMF in patients with EGPA apart from case reports and a recent retrospective study.[71,72] In remission maintenance studies in GPA and MPA, there were more relapses seen with MMF compared with AZA.[73] MMF is dosed at 750 to 1500 mg by mouth twice daily, usually during a couple weeks to alleviate gastrointestinal upset. Along with gastrointestinal symptoms, possible adverse effects of MMF include increased infections, cytopenias, teratogenicity, and malignancy.

Interleukin-5 inhibitors

During the last 7 years, there has been an emergence of a new class of therapies targeting interleukin-5 (IL-5; **Fig. 2**).[74] IL-5 is a cytokine that specifically affects eosinophil maturation, proliferation, activation, migration to blood and tissues, and survival. Thus, by interrupting IL-5 signaling, the number of eosinophils in blood and tissue may be greatly reduced. Although this could potentially put individuals at increased risk of parasitic infection, there have been no reports of such cases. Side effects can include injection site reactions, hypersensitivity, and a possible increased risk for Herpes zoster. The most prominent anti-IL-5 therapy is mepolizumab, an anti-IL-5 monoclonal antibody targeting peripheral eosinophils, which is administered as a subcutaneous injection. Mepolizumab was first approved by the United States Food and Drug Administration (FDA) in 2015 at a dose of 100 mg/mo for use in patients 12 years and older with severe eosinophilic asthma (and later for children aged 6–12 years in

2019) because it significantly reduced asthma exacerbations and hospitalizations. In 2017, mepolizumab gained FDA approval to treat adults with EGPA because of a multicenter, double-blind, parallel-group, phase 3 trial that assigned patients with relapsing or refractory EGPA to receive 300 mg of mepolizumab or placebo every 4 weeks for 52 weeks.[75] Patients had already received treatment for at least 4 weeks and were on stable doses of glucocorticoids and standard of care therapies. The results demonstrated a significantly greater number of weeks of remission in the mepolizumab group than the placebo group (28% vs 3% accrued >24 weeks). More than half of patients on mepolizumab achieved remission, and the mepolizumab treated group had a decreased annualized relapse rate versus placebo (1.14 compared to 2.27). Significantly more patients on mepolizumab reached the daily low-dose glucocorticoid average compared with the placebo group (44% vs 7%) and mepolizumab treated patients achieved a 50% reduction in prednisone dosing by the end of the study compared with placebo.[76] As both groups had similar safety profiles in this first randomized controlled trial completed in EGPA, mepolizumab became the first drug approved by the FDA for EGPA.

Notably, the dose for severe eosinophilic asthma is 100 mg every 4 weeks as opposed to the 300 mg for EGPA striking debate as to whether a lower dose could be effective in patients with EGPA. Bettiol and colleagues compared the effectiveness of these doses in 191 patients with EGPA: 158 received 100 mg mepolizumab every 4 weeks, while 33 received mepolizumab 300 mg every 4 weeks. There were no significant differences observed in their Birmingham vasculitis activity score, prednisone dose, or eosinophil counts between 3 and 24 months.[77] Although this study suggests similar efficacy, others question whether the higher doses are needed for extrapulmonary and/or vasculitic manifestations. Additional anti-IL-5 agents have also showed promise and are discussed further below. Because patients with both severe disease and new onset disease were excluded from the mepolizumab trial, its efficacy in these settings is unknown; EGPA patients with new onset organ-threatening or life-threatening disease should receive a remission induction regimen with CYC or rituximab and glucocorticoids as previously described.

Therapies Under Active Investigation

Additional anti-IL-5 therapies that have been approved for eosinophilic asthma are currently under investigation for use in EGPA. In 2016, the monoclonal antibody against IL-5, reslizumab, was FDA approved for use in severe eosinophilic asthma in adults. In 2018, Kent and colleagues reported on 9 patients with treatment-refractory, glucocorticoid-dependent EGPA with severe eosinophilic asthma and extrapulmonary involvement treated with 3 mg/kg IV reslizumab every 4 weeks for 48 weeks. All patients tolerated more than a 50% reduction in glucocorticoid dose without deterioration in disease control as well as improved patient-reported outcomes.[78] Manka and colleagues assessed the safety and efficacy of reslizumab in an open-label study of 10 adults with EGPA and found it to be both safe and effective.[79]

A third anti-IL-5 agent, benralizumab, gained FDA-approval in 2017 for severe eosinophilic asthma in patients aged older than 12 years due to significant reductions in asthma exacerbations and glucocorticoid use and a strong safety profile. Benralizumab is an anti-IL-5 receptor-alpha monoclonal antibody that affects both peripheral and tissue eosinophils through antibody-dependent cell-mediated cytotoxicity. It is administered in asthma as a 30-mg subcutaneous injection every 4 weeks for 3 doses followed by every 8 weeks. In 2018, benralizumab was deemed an orphan drug by the FDA for treatment of EGPA. In 2020, a prospective 40-week open-label pilot study of benralizumab in 10 adults with EGPA showed that benralizumab allowed for a greater than 50% reduction in oral glucocorticoid use and fewer EGPA exacerbations. A Phase 3, randomized, double blind multicenter clinical trial is currently underway to examine the efficacy and safety of monthly benralizumab versus mepolizumab in patients with relapsing or refractory EGPA.[80]

Depemokimab is a novel experimental long-acting anti-IL-5 therapy that can be administered every 6 months. It lowers eosinophil counts and is currently being evaluated in a phase 3 study in comparison to mepolizumab in both eosinophilic asthma as well as in relapsing and refractory EGPA.[81]

Possible Future Investigational Targets

With the development of so many novel biologic agents in the last decade for more common diseases such as asthma, it is not surprising that several new therapies could be on the horizon to investigate in EGPA based on their mechanism of action (see **Fig. 2**). To date, there remains no information on their efficacy and safety in this setting such that these should not be used in the clinical care of patients with EGPA.

- Although anti-IL-4/IL-13 therapy with dupilumab may prevent eosinophilic trafficking from blood into tissue, and has been approved for eosinophilic asthma, chronic rhinosinusitis, eosinophilic esophagitis and atopic dermatitis, concerns regarding increasing eosinophil counts and rare systemic eosinophilic manifestations have precluded its being studied in EGPA and thus a role in this disease is unknown.[82]
- Targeting of epithelial cytokines known as alarmins that are upstream to Th2 and ILC2 mediated cytokines such as IL4, IL5, and IL13 has been a strategy used in severe asthma with good success. Tezepelumab is an antithymic stromal lymphopoietin (TSLP) monoclonal antibody approved by the FDA for severe asthma in 2021. Because it lowers eosinophil counts, IgE and exhaled nitric oxide, it may be an effective strategy worth studying in EGPA.[83] Anti-IL33 targeted therapies such as itepekimab and astegolimab also work upstream, preventing IL33 from activating ILC2 cells from producing IL5. Anti-IL33 therapies are showing promise in both asthma and chronic obstructive pulmonary disease and therefore could be an attractive target to explore in EGPA as well.[84,85]
- Dexpramipexole is an oral investigational therapy first developed as a treatment of amyotrophic lateral sclerosis (ALS). Although it failed to meet its primary end point in ALS, dexpramipexole was observed to produce a significant and targeted depletion of eosinophils in the blood of ALS patients, making it a potential oral option for future investigation in EGPA, and in asthma, for which it is being actively studied.[86,87]
- Another eosinophil targeted therapy is lirentelimab, an anti-Siglec-8 antibody that depletes eosinophils and inhibits mast cells and that has shown potential in animal models and humans as a treatment of eosinophilic gastritis and duodenitis.[88] This oral therapy could also be an attractive option to study in patients with EGPA.
- Based on the complexity of EGPA pathophysiology, there is a strong rationale to target a variety of type 2 and nontype 2 cytokines and mediators in EGPA. Although chemokine receptor antagonists that bind CCR3 or therapies that target prostaglandins (CRTH2 antagonists such as fevipiprant) have not been shown to be effective in asthma, there still remains potential that these drugs, and others that target EMR1 or the cysteinyl leukotriene receptors, could be beneficial in EGPA, warranting further study.
- Avacopan, an oral anti-C5a receptor antagonist, is indicated as an adjunctive treatment of adults with severe GPA and MPA in combination with standard

therapy. It was safe and well tolerated in comparison to glucocorticoids.[89] Although EGPA is also considered to be within the family of AAV, there have been no data to date with the use of avacopan in EGPA.

MONITORING AND PROPHYLAXIS

Patients with EGPA require close monitoring for disease activity and medication safety. Ideally, patients will acquire a multidisciplinary team of providers most relevant to their needs, including (but not limited to) a pulmonologist, rheumatologist, allergy/immunologist, otolaryngologist, cardiologist, dermatologist, gastroenterologist, neurologist, and/or mental health professional. We recommend visits every 2 to 4 weeks for the first 3 months spaced out to 3-month intervals once disease control is obtained. Laboratory monitoring should include a complete blood cell count with differential (including eosinophils), complete chemistries, ESR and/or CRP, and urinalysis at an interval based on the disease activity status and medication. Immunoglobulin E monitoring may be useful in selected patients. Patients should undergo frequent pulmonary function testing. We also recommend vaccinating all patients against pneumococcal pneumonia, influenza, and SARS-CoV-2 according to published guidelines as well as providing any other nonlive vaccines recommended by current published guidelines for immunosuppressed hosts. Recombinant zoster (shingles) vaccine, for instance, is appropriate for patients receiving mepolizumab while prophylaxis against Pneumocystis jiroveci is recommended to patients on high doses of glucocorticoids in combination with additional immunosuppressive therapies. Prophylaxis against osteoporosis should be implemented and monitoring should be done annually with bone densitometry in patients on systemic glucocorticoids.

PROGNOSIS

EGPA carries significant risk of morbidity and potential mortality. Morbidity from EGPA may be related to the disease itself but also to toxicity from medications and the psychosocial burden of chronic disease. Although largely fatal initially, the use of glucocorticoids and other immunosuppressive therapies in patients with EGPA has improved mortality rates to roughly 10% with 5-year-survival rates of more than 90%.[9] Cardiac involvement represents the greatest cause of mortality.[7,9] Factors that attribute to a poor prognosis include age greater than or equal to 65 years old, renal failure, gastrointestinal bleeding, cerebral hemorrhage, and severe asthma.[9] Puechal and colleagues showed that the presence of anti-MPO antibodies at baseline is associated with shorter disease-free survival and higher risk of relapse, though overall survival rates were no different between groups, while Doubelt and colleagues did not find a difference in relapse or death rates based on ANCA status.[37,90] Infections in the setting of immunosuppressive therapies also contribute to mortality. Finally, a higher FFS (0 vs 1 vs 2) correlates with increasing 5-year mortality rates (9% vs 21% vs 40%), though anecdotally, many providers solely use these scores as a reminder of the most severe features of disease.[53]

EOSINOPHILIC GRANULOMATOSIS WITH POLYANGIITIS IN CHILDREN

The incidence of all AAV in children is 0.45 to 6.4 cases per million children per year; as the smallest subset, EGPA is extremely rare in the pediatric age range.[91,92] Diagnosing EGPA in children is challenging, in part because classification and diagnostic criteria are based on adult patients. The mean age of onset in a systematic review of published pediatric EGPA cases was 12 years old with a male-to-female ratio of 0.74.[93]

Table 2
Current and emerging therapies in eosinophilic granulomatosis with polyangiitis

Class	Examples
Current Therapies	
Alkylating agent	Cyclophosphamide
Anti-CD20	Rituximab
Anti-IL-5	Mepolizumab[a]
Antimetabolite	Azathioprine
Antimetabolite	Methotrexate
Antimetabolite	Mycophenolate Mofetil
Therapies under active investigation	
Anti-IL-5	Depemokimab
Anti-IL-5	Benralizumab
Anti-IL-5	Reslizumab
Possible Future Investigational Targets	
Anti-EMR1	N/A
Anti-CRTH2	Fevipiprant
Anti-CCR3	N/A
Anticysteinyl leukotriene receptors	Montelukast
Anti-IL-4/IL-13	Dupilumab
Anti-interleukin 33	Astegolimab Itepekimab
Antithymic stromal lymphopoietin	Tezepelumab
Antisiglec-8	Lirentelimab
Small molecule	Dexpramipexole

Abbreviation: N/A, not applicable.
[a] Currently approved for use in adults with EGPA by the FDA and European Commission.

Fewer than one-third of children with EGPA have positive ANCA antibodies, although when present, they are often directed at MPO.[6,7,93,94] Overall, EGPA in pediatrics is thought to be quite aggressive and often involves the heart and lungs.[6,7,95] A review of 47 published pediatric cases reported 13% mortality while relapse rates in 2 pediatric EGPA series were 46% and 64% during 12 to 18 months.[93,94]

Given its rarity, EGPA is greatly understudied in children, as is AAV in general, with no randomized controlled trials or observational studies involving children. Therefore, pediatric providers largely base their management principles from the adult strategies outlined above, considering that children metabolize medications differently and could be exposed to larger cumulative doses during their lifetime. Pediatric providers are especially interested in glucocorticoid-sparing therapies given the adverse effects of glucocorticoids on growth in childhood as well as their long-term sequalae.

In 2019, rituximab received FDA approval for GPA and MPA in children aged 2 years and older.[96] More recently, pediatric providers have been exploring the use of anti-IL-5 therapies such as mepolizumab and benralizumab in children with EGPA.[97,98] Although providers typically follow similar approaches to treatment in children with EGPA as described in this article, insurance approvals provide significant barriers given the lack of rigorous pediatric studies available. We encourage the medical community to report cases highlighting the clinical presentation, treatment, complications, and outcomes of children with EGPA in order to increase pediatric patients' access to glucocorticoid-sparing agents.

FUTURE DIRECTIONS

The future is bright for the management of EGPA; however, collaborative multidisciplinary care and rigorous research must be prioritized to advance outcomes in this rare disease. The ability to conduct multicenter studies on EGPA as its own entity separate from other forms of vasculitis together with further investigation of the immunologic pathways involved in EGPA will allow for a greater focus on potential therapeutic targets unique to the disease. Identification of novel predictive and response biomarkers will be critical to advance the science and treatment of EGPA. In the meantime, expanding investigations of emerging therapies (**Table 2**) in EGPA will be critical to inform discussions with patients and their families regarding the risks and benefits of management decisions. Our community is also learning more about the ways in which EGPA presents and progresses in children and young adults and we hope to expand the toolbox of therapeutics available to pediatric patients. Ultimately, we aim to progress toward a more personalized approach to care for patients with EGPA, including best practices for ANCA-positive and ANCA-negative patients as well as organ-specific manifestations.

CLINICS CARE POINTS

- EGPA can be a difficult diagnosis to establish. Consideration of EGPA should be prompted by the constellation of allergic rhinitis, asthma, hypereosinophilia, and features of a systemic vasculitis although these features may not be present in sequence or at the same time.

- Patients receiving prednisone may not have hypereosinophilia and yet still have an underlying diagnosis of EGPA because the eosinophil count will normalize with glucocorticoid treatment.

- Patients with organ-threatening or life-threatening vasculitic disease should be treated by clinicians with experience managing vasculitis; glucocorticoids combined with rituximab or CYC should be used in most severe patients while milder patients may be treated with glucocorticoids alone.

- Consider anti-IL-5 therapy with mepolizumab for patients with relapsing or refractory disease; it has been shown to reduce exacerbations and glucocorticoid dose by 50% or more.

DISCLOSURE

Dr J.L. Bloom has nothing to disclose. Dr C.A. Langford has received research grants from GlaxoSmioth Kline, AstraZeneca, Bristol-Myers Squibb, ChemoCentryx. Dr M. Wechsler has received consulting, advisory, or speaking honoraria from the following: Amgen, AstraZeneca, Avalo Therapeutics, Boehringer Ingelheim, Cerecor, Cohero Health, Cytoreason, Eli Lilly, Equillium, Glaxosmithkline, Incyte, Kinaset, Novartis, Om Pharma, Phylaxis, Pulmatrix, Rapt Therapeutics, Regeneron, Restorbio, Roche/Genentech, Sanofi/Genzyme, Sentien, Sound Biologics, Tetherex Pharmaceuticals, Teva, Upstream Bio.

REFERENCES

1. Lie J. Illustrated histopathologic classification criteria for selected vasculitis syndromes. American College of Rheumatology Subcommittee on Classification of Vasculitis. Arthritis Rheum 1990;33(8):1074–87.

2. Jennette J. Overview of the 2012 revised International Chapel Hill Consensus Conference nomenclature of vasculitides. Clin Exp Nephrol 2013;17(5):603–6.
3. Masi AT, Hunder GG, Lie JT, et al. The American College of Rheumatology 1990 criteria for the classification of Churg-Strauss syndrome (allergic granulomatosis and angiitis). Arthritis Rheum 1990;33(8):1094–100.
4. Sablé-Fourtassou R, Cohen P, Mahr A, et al. Antineutrophil cytoplasmic antibodies and the Churg-Strauss syndrome. Ann Intern Med 2005;143(9):632–8.
5. Sinico RA, Di Toma L, Maggiore U, et al. Prevalence and clinical significance of antineutrophil cytoplasmic antibodies in Churg-Strauss syndrome. Arthritis Rheum 2005;52(9):2926–35.
6. Gendelman S, Zeft A, Spalding SJ. Childhood-onset eosinophilic granulomatosis with polyangiitis (formerly Churg-Strauss syndrome): a contemporary single-center cohort. J Rheumatol 2013;40(6):929–35.
7. Zwerina J, Eger G, Englbrecht M, et al. Churg-Strauss syndrome in childhood: a systematic literature review and clinical comparison with adult patients. Semin Arthritis Rheum 2009;39(2):108–15.
8. Mouthon L, Dunogue B, Guillevin L. Diagnosis and classification of eosinophilic granulomatosis with polyangiitis (formerly named Churg-Strauss syndrome). J Autoimmunr 2014;48-49:99–103.
9. Comarmond C, Pagnoux C, Khellaf M, et al. Eosinophilic granulomatosis with polyangiitis (Churg-Strauss): clinical characteristics and long-term followup of the 383 patients enrolled in the French Vasculitis Study Group cohort. Arthritis Rheum 2013;65(1):270–81.
10. Gómez-Puerta JA, Gedmintas L, Costenbader KH. The association between silica exposure and development of ANCA-associated vasculitis: systematic review and meta-analysis. Autoimmun Rev 2013;12(12):1129–35.
11. Pagnoux C, Guilpain P, Guillevin L. Churg-Strauss syndrome. Curr Opin Rheumatol 2007;19(1):25–32.
12. Williams M, Li J, Talbot P. Effects of Model, Method of Collection, and Topography on Chemical Elements and Metals in the Aerosol of Tank-Style Electronic Cigarettes. Sci Rep 2019;9(1):13969.
13. Detoraki A, Di Capua L, Varricchi G, et al. Omalizumab in patients with eosinophilic granulomatosis with polyangiitis: a 36-month follow-up study. J Asthma 2016;53(2):201–6.
14. Jachiet M, Samson M, Cottin V, et al. Anti-IgE Monoclonal Antibody (Omalizumab) in Refractory and Relapsing Eosinophilic Granulomatosis With Polyangiitis (Churg-Strauss): Data on Seventeen Patients. Arthritis Rheumatol 2016;68(9):2274–82.
15. Weller PF, Plaut M, Taggart V, et al. The relationship of asthma therapy and Churg-Strauss syndrome: NIH workshop summary report. J Allergy Clin Immunol 2001;108(2):175–83.
16. Celebi Sozener Z, Gorgulu B, Mungan D, et al. Omalizumab in the treatment of eosinophilic granulomatosis with polyangiitis (EGPA): single-center experience in 18 cases. World Allergy Organ J 2018;11(1):39.
17. Vaglio A, Martorana D, Maggiore U, et al. HLA-DRB4 as a genetic risk factor for Churg-Strauss syndrome. Arthritis Rheum 2007;56(9):3159–66.
18. Wieczorek S, Hellmich B, Gross WL, et al. Associations of Churg-Strauss syndrome with the HLA-DRB1 locus, and relationship to the genetics of antineutrophil cytoplasmic antibody-associated vasculitides: comment on the article by Vaglio et al. Arthritis Rheum 2008;58(1):329–30.

19. Wieczorek S, Hellmich B, Arning L, et al. Functionally relevant variations of the interleukin-10 gene associated with antineutrophil cytoplasmic antibody-negative Churg-Strauss syndrome, but not with Wegener's granulomatosis. Arthritis Rheum 2008;58(6):1839–48.

20. Gioffredi A, Maritati F, Oliva E, et al. Eosinophilic granulomatosis with polyangiitis: an overview. Front Immunol 2014;5:549.

21. Saito H, Tsurikisawa N, Tsuburai T, et al. Cytokine production profile of CD4+ T cells from patients with active Churg-Strauss syndrome tends toward Th17. Int Arch Allergy Immunol 2009;149(Suppl 1):61–5.

22. Saito H, Tsurikisawa N, Tsuburai T, et al. The proportion of regulatory T cells in the peripheral blood reflects the relapse or remission status of patients with Churg-Strauss syndrome. Int Arch Allergy Immunol 2011;155(Suppl 1):46–52.

23. Tsurikisawa N, Saito H, Oshikata C, et al. Decreases in the numbers of peripheral blood regulatory T cells, and increases in the levels of memory and activated B cells, in patients with active eosinophilic granulomatosis and polyangiitis. J Clin Immunol 2013;33(5):965–76.

24. Hellmich B, Csernok E, Gross WL. Proinflammatory cytokines and autoimmunity in Churg-Strauss syndrome. Ann N Y Acad Sci 2005;1051:121–31.

25. Akuthota P, Weller PF. Spectrum of Eosinophilic End-Organ Manifestations. Immunol Allergy Clin North Am 2015;35(3):403–11.

26. Roufosse F. L4. Eosinophils: how they contribute to endothelial damage and dysfunction. Presse Med 2013;42(4 Pt 2):503–7.

27. Tai PC, Holt ME, Denny P, et al. Deposition of eosinophil cationic protein in granulomas in allergic granulomatosis and vasculitis: the Churg-Strauss syndrome. Br Med J 1984;289(6442):400–2.

28. Wechsler ME, Fulkerson PC, Bochner BS, et al. Novel targeted therapies for eosinophilic disorders. J Allergy Clin Immunol 2012;130(3):563–71.

29. Vaglio A, Strehl JD, Manger B, et al. IgG4 immune response in Churg-Strauss syndrome. Ann Rheum Dis 2012;71(3):390–3.

30. Fagni F, Bello F, Emmi G. Eosinophilic Granulomatosis With Polyangiitis: Dissecting the Pathophysiology. Front Med 2021;8:627776.

31. Makiya MA, Khoury P, Kuang FL, et al. Urine eosinophil-derived neurotoxin: A potential marker of activity in select eosinophilic disorders. Allergy 2022. https://doi.org/10.1111/all.15481.

32. Lanham JG, Elkon KB, Pusey CD, et al. Systemic vasculitis with asthma and eosinophilia: a clinical approach to the Churg-Strauss syndrome. Medicine (Baltim) 1984;63(2):65–81.

33. Baldini C, Talarico R, Della Rossa A, et al. Clinical manifestations and treatment of Churg-Strauss syndrome. Rheum Dis Clin North Am 2010;36(3):527–43.

34. Chumbley LC, Harrison EG Jr, DeRemee RA. Allergic granulomatosis and angiitis (Churg-Strauss syndrome). Report and analysis of 30 cases. Mayo Clin Proc 1977;52(8):477–84.

35. Vaglio A, Buzio C, Zwerina J. Eosinophilic granulomatosis with polyangiitis (Churg-Strauss): state of the art. Allergy 2013;68(3):261–73.

36. Kallenberg CG. Churg-Strauss syndrome: just one disease entity? Arthritis Rheum 2005;52(9):2589–93.

37. Doubelt I, Cuthbertson D, Carette S, et al. Clinical Manifestations and Long-Term Outcomes of Eosinophilic Granulomatosis With Polyangiitis in North America. ACR Open Rheumatol 2021;3(6):404–12.

38. Sinico RA, Bottero P. Churg-Strauss angiitis. Best Pract Res Clin Rheumatol 2009;23(3):355–66.

39. Szczeklik W, Sokołowska B, Mastalerz L, et al. Pulmonary findings in Churg-Strauss syndrome in chest X-rays and high resolution computed tomography at the time of initial diagnosis. Clin Rheumatol 2010;29(10):1127–34.

40. Dennert RM, van Paassen P, Schalla S, et al. Cardiac involvement in Churg-Strauss syndrome. Arthritis Rheum 2010;62(2):627–34.

41. Dunogué B, Terrier B, Cohen P, et al. Impact of cardiac magnetic resonance imaging on eosinophilic granulomatosis with polyangiitis outcomes: A long-term retrospective study on 42 patients. Autoimmun Rev 2015;14(9):774–80.

42. Fijolek J, Wiatr E, Gawryluk D, et al. The significance of cardiac magnetic resonance imaging in detection and monitoring of the treatment efficacy of heart involvement in eosinophilic granulomatosis with polyangiitis patients. Sarcoidosis Vasc Diffuse Lung Dis 2016;33(1):51–8.

43. Marmursztejn J, Guillevin L, Trebossen R, et al. Churg-Strauss syndrome cardiac involvement evaluated by cardiac magnetic resonance imaging and positron-emission tomography: a prospective study on 20 patients. Rheumatology 2013;52(4):642–50.

44. Sauvetre G, Fares J, Caudron J, et al. [Usefulness of magnetic resonance imaging in Churg-Strauss syndrome related cardiac involvement. A case series of three patients and literature review]. *Rev Med Interne*. Sep 2010;31(9):600–5 [Intérêt de l'imagerie par résonance magnétique nucléaire au cours de l'atteinte cardiaque du syndrome de Churg-Strauss. Trois observations et revue de la littérature].

45. Grayson PC, Ponte C, Suppiah R, et al. American College of Rheumatology/European Alliance of Associations for Rheumatology Classification Criteria for Eosinophilic Granulomatosis with Polyangiitis. Ann Rheum Dis 2022;81(3): 309–14.

46. Groh M, Pagnoux C, Baldini C, et al. Eosinophilic granulomatosis with polyangiitis (Churg-Strauss) (EGPA) Consensus Task Force recommendations for evaluation and management. Eur J Intern Med 2015;26(7):545–53.

47. Wechsler ME. Pulmonary eosinophilic syndromes. Immunol Allergy Clin North Am 2007;27(3):477–92.

48. Nguyen Y, Guillevin L. Eosinophilic Granulomatosis with Polyangiitis (Churg-Strauss). Semin Respir Crit Care Med 2018;39(4):471–81.

49. Valent P, Klion AD, Horny HP, et al. Contemporary consensus proposal on criteria and classification of eosinophilic disorders and related syndromes. J Allergy Clin Immunol 2012;130(3):607–12.e9.

50. Cruz T, Reboucas G, Rocha H. Fatal strongyloidiasis in patients receiving corticosteroids. N Engl J Med 1966;275(20):1093–6.

51. Chung SA, Langford CA, Maz M, et al. American College of Rheumatology/Vasculitis Foundation Guideline for the Management of Antineutrophil Cytoplasmic Antibody-Associated Vasculitis. Arthritis Care Res 2021;73(8): 1088–105.

52. Guillevin L, Lhote F, Gayraud M, et al. Prognostic factors in polyarteritis nodosa and Churg-Strauss syndrome. A prospective study in 342 patients. Medicine (Baltim) 1996;75(1):17–28.

53. Guillevin L, Pagnoux C, Seror R, et al. The Five-Factor Score revisited: assessment of prognoses of systemic necrotizing vasculitides based on the French Vasculitis Study Group (FVSG) cohort. Medicine (Baltim) 2011;90(1):19–27.

54. Gayraud M, Guillevin L, le Toumelin P, et al. Long-term followup of polyarteritis nodosa, microscopic polyangiitis, and Churg-Strauss syndrome: analysis of

four prospective trials including 278 patients. Arthritis Rheum 2001;44(3): 666–75.

55. Jones RB, Tervaert JW, Hauser T, et al. Rituximab versus cyclophosphamide in ANCA-associated renal vasculitis. N Engl J Med 2010;363(3):211–20.

56. Stone JH, Merkel PA, Spiera R, et al. Rituximab versus cyclophosphamide for ANCA-associated vasculitis. N Engl J Med 2010;363(3):221–32.

57. Menditto VG, Rossetti G, Olivari D, et al. Rituximab for eosinophilic granulomatosis with polyangiitis: a systematic review of observational studies. Rheumatology 2021;60(4):1640–50.

58. Mohammad AJ, Hot A, Arndt F, et al. Rituximab for the treatment of eosinophilic granulomatosis with polyangiitis (Churg-Strauss). Ann Rheum Dis 2016;75(2): 396–401.

59. Casal Moura M, Berti A, Keogh KA, et al. Asthma control in eosinophilic granulomatosis with polyangiitis treated with rituximab. Clin Rheumatol 2020;39(5): 1581–90.

60. Wang CR, Tsai YS, Tsai HW, et al. B-Cell-Depleting Therapy Improves Myocarditis in Seronegative Eosinophilic Granulomatosis with Polyangiitis. J Clin Med 2021;(19):10.

61. Teixeira V, Mohammad AJ, Jones RB, et al. Efficacy and safety of rituximab in the treatment of eosinophilic granulomatosis with polyangiitis. RMD Open 2019;5(1):e000905.

62. Puéchal X, Pagnoux C, Baron G, et al. Adding Azathioprine to Remission-Induction Glucocorticoids for Eosinophilic Granulomatosis With Polyangiitis (Churg-Strauss), Microscopic Polyangiitis, or Polyarteritis Nodosa Without Poor Prognosis Factors: A Randomized, Controlled Trial. Arthritis Rheumatol 2017;69(11):2175–86.

63. Ribi C, Cohen P, Pagnoux C, et al. Treatment of Churg-Strauss syndrome without poor-prognosis factors: a multicenter, prospective, randomized, open-label study of seventy-two patients. Arthritis Rheum 2008;58(2):586–94.

64. Metzler C, Csernok E, Gross WL, et al. Interferon-alpha for maintenance of remission in Churg-Strauss syndrome: a long-term observational study. Clin Exp Rheumatol 2010;28(1 Suppl 57):24–30.

65. Metzler C, Schnabel A, Gross WL, et al. A phase II study of interferon-alpha for the treatment of refractory Churg-Strauss syndrome. Clin Exp Rheumatol 2008; 26(3 Suppl 49):S35–40.

66. Jayne D, Rasmussen N, Andrassy K, et al. A randomized trial of maintenance therapy for vasculitis associated with antineutrophil cytoplasmic autoantibodies. N Engl J Med 2003;349(1):36–44.

67. Karras A, Pagnoux C, Haubitz M, et al. Randomised controlled trial of prolonged treatment in the remission phase of ANCA-associated vasculitis. Ann Rheum Dis 2017;76(10):1662–8.

68. Guillevin L, Pagnoux C, Karras A, et al. Rituximab versus azathioprine for maintenance in ANCA-associated vasculitis. N Engl J Med 2014;371(19):1771–80.

69. Metzler C, Hellmich B, Gause A, et al. Churg Strauss syndrome–successful induction of remission with methotrexate and unexpected high cardiac and pulmonary relapse ratio during maintenance treatment. Clin Exp Rheumatol 2004;22(6 Suppl 36):S52–61.

70. Pagnoux C, Mahr A, Hamidou MA, et al. Azathioprine or methotrexate maintenance for ANCA-associated vasculitis. N Engl J Med 2008;359(26):2790–803.

71. Assaf C, Mewis G, Orfanos CE, et al. Churg-Strauss syndrome: successful treatment with mycophenolate mofetil. Br J Dermatol 2004;150(3):598–600.

72. Philobos M, Perkins A, Karabayas M, et al. A real-world assessment of mycophenolate mofetil for remission induction in eosinophilic granulomatosis with polyangiitis. Rheumatol Int 2021;41(10):1811–4.

73. Hiemstra TF, Walsh M, Mahr A, et al. Mycophenolate mofetil vs azathioprine for remission maintenance in antineutrophil cytoplasmic antibody-associated vasculitis: a randomized controlled trial. JAMA 2010;304(21):2381–8.

74. Roufosse F. Targeting the Interleukin-5 Pathway for Treatment of Eosinophilic Conditions Other than Asthma. Front Med 2018;5:49.

75. FDA approves first drug for Eosinophilic Granulomatosis with Polyangiitis, a rare disease formerly known as the Churg-Strauss Syndrome. 2017. Avilable at: https://www.fda.gov/news-events/press-announcements/fda-approves-first-drug-eosinophilic-granulomatosis-polyangiitis-rare-disease-formerly-known-churg.

76. Wechsler ME, Akuthota P, Jayne D, et al. Mepolizumab or Placebo for Eosinophilic Granulomatosis with Polyangiitis. N Engl J Med 2017;376(20):1921–32.

77. Bettiol A, Urban ML, Dagna L, et al. Mepolizumab for Eosinophilic Granulomatosis With Polyangiitis: A European Multicenter Observational Study. Arthritis Rheumatol 2022;74(2):295–306.

78. Kent B, d'Ancona G, Fernandes M, et al. Glucocorticoid sparing effects of reslizumab in the treatment of eosinophilic granulomatosis with polyangiitis. Thorax 2018;73(Suppl 4):A1–28.

79. Manka LA, Guntur VP, Denson JL, et al. Efficacy and safety of reslizumab in the treatment of eosinophilic granulomatosis with polyangiitis. Ann Allergy Asthma Immunol 2021;126(6):696–701.e1.

80. Efficacy and Safety of Benralizumab in EGPA Compared to Mepolizumab. (MANDARA). ClinicalTrials.gov Identifier: NCT04157348. Updated September 2, 2022. Available at: https://clinicaltrials.gov/ct2/show/NCT04157348. Accessed September 25, 2022.

81. Efficacy and Safety of Depemokimab Compared With Mepolizumab in Adults With Relapsing or Refractory Eosinophilic Granulomatosis With Polyangiitis (EGPA) (OCEAN). ClinicalTrials.gov Identifier: NCT05263934. Updated September 16, 2022. Available at: https://clinicaltrials.gov/ct2/show/NCT05263934. Accessed September 25, 2022.

82. Wechsler ME, Ford LB, Maspero JF, et al. Long-term safety and efficacy of dupilumab in patients with moderate-to-severe asthma (TRAVERSE): an open-label extension study. Lancet Respir Med 2022;10(1):11–25.

83. Menzies-Gow A, Corren J, Bourdin A, et al. Tezepelumab in Adults and Adolescents with Severe, Uncontrolled Asthma. N Engl J Med 2021;384(19):1800–9.

84. Rabe KF, Celli BR, Wechsler ME, et al. Safety and efficacy of itepekimab in patients with moderate-to-severe COPD: a genetic association study and randomised, double-blind, phase 2a trial. Lancet Respir Med 2021;9(11):1288–98.

85. Wechsler ME, Ruddy MK, Pavord ID, et al. Efficacy and Safety of Itepekimab in Patients with Moderate-to-Severe Asthma. N Engl J Med 2021;385(18):1656–68.

86. Panch SR, Bozik ME, Brown T, et al. Dexpramipexole as an oral steroid-sparing agent in hypereosinophilic syndromes. Blood 2018;132(5):501–9.

87. Dworetzky SI, Hebrank GT, Archibald DG, et al. The targeted eosinophil-lowering effects of dexpramipexole in clinical studies. Blood Cells Mol Dis 2017;63:62–5.

88. Dellon ES, Peterson KA, Murray JA, et al. Anti-Siglec-8 Antibody for Eosinophilic Gastritis and Duodenitis. N Engl J Med 2020;383(17):1624–34.

89. Jayne DRW, Merkel PA, Schall TJ, et al. Avacopan for the Treatment of ANCA-Associated Vasculitis. N Engl J Med 2021;384(7):599–609.

90. Puéchal X, Iudici M, Pagnoux C, et al. Comparative study of granulomatosis with polyangiitis subsets according to ANCA status: data from the French Vasculitis Study Group Registry. RMD Open 2022;8(1). https://doi.org/10.1136/rmdopen-2021-002160.

91. Jariwala MP, Laxer RM. Primary Vasculitis in Childhood: GPA and MPA in Childhood. Front Pediatr 2018;6:226.

92. Petty R, Laxer R, Lindsley C, et al. In: *Textbook of Pediatric Rheumatology.* 8th edition. Philadelphia, PA: Elsevier; 2021.

93. Fina A, Dubus JC, Tran A, et al. Eosinophilic granulomatosis with polyangiitis in children: Data from the French RespiRare® cohort. *Pediatr Pulmonol.* Dec 2018; 53(12):1640–50.

94. Eleftheriou D, Gale H, Pilkington C, et al. Eosinophilic granulomatosis with polyangiitis in childhood: retrospective experience from a tertiary referral centre in the UK. Rheumatology 2016;55(7):1263–72.

95. Iudici M, Puéchal X, Pagnoux C, et al. Brief Report: Childhood-Onset Systemic Necrotizing Vasculitides: Long-Term Data From the French Vasculitis Study Group Registry. *Arthritis Rheumatol.* Jul 2015;67(7):1959–65.

96. FDA approves first treatment for children with rare diseases that cause inflammation of small blood vessels. 2019. Available at: https://www.fda.gov/news-events/press-announcements/fda-approves-first-treatment-children-rare-diseases-cause-inflammation-small-blood-vessels.

97. Hinds DM, Bloom JL, Cooper JC, et al. Pulmonary eosinophilic vasculitis with granulomas and benralizumab in children. Pediatr Pulmonol 2021;56(6): 1789–92.

98. Nara M, Saito M, Abe F, et al. A Pediatric Case of Relapsing Eosinophilic Granulomatosis with Polyangiitis Successfully Treated with Mepolizumab. Intern Med 2019;58(24):3583–7.

99. Guillevin L, Cohen P, Gayraud M, et al. Churg-Strauss syndrome. Clinical study and long-term follow-up of 96 patients. Medicine (Baltim) 1999;78(1):26–37.

100. Bacciu A, Bacciu S, Mercante G, et al. Ear, nose and throat manifestations of Churg-Strauss syndrome. Acta Otolaryngol 2006;126(5):503–9.

Behçet Syndrome

Gülen Hatemi, MD[a,b,*], Didar Uçar, MD[b,c], Uğur Uygunoğlu, MD[b,d],
Hasan Yazici, MD[e], Yusuf Yazici, MD[f]

KEYWORDS

- Behçet's syndrome • Epidemiology • Pathogenesis • Clinical findings • Diagnosis
- Outcome measures • Management

KEY POINTS

- Diagnosis of Behçet syndrome is made by recognizing the clinical manifestations, since laboratory tests, biomarkers, or genetic tests are not diagnostic.
- Imaging modalities including fundus fluorescein angiograms, MRI, MR angiograms, CT, CT angiograms, and PET scans help to diagnose different manifestations and to monitor the treatment.
- Criteria sets are not ideal because during their development several diseases were not adequately included as controls and disease prevalence were not taken into account.
- Management should be planned by a multidisciplinary team according to activity and severity of organ involvement, prognostic factors such as disease duration, age, and sex, and patients' preferences.
- A treat-to-target approach is desirable in BS. Further research is needed to identify the best targets that predict a good long-term outcome for each organ.

INTRODUCTION

Behçet syndrome (BS) is unique among the systemic vasculitides for causing arterial and venous inflammation, affecting vessels of all sizes, and additional recurrent, self-limiting skin and mucosa lesions that occur in almost all patients.[1] The affected vessels range from the aorta and pulmonary arteries to retinal arteries on the arterial side and from the superior and inferior vena cava to superficial veins on the venous side.[2] This may result in damage and loss of function in several organs and systems

[a] Division of Rheumatology, Department of Internal Medicine, Istanbul University – Cerrahpasa, School of Medicine, Istanbul, Turkey; [b] Behçet's Disease Research Center, Istanbul University - Cerrahpasa, Istanbul, Turkey; [c] Department of Ophthalmology, Istanbul University – Cerrahpasa, School of Medicine, Istanbul, Turkey; [d] Department of Neurology, Istanbul University – Cerrahpasa, School of Medicine, Istanbul, Turkey; [e] Rheumatology, Academic Hospital, Istanbul, Turkey; [f] Division of Rheumatology, New York University School of Medicine, New York, NY, USA
* Corresponding author. Istanbul University—Cerrahpaşa Medical School, Kocamustafapaşa, Istanbul 34093, Turkey.
E-mail address: gulenhatemi@yahoo.com

Rheum Dis Clin N Am 49 (2023) 585–602
https://doi.org/10.1016/j.rdc.2023.03.010
0889-857X/23/© 2023 Elsevier Inc. All rights reserved.

including the eyes, central nervous system, and gastrointestinal system. The mucosal lesions, including oral and genital ulcers, skin lesions including nodular and papulo-pustular lesions, and musculoskeletal involvement including arthritis and enthesitis, may recur frequently impairing quality of life and daily living activities.[3] These manifestations can be present in various combinations and sequences over time. This may cause difficulty in diagnosing BS, especially in settings where it has a low prevalence. The diagnosis is made by recognizing the manifestations and bringing them together, as laboratory tests, biomarkers, or genetic tests are not diagnostic. A number of disease criteria have been developed and used over the years including the International Study Group criteria and the more recent International Criteria for Behçet's Disease.[4,5] However, none of these criteria sets are ideal because during the development process several diseases that are important in the differential diagnosis of BS were not adequately included as controls and because disease prevalence were not taken into account. The heterogeneity in disease manifestations makes it difficult to develop a standard treatment strategy that would be useful for most of the patients. The choice of treatment modalities differs according to the severity and activity of each organ involvement as well as prognostic factors including age, sex, and disease duration.[6] BS is more active during the early years of the disease and uveitis, central nervous system lesions, arterial aneurysms, and venous thrombosis are more common among men.[7,8] In this review, the authors aimed to give an overview based on the most recent evidence on the epidemiology, pathogenesis, clinical manifestations, and management of BS.

Epidemiology

BS was first described by Hulusi Behçet, a Turkish dermatologist. Patients are most commonly from the Middle East, the Mediterranean region, and the Far East with Japan and South Korea leading the list. It is most prevalent in Turkey, with a prevalence of one in 250 adults[9]; it is rare in northern Europe and Africa. BS has a unique geographical distribution of incidence and prevalence and is sometimes referred to as the Silk Route disease because of its increased frequency in the Middle East and far-East Asia. It is relatively rare before late teens and after age 50 years and most commonly seen in patients in their second and third decades.

Males and females are equally affected, but males frequently have more severe disease and poorer outcomes.[10] Some manifestations may show regional differences; for example, gastrointestinal involvement, rare in Turkey, is more common in Japan and is seen in about 30% of patients in the United States[11,12] Pathergy (subcutaneous skin hyperactivity to needle prick) is more common in the Middle East than in the United States and northern Europe.

Pathogenesis

Although our understanding of pathogenetic mechanisms underlying BS is still limited, current knowledge points to the role of environmental factors including infections that activate the adaptive immune system in the presence of an active innate immune system, driven by a complex genetic background. The strongest genetic association is with human leuhocyte antigen B51 (HLA B51), and carrying HLA B5/B*51 alleles increases the risk of developing BS more than 5.8 times.[13] However, this locus is considered to explain less than 20% of the genetic predisposition to BS.[14] The epistasis with endoplasmic reticulum amino peptidase1 (ERAP1) which trims peptides that can be loaded onto major histocompatibility complex - 1 (MHC-1) and the increased risk for developing BS in individuals carrying the ERAP1-Hap10 variant is interesting.[15] It was recently suggested that ERAP1-Hap10 plays role in BS pathogenesis through generation of HLAB51-restricted peptides, causing a change in CD8 T-cell response.[16] GWAS studies additionally suggested association with non-HLA genes including interleukin (IL)10, IL12A, IL23R, FUT2, and STAT.[17] Microorganisms including streptococci and Herpes simplex virus were thought to play a role as environmental triggers through molecular mimicry.[16] It was hypothesized that the homology between microorganism and human proteins such as mycobacterial heat shock protein (HSP) 65 and human HSP 60 may cause stimulation of γδ T cells. Studies on the saliva and the gut microbiome of active BS patients showed differences from inactive BS patients, healthy and diseased controls.[18–25] Interestingly, inoculating the pathergy site with patients' own saliva increased pathergy positivity and a previous study had shown that surgical cleaning decreases the pathergy reaction.[26,27] The skin microbiome has not been studied adequately in BS, but the association of arthritis with papulopustular lesions which were infected with various bacteria including staphylococci and *Prevotella*, the increased frequency of this association in familial BS patients, and concurrence of enthesopathy suggested a reactive arthritis like mechanism in this subgroup of BS patients.[28–31] Studies of gut microbiome showed a reduction in short-chain fatty acid butyrate-producing species.[32] This was suggested to cause an increase in Th17 cells and decrease in Tregs. A butyrate-enriched diet was proposed for controlling disease activity.[33]

Thrombosis seems to be induced by inflammation in BS.[34] Neutrophil hyperactivation and neutrophil-mediated damage is thought to cause endothelial dysfunction, platelet activation, and thrombogenesis. Butyrate-rich diets were proposed to reduce reactive oxygen species production through hyperactive neutrophils which are thought to be responsible for alterations in fibrinogen structure and impaired function. Neutrophil extracellular traps (NETs) were shown to activate macrophages, induce pro-inflammatory cytokine production, activate intrinsic and extrinsic coagulation pathways, and induce thrombin production.[35,36] NETs levels were increased in patients with BS, especially in those with vascular involvement.[37]

Clinical Findings, Laboratory, and Imaging

Skin, mucosa, and joint involvement

Various mucocutaneous manifestations are the most common clinical presentation of BS (**Fig. 1**). None of the skin or mucosa lesions that patients present with are highly specific for BS by themselves, but the recurrent nature, occurrence of different types of lesions in the same patient, and the presence of organ involvement may lead to the diagnosis. Oral ulcers are seen in virtually all patients and are commonly the first manifestation. They can be present years before other findings of BS develop. Commonly, like ordinary cancer sores, they are usually multiple. Unlike herpes ulcers, these lesions are virtually always in the moist mucosal surfaces inside the mouth such as the mucosal lining of the cheeks, lips, the tongue, and the gingiva and do not occur on the outer surfaces of the lips. They are not distinguishable from ordinary oral ulcers.[38] They last around 7 days to 2 weeks and tend to recur unless treated. Only major ulcers, which are rare, leave scars.

Genital ulcers are the most specific lesions, most commonly occurring on the scrotum in men and major labia in women; shaft and the glans penis are usually spared. They are usually larger and deeper and take longer to heal than oral ulcers. These lesions tend to get infected, which potentially interferes with the healing process. About 80% of BS patients have genital ulcers. Genital ulcers tend to lead to scarring in about two-third of patients; scrotal scarring in males is quite specific.[39]

Also seen in most of the BS patients are acne-like or papulopustular lesions that are indistinguishable from acne vulgaris in appearance and pathology. They are seen both

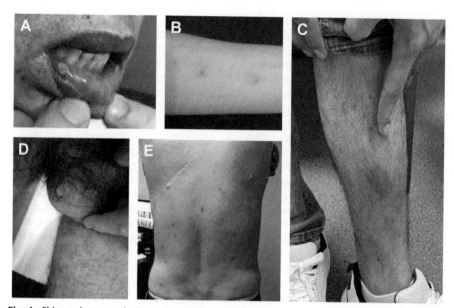

Fig. 1. Skin and mucosa lesions of Behçet syndrome: (A) oral ulcer; (B) pathergy test that resulted in papules on two of the three skin prick sites, 48 hours after the prick; (C) nodular lesion on the tibial surface, differentiating erythema npdpsum like lesions from superficial thrombophlebitis may be difficult on clinical examination and may require ultrasonographic examination; (D) genital ulcer that is already healing with a hypopigmented scar; (E) papulopustular lesions on the back of a patient with Behçet syndrome.

at the usual acne sites and uncommon sites such as lower extremities. Other skin findings are the nodular lesions which are of two types: erythema nodosum like lesions due to panniculitis and superficial vein thromboses.[40] Superficial thrombophlebitis often occurs in men and is associated with deep vein thrombosis, which should trigger workup for other vascular involvement, including pulmonary artery aneurysms.

Arthritis in BS is usually a recurrent, nondeforming, monoarthritis or oligoarthritis usually of lower extremities.[41] Polyarticular involvement of small joints is rare.

Eye involvement

Ocular involvement is one of the major manifestations of the disease and greatly helps diagnosis when present. It affects 50% to 70% of patients, showing higher frequency and increased severity in male patients.[42]

Characteristic ocular involvement is recurrent uveitis attacks with spontaneous resolution. Uveitis in BS most commonly presents with recurrent bilateral nongranulomatous panuveitis and retinal vasculitis. Anterior involvement shows a nongranulomatous pattern. It may be unilateral, bilateral, or alternating. The classic form is iridocyclitis with hypopyon. Hypopyon in Behçet's uveitis usually presents with mild ciliary injection (cold appearance) and is mobile depending on the patients' position. Even though hypopyon is a very typical anterior sign of Behçet's uveitis, it is not common after the implementation of immunomodulatory treatment. However, its presence almost always indicates a severe posterior involvement.[42]

Diffuse vitritis, retinal infiltrates, and occlusive retinal vasculitis are the common findings of posterior involvement (**Fig. 2**). Diffuse vitritis is a consequence of diffuse retinal vasculitis and its severity correlates with the activity of inflammation. In severe cases, it might prevent visualization of the fundus and cause severe visual loss. Retinal infiltrates

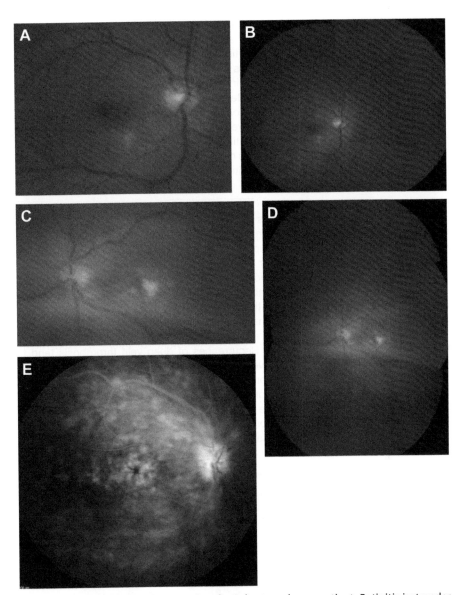

Fig. 2. (*A–D*) Color fundus photographs of a Behçet syndrome patient. Retinitis just underneath the fovea in the right eye and a huge retinitis with hemorrhage in the left eye. (*E*) Fundus fluorescein angiography showing diffuse capillary leakage with macular edema and optic nerve dyeing.

are common, affect inner retinal layers and always indicate active uveitis. They may be numerous, in any form and/or location. They quickly resolve with or without treatment.[42]

Fluorescein angiography is the gold-standard technique in detecting and monitoring retinal vascular involvement. The most common fluorescein angiographic finding in BS is diffuse "fern-like" capillary leakage.

Uveitis may be the initial manifestation in up to 20% of patients with BS or it may be the first manifestation that causes the patient to seek medical attention.[43,44] Taking a good medical history for other BS manifestations is essential. A number of ocular features strongly suggested Behçet's uveitis even in the absence of other BS features.[45] Smooth-layered hypopyon, superficial retinal infiltrate with retinal hemorrhages, and branch retinal vein occlusion with vitreous haze were recognized as features of Behçet's uveitis by majority of experts reviewing ocular photographs, blinded to patients' diagnoses. The differential diagnosis of Behçet's uveitis includes both infectious and noninfectious causes of acute non-granulomatous anterior uveitis, retinitis, and retinal vasculitis. A diagnostic algorithm was developed, which included superficial retinal infiltrates, signs of occlusive retinal vasculitis, diffuse retinal capillary leakage, and the absence of granulomatous anterior uveitis or choroiditis as predictors of Behçet's uveitis among patients who present with vitritis.[46]

Vascular involvement

Some form of vascular involvement is reported in 15% to 40% of the patients and is more frequent among men. Venous thrombosis is more common and tends to occur earlier than arterial involvement. Superficial thrombophlebitis usually presents as recurrent nodular lesions on the lower and less commonly upper extremities. Ultrasonography examination of these lesions shows venous wall inflammation with or without thrombosis. Deep vein thrombosis of the extremities shows frequent recurrences, reported in up to 45% of patients despite immunosuppressive treatment.[47] Moreover, recanalization is not optimal in around half of the patients. These factors lead to the frequent development of post-thrombotic syndrome in patients with BS that are very resistant to treatment. Recurrences of deep vein thrombosis tend to extend to larger veins including iliac veins, inferior and superior vena cavae[2] (**Fig. 3**). Inferior vena cava thrombosis with or without hepatic vein involvement may cause Budd–Chiari syndrome that has a poor prognosis in around half of the patients. Intracardiac thrombosis usually affects the right side of the heart and may accompany superior vena cava thrombosis and pulmonary artery aneurysms. Overall, different venous lesions tend to occur in the same patient and may precede arterial lesions.[2]

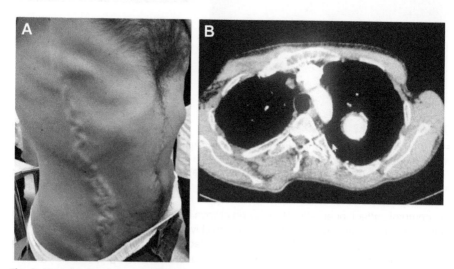

Fig. 3. Vascular involvement affects both arteries and veins. (A) Venous collaterals in a patient with inferior vena cava thrombosis. (B) Computed tomography scan of a patient with a large pulmonary artery aneurysm.

Most of the arterial lesions occur in men. Pulmonary artery aneurysms occur in up to 3% of patients, and despite this low frequency, they are an important cause of mortality due to massive hemoptysis (see **Fig. 3**). In situ thrombosis of pulmonary arteries may accompany or develop after pulmonary artery aneurysms or occur without aneurysms.[48] Pulmonary hypertension due to chronic thrombosis may result in severe right heart failure. Aneurysms may also develop in other arteries including extremity arteries, carotid and coronary arteries, and the abdominal aorta.[2]

Venous wall thickening observed with MR angiography and ultrasonography as well as thickening of the arterial wall with adjacent fibrosis and lymph node enlargement point to inflammation of the vessel wall.[49–51] The use of vein wall thickness as a diagnostic tool was proposed, but it was suggested that there may be an overestimation of diagnostic accuracy because these studies included convenient samples of patients with various inflammatory and thrombotic conditions instead of patients who are being evaluated with a suspicion of BS and that an external validation is lacking.[52] Histologic and immunological studies of the inflammation in the vessel walls may provide important findings for our understanding of BS. Systemic inflammation is also prevalent during active vascular involvement. Patients may present with fever and acute phase response. Vascular and gastrointestinal involvement should be evaluated for in BS patients with elevated acute phase reactants or fever of unknown origin.

Nervous system involvement

Patients with BS may present with different neurologic problems related either directly (primary) or indirectly (secondary) to the disease.[53] Direct neurologic involvement of BS can be classified into two: (1) parenchymal neuro-BS (p-NBS) and (2) cerebral venous sinus thrombosis (CVST).

Parenchymal NBS: The onset of a subacute brainstem syndrome in a young man, particularly of Mediterranean, Middle Eastern, or Asian origin presenting with cranial nerve findings, dysarthria, unilateral, or bilateral corticospinal tract signs with or without weakness, ataxia, and mild confusion should raise the possibility of NBS.[54] Considering that dysarthria, ataxia, and hemiparesis are the major clinical features of NBS accompanying headache in almost all cases, MRI might help clinicians to differentiate the headache occurring in NBS from the nonstructural headache of BS.[55] The most commonly affected areas in p-NBS are the mesodiencephalic junction (MDJ), pons, and medulla oblongata.[56] MDJ lesions tend to extend upward to involve the diencephalic structures and downward to involve the pontobulbar region—the most common radiological finding observed in p-NBS (**Fig. 4**). Apart from the brainstem, spinal cord involvement is also observed in p-NBS. A long-segment myelopathy occurs in most cases, mimicking neuromyelitis optica spectrum disorder (NMOSD) and myelin oligodendrocyte glycoprotein (MOG) antibody-associated disorders (MOGAD). However, the recently described "Bagel Sign" pattern of spinal cord involvement in BS may help differentiate NMOSD and MOGAD from p-NBS.[57] The "Bagel Sign" pattern is characterized by a central lesion with a hypointense core and a hyperintense rim, with or without contrast enhancement.

Cerebral venous sinus thrombosis: CVST occurs in up to 20% of BS patients with neurologic involvement. The principal clinical features of CVST, including the severe headache, papilledema, and sixth-nerve palsy on neurologic examination, are compatible with intracranial hypertension, and these clinical manifestations vary by the site and extension of venous thrombosis.[58] BS-associated CVST is associated with a better prognosis than p-NBS and is more likely to show a good prognosis in contrast to other etiologies causing CVST.[59]

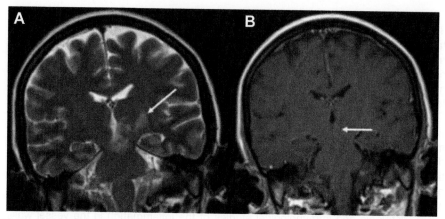

Fig. 4. Cranial MRI of a patient with brainstem syndrome. (*A*) Coronal T2W image reveals an extending lesion from the left thalamus to the mesencephalon. (*B*) Coronal T1W gd (+) image illustrates the contrast enhancement pattern in parenchymal neuro-Behçet syndrome (*arrows*). T1W, T1 weighted; T2W, T2 weighted.

Cerebrospinal fluid findings: During the acute phase of p-NBS, inflammatory changes are seen in the CSF of most cases with p-NBS, with an increased number of cells (up to ≥ 100/mL), predominantly neutrophils, and modestly elevated protein levels.[60] However, early lymphocytic pleocytosis is not unusual.[61] Also, the neutrophilic pleocytosis may later be replaced by lymphocytes. Oligoclonal band positivity is not common, seen in ≤20% of the cases.[62] BS patients with CVST do not exhibit any remarkable CSF findings except for the increased pressure.

Gastrointestinal involvement

BS patients with gastrointestinal involvement may be misdiagnosed as Crohn's disease when more specific findings such as genital ulcers or pathergy phenomenon are not present or are not recognized. Patients usually present with abdominal pain, diarrhea, weight loss, and rectal bleeding.[63] Endoscopy shows intestinal ulcers most commonly in the terminal ileum, cecum, or other parts of the colon. Small intestinal and esophageal involvement are much less common. A typical Behçet's ulcer is round or oval in shape with distinct borders, single or few in number, large and deep (**Fig. 5**). Multiple ulcers that are irregular in shape, small aphtous ulcers and

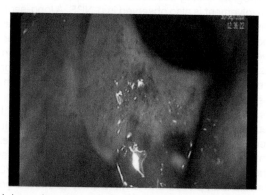

Fig. 5. A large and deep ulcer detected at the terminal ileum during colonoscopy.

multisegmental involvement of the bowel can also occur but are less frequent. Computerized tomography (CT) scans may show thickening of the bowel wall and enlarged lymph nodes around the involved area and PET scans can show inflammatory activity.[64]

Perforation, fistula formation, and major bleeding may be more common compared with other inflammatory diseases of the bowel due to the large and deep nature of the ulcers. Intestinal ulcers are one of the most refractory lesions of BS. They may persist despite aggressive treatment, even when there are no clinical signs of disease activity. In addition to clinical remission, mucosal healing should be achieved, as this is the strongest predictor of gastrointestinal relapses in BS.[65] Repeat colonoscopies used to be performed during follow-up. More recently, fecal calprotectin has been proposed as a biomarker that could predict endoscopic activity with good sensitivity and specificity.[66]

OUTCOME MEASURES

As BS involves multiple organ systems and with differing severity, it has been challenging to develop universally applicable outcome measures for disease assessment. Tools have been developed for overall disease activity levels for use in clinical trials. The Behcet's Disease Current Activity Form (BDCAF) is the most commonly used assessment tool and assesses disease activity over the last month of the period being measured.[67] BDCAF has both patient-reported and physician-reported components. It is not body system-specific and is an overall disease activity measure. Another composite index finding more use in clinical trials is the Behcet's Syndrome Activity Score, which was derived from the Multi-Dimensional Health Assessment Questionnaire as a model for patient-reported outcome measure collection tool. The questionnaire asks about various symptoms over the previous month before the clinic visit and is completed by the patient at the time of visit. It has been shown to be strongly correlated with the BDCAF and less so with quality of life assessments.[68]

Other disease manifestation-specific measures are available, such as the Composite Index for Oral Ulcer Activity,[69] Genital Ulcer Severity Score,[70] and Disease Activity Index for Intestinal Behcet's Disease,[71] to name a few, which focus on one specific aspect of BS involvement. For the assessment of quality of life, the Behçet's Disease Quality of Life Index, a Behçet-specific instrument is available and has been used in many clinical trials.[72]

MANAGEMENT

Management of BS should be planned by a multidisciplinary team according to the organs that are involved, activity and severity of organ involvement, prognostic factors such as disease duration, age, and sex, and patients' preferences. Treatment response to each drug may be different for different types of organ involvement (**Fig. 6**). Patients should be followed carefully, as they may develop organ involvement over time, even if they have only mucocutaneous disease during the first few years.[8]

Skin, Mucosa, and Joint Involvement

Management of mucocutaneous involvement in BS is determined by the extent of involvement and the presence or absence of more serious organ involvement such as eye or gastrointestinal disease. If there is no systemic organ involvement, topical steroids can be tried for oral and genital ulcers. If these do not help, colchicine is the usually preferred first agent.[6]

	Skin and mucosa	Arthritis	Uveitis	Vascular involvement	CNS invovlement	Gastrointest involvement
Colchicine						
Apremilast						
Azathioprine						
Cyclosporine-A						
Cyclophosphamide						
Interferon-alpha						
TNF inhibitors						
IL-1 inhibitors			ANA CAN / GEV			
IL-6 inhibitor						
IL-17 inhibitor						
IL-23 inhibitor						

	Effective based on RCTs		Contraversial / inconclusive data
	Beneficial based on non-randomized data		Reported to cause relapses
	Not effective		Not evaluated

Fig. 6. Evidence on treatment modalities for different types of organ/system involvement in Behçet syndrome. ANA, Anakinra; CAN, Canakinumab; GEV, Gevokizumab; RCT, Randomized controlled trial.

If an adequate trial of colchicine does not provide benefit, apremilast is a good option.[73] Apremilast has been shown to control oral ulcers in BS clinical trials and potentially help with genital ulcers, skin lesions, and arthritis in clinical experience from patient registries and uncontrolled studies. For patients who continue to have significant symptoms of mucocutaneous manifestations, azathioprine, and biologic agents can be considered, either alone or in combination. Low-dose glucocorticoids can be used as needed for flares of lesions.

Non-steroidal antiinflammatory drugs (NSAIDs) and colchicine are usually enough to control arthralgia and arthritis; however, some patients may require more potent treatments. Most patients are able to stop their drugs in 2 to 5 years as the natural history of BS is one of undulating activity that gets milder over time.[74]

Eye Involvement

The aim of treatment in Behçet's uveitis is to suppress active inflammation and prevent recurrent attacks. Because of the recurrent course of the disease and risk of visual loss in each attack and/or cumulative tissue damage, Behçet's uveitis should be treated with immunosuppressives.

Systemic corticosteroids cannot be used as monotherapy and should only be applied as an adjunctive treatment during active inflammation, along with immunosuppressives. After active disease is controlled, corticosteroids should be tapered slowly to a dose of ≤10 mg/d within 3 months. The effectiveness of azathioprine and cyclosporine-A in Behçet's uveitis have been shown in controlled trials, and these have been successfully used in the majority of cases before the biologic era.[75,76] According to the European League Against Rheumatism (EULAR) 2018 recommendations, conventional therapies may still be a choice in mild cases, but if the inflammation is severe and there is a risk for visual loss, especially in high-risk patients such as young males, biologic therapies should be used as first line. Biologic agents, including interferon-alpha and tumor necrosis factor (TNF) inhibitors, are effective and safe in most of the resistant cases. Tuberculosis screening should be conducted before the administration of TNF inhibitors and latent tuberculosis should be treated, if detected. IL-6 and IL-1 inhibitors may be alternatives in patients who are refractory to TNF inhibitors.[77–79]

Fundus fluorescein angiography should be performed to assess the efficacy of treatment and when making treatment decisions. It should be repeated regularly at 3 to 6 month intervals depending on the severity of involvement after complete control of the inflammation.

There is no consensus about the frequency of follow-up visits and treatment cessation in patients with uveitis. Frequency of follow-up and treatment modalities should be individualized according to anatomic involvement, severity of inflammation, and presence of macula, and/or optic nerve involvement. Treatment cessation can be tried after a sustained period of complete remission with close monitoring.

Vascular Involvement

Treatment with high-dose glucocorticoids and immunosuppressives should be started immediately in BS patients with arterial aneurysms due to the risk of rupture and fatal bleeding. Methylprednisolone pulses followed by prednisolone 1 mg/kg in addition to cyclophosphamide have been the traditional induction regimen. Prednisolone is gradually tapered over 6 to 12 months. Cyclophosphamide use may be limited to 6 months to avoid long-term adverse events. Azathioprine may be used for maintenance after remission. Deciding whether remission has been obtained may not be easy as aneurysms do not completely resolve on imaging in around 40% of the patients, the role of PET scan in monitoring inflammation of the vessel wall is not clear in BS, acute phase reactants may be elevated due to other causes, and hemoptysis may occur due to enlargement of bronchial arteries in patients with pulmonary artery thrombosis. Monoclonal TNF inhibitors have been used with success as induction treatment in refractory patients and maintenance treatment instead of azathioprine in high-risk patients such as those with previous relapses or life-threatening aneurysms. The outcome of surgical interventions has been poor in pulmonary aneurysms.[80] On the other hand, peripheral artery and aortic aneurysms may require surgical or endovascular interventions such as graft insertion, ligation, or bypass.[80] Glucocorticoid (GC) and immunosuppressive treatment, ideally started before the intervention, is important to reduce the risk of anastomotic leakage, pseudoaneurysms, or occlusions.[80] Synthetic grafts should be preferred to venous grafts that carry a higher risk of occlusion.

A similar treatment protocol with high-dose GCs, cyclophosphamide, and/or TNF inhibitors may be preferred in patients with organ-threatening venous thrombosis such as inferior or superior vena cava thrombosis, hepatic vein thrombosis causing Budd–Chiari syndrome, or intracardiac thrombosis.[6] Patients with refractory CVST who carry risk of visual loss due to optic nerve compression should also be treated aggressively, with interventions such as lumboperitoneal shunts if necessary. Initial treatment choice for deep vein thrombosis of the lower extremities may be azathioprine together with short-term moderate-dose GCs. However, relapses and lack of good recanalization have been observed in almost half of the patients treated with azathioprine.[47] Interferon-alpha and TNF inhibitors may be preferred in such patients. Anticoagulant treatment did not seem effective for preventing relapses or post-thrombotic syndrome in retrospective studies.[80] Prospective data are needed regarding the benefit and if there is any, the optimal duration and type of anticoagulant therapy. In patients that have already developed post-thrombotic syndrome, stockings may help to decrease pain and swelling and reduce the risk of leg ulcers.

Nervous System Involvement

The first goal of treatment in NBS is to suppress the acute episode and to shorten the recovery time with minimal irreversible disability. The second goal is to prevent further attacks. High-dose intravenous methylprednisolone pulses for 5 to 10 days, followed by slow oral tapering, are the first choice for treating acute episodes.[81] The preferred dose and duration of GC treatment vary among centers. Colchicine, azathioprine, cyclophosphamide, methotrexate, chlorambucil, thalidomide, interferon alpha, TNF inhibitors, and IL-6 blockers are among the drugs used for the treatment of the systemic features of BS, which have been tried for central nervous system (CNS) involvement as well.[82]

Azathioprine is preferred as the first-line drug in many centers, as also suggested by 2018 updated EULAR recommendations.[6] We tend to start infliximab in patients in whom azathioprine fails and as first-line therapy in patients who present with a severe acute attack of p-NBS with poor prognostic factors.[83] Cyclophosphamide in addition to steroid treatment was not superior to steroids alone in a retrospective study.[82] Given that cyclosporine-A use is associated with increased risk of neurologic involvement, it should be avoided in patients who have NBS and immediately stopped in patients developing NBS under cyclosporine-A.[84]

Gastrointestinal Involvement

The choice of treatment depends on the extent and size of intestinal ulcers and severity of clinical manifestations. Patients with small aphthous ulcers and mild symptoms may be treated with 5-ASA, whereas patients with larger ulcers, moderate to severe symptoms, and those who are refractory to 5-ASA treatment are prescribed azathioprine. Monoclonal TNF inhibitors are preferred in refractory patients who have persistent diarrhea and bleeding and those who carry a high risk of perforation. Adding thalidomide may be beneficial when remission cannot be obtained with TNF inhibitors.[85]

An interesting association is between myelodysplastic syndrome and gastrointestinal involvement of BS.[86] Gastrointestinal involvement is quite severe and refractory to immunosuppressives in these patients, whereas bone marrow transplantation or other treatment modalities targeting myelodysplastic syndrome may alleviate BS manifestations.[87,88]

FUTURE PERSPECTIVES

A treat-to-target approach is desirable in BS, but a single-standard treat-to-target strategy applicable to all patients may not be possible due to heterogeneity of manifestations and disease course. The recurrent course impairs quality of life in patients with only mucocutaneous involvement, whereas it causes damage and disability in patients with organ involvement. Research is needed to identify the best targets that predict a good long-term outcome for each organ, compare step-up versus step-down treatment for major organ involvement, determine predictors of refractoriness to conventional modalities, and develop a feasible approach for treatment cessation once sustained remission is achieved.

CLINICS CARE POINTS

- The choice of treatment modalities differs according to severity and activity of each organ involvement as well as prognostic factors including age, sex, and disease duration.

- Management of mucosal, skin, and musculoskeletal manifestations is determined by patients' preferences. To prevent new lesions colchicine, apremilast, azathioprine, or biologic agents may be used depending on disease severity. Topical agents and short-term, low-dose glucocorticoids may be used for active lesions.

- First-line treatment with TNF inhibitors may be preferred in patients with severe disease such as sight-threatening uveitis, severe parenchymal nervous system involvement, arterial aneurysms, major venous thrombosis, and intestinal ulcers carrying a high risk of perforation. In addition, high-dose glucocorticoids may be used for rapidly suppressing disease flares and tapered over 3 to 6 months.

- A step-up strategy starting with conventional immunosuppressives such as azathioprine may be used in patients with mild-to-moderate organ involvement.

- Long-term maintenance treatment with immunosuppressives is required to prevent relapses or organ involvement.

DISCLOSURE

G. Hatemi has received grant/research support from Celgene, United States, Amgen and Silk Road Therapeutics and has served as a speaker for AbbVie, Boehringer Ingelheim, Novartis, and UCB Pharma. D. Ucar has received honoraria from AbbVie. U. Uygunoğlu has received advisory board honorariums and speaker fees from F Hoffmann La-Roche, Bayer, Merck-Serono, Novartis, Teva, and Biogen Idec/Gen Pharma of Turkey. H. Yazici has no financial disclosures. Y. Yazici has served as a consultant for Amgen, Bristol Myers Squibb, Celgene, Genentech, and Sanofi.

REFERENCES

1. Yazici Y, Hatemi G, Bodaghi B, et al. Behçet syndrome. Nat Rev Dis Primers 2021;7(1):67.
2. Tascilar K, Melikoglu M, Ugurlu S, et al. Vascular involvement in Behçet's syndrome: a retrospective analysis of associations and the time course. Rheumatology 2014;53(11):2018–22.
3. Ozguler Y, Merkel PA, Gurcan M, et al. Patients' experiences with Behçet's syndrome: structured interviews among patients with different types of organ involvement. Clin Exp Rheumatol 2019;37(Suppl 121):28–34.
4. Criteria for diagnosis of Behçet's disease. International Study Group for Behçet's Disease. Lancet 1990;335(8697):1078–80.
5. Davatchi F, Assaad-Khalil S, Calamia KT, et al. The International Criteria for Behcet's Disease (ICBD): a collaborative study of 27 countries on the sensitivity and specificity of the new criteria. J Eur Acad Dermatol Venereol 2014;28:338–47.
6. Hatemi G, Christensen R, Bang D, et al. 2018 update of the EULAR recommendations for the management of Behçet's syndrome. Ann Rheum Dis 2018;77(6): 808–18.
7. Yazici H, Tüzün Y, Pazarli H, et al. Influence of age of onset and patient's sex on the prevalence and severity of manifestations of Behçet's syndrome. Ann Rheum Dis 1984;43(6):783–9.
8. Hamuryudan V, Hatemi G, Tascilar K, et al. Prognosis of Behcet's syndrome among men with mucocutaneous involvement at disease onset: long-term outcome of patients enrolled in a controlled trial. Rheumatology 2010;49(1): 173–7.
9. Yurdakul S, Gunaydin I, Tuzun Y, et al. The prevalence of Behcet's syndrome in a rural area in northern Turkey. J Rheumatol 1988;15:820–2.

10. Kural-Seyahi E, Fresko I, Seyahi N, et al. The long-term mortality and morbidity of Behcet's syndrome: a 2-decade outcome survey of 387 patients followed at a dedicated center. Medicine (Baltim) 2003;82:60–76.

11. Yurdakul S, Tuzuner N, Yurdakul I, et al. Gastrointestinal involvement in Behcet's syndrome: a controlled study. Ann Rheum Dis 1996;55:208–10.

12. Yazici Y, Adler NM. Clinical manifestations and ethnic background of patients with Behcet's syndrome in a US cohort. Arthritis Rheum 2007;56(suppl):S502.

13. de Menthon M, Lavalley MP, Maldini C, et al. HLA-B51/B5 and the risk of Behçet's disease: a systematic review and meta-analysis of case-control genetic association studies. Arthritis Rheum 2009;61(10):1287–96.

14. Gül A, Hajeer AH, Worthington J, et al. Evidence for linkage of the HLA-B locus in Behçet's disease, obtained using the transmission disequilibrium test. Arthritis Rheum 2001;44(1):239–40.

15. Kirino Y, Bertsias G, Ishigatsubo Y, et al. Genome-wide association analysis identifies new susceptibility loci for Behçet's disease and epistasis between HLA-B*51 and ERAP1. Nat Genet 2013;45(2):202–7.

16. Cavers A, Kugler MC, Ozguler Y, et al. Behçet's disease risk-variant HLA-B51/ERAP1-Hap10 alters human CD8 T cell immunity. Ann Rheum Dis 2022;81(11):1603–11.

17. Gül A. Genetics of Behçet's disease: lessons learned from genomewide association studies. Curr Opin Rheumatol 2014;26(1):56–63.

18. Hatemi G, Yazici H. Behçet's syndrome and micro-organisms. Best Pract Res Clin Rheumatol 2011;25(3):389–406.

19. Seoudi N, Bergmeier LA, Drobniewski F, et al. The oral mucosal and salivary microbial community of Behçet's syndrome and recurrent aphthous stomatitis. J Oral Microbiol 2015;7:27150.

20. Shimizu J, Kubota T, Takada E, et al. Bifidobacteria Abundance-Featured Gut Microbiota Compositional Change in Patients with Behcet's Disease. PLoS One 2016;11(4):e0153746.

21. Coit P, Mumcu G, Ture-Ozdemir F, et al. Sequencing of 16S rRNA reveals a distinct salivary microbiome signature in Behçet's disease. Clin Immunol 2016;169:28–35.

22. Ye Z, Zhang N, Wu C, et al. A metagenomic study of the gut microbiome in Behcet's disease. Microbiome 2018;6(1):135.

23. van der Houwen TB, van Laar JAM, Kappen JH, et al. Behçet's Disease Under Microbiotic Surveillance? A Combined Analysis of Two Cohorts of Behçet's Disease Patients. Front Immunol 2020;11:1192.

24. Yasar Bilge NS, Pérez Brocal V, Kasifoglu T, et al. Intestinal microbiota composition of patients with Behçet's disease: differences between eye, mucocutaneous and vascular involvement. The Rheuma-BIOTA study. Clin Exp Rheumatol 2020;38(Suppl 127):60–8.

25. Tecer D, Gogus F, Kalkanci A, et al. Succinivibrionaceae is dominant family in fecal microbiota of Behçet's Syndrome patients with uveitis. PLoS One 2020;15(10):e0241691.

26. Kaneko F, Togashi A, Nomura E, et al. A New Diagnostic Way for Behcet's Disease: Skin Prick with Self-Saliva. Genet Res Int 2014;2014:581468.

27. Fresko I, Yazici H, Bayramiçli M, et al. Effect of surgical cleaning of the skin on the pathergy phenomenon in Behçet's syndrome. Ann Rheum Dis 1993;52(8):619–20.

28. Tunc R, Keyman E, Melikoglu M, et al. Target organ associations in Turkish patients with Behçet's disease: a cross sectional study by exploratory factor analysis. J Rheumatol 2002;29(11):2393–6.
29. Hatemi G, Bahar H, Uysal S, et al. The pustular skin lesions in Behcet's syndrome are not sterile. Ann Rheum Dis 2004;63(11):1450–2.
30. Karaca M, Hatemi G, Sut N, et al. The papulopustular lesion/arthritis cluster of Behçet's syndrome also clusters in families. Rheumatology 2012;51(6):1053–60.
31. Hatemi G, Fresko I, Tascilar K, et al. Increased enthesopathy among Behçet's syndrome patients with acne and arthritis: an ultrasonography study. Arthritis Rheum 2008;58(5):1539–45.
32. Consolandi C, Turroni S, Emmi G, et al. Behçet's syndrome patients exhibit specific microbiome signature. Autoimmun Rev 2015;14:269–76.
33. Emmi G, Bettiol A, Niccolai E, et al. Butyrate-Rich Diets Improve Redox Status and Fibrin Lysis in Behçet's Syndrome. Circ Res 2021;128(2):278–80.
34. Emmi G, Becatti M, Bettiol A, et al. Behçet's Syndrome as a Model of Thrombo-Inflammation: The Role of Neutrophils. Front Immunol 2019;10:1085.
35. Li L, Yu X, Liu J, et al. Neutrophil Extracellular Traps Promote Aberrant Macrophages Activation in Behçet's Disease. Front Immunol 2021;11:590622.
36. Folco EJ, Mawson TL, Vromman A, et al. Neutrophil Extracellular Traps Induce Endothelial Cell Activation and Tissue Factor Production Through Interleukin-1α and Cathepsin G. Arterioscler Thromb Vasc Biol 2018;38(8):1901–12.
37. Le Joncour A, Martos R, Loyau S, et al. Critical role of neutrophil extracellular traps (NETs) in patients with Behcet's disease. Ann Rheum Dis 2019;78(9):1274–82.
38. Main DM, Chamberlain MA. Clinical differentiation of oral ulceration in Behçet's disease. Br J Rheumatol 1992;31:767–70.
39. Mat MC, Goksugur N, Engin B, et al. The frequency of scarring after genital ulcers in Behçet's syndrome: a prospective study. Int J Dermatol 2006;45:554–6.
40. Demirkesen C, Tuzuner N, Mat C, et al. Clinicopathologic evaluation of nodular cutaneous lesions of Behçet syndrome. Am J Clin Pathol 2001;116:341–6.
41. Fatemi A, Shahram F, Akhlaghi M, et al. Prospective study of articular manifestations in Behçet's disease: five-year report. Int J Rheum Dis 2017;20:97–102.
42. Ozyazgan Y, Ucar D, Hatemi G, et al. Ocular Involvement of Behçet's Syndrome: a Comprehensive Review. Clin Rev Allergy Immunol 2015;49(3):298–306.
43. Mishima S, Masuda K, Izawa Y, et al. The eighth Frederick H. Verhoeff Lecture, presented by Saiichi Mishima, MD. Behcet's disease in Japan: ophthalmologic aspects. Trans Am Ophthalmol Soc 1979;77:225–79.
44. Deuter CM, Kotter I, Wallace GR, et al. Behcet's disease: ocular effects and treatment. Prog Retin Eye Res 2008;27:111–36.
45. Tugal-Tutkun I, Onal S, Ozyazgan Y, et al. Validity and agreement of uveitis experts in interpretation of ocular photographs for diagnosis of Behçet uveitis. Ocul Immunol Inflamm 2014;22(6):461–8.
46. Tugal-Tutkun I, Onal S, Stanford M, et al. An Algorithm for the Diagnosis of Behçet Disease Uveitis in Adults. Ocul Immunol Inflamm 2021;29(6):1154–63.
47. Ozguler Y, Hatemi G, Cetinkaya F, et al. Clinical course of acute deep vein thrombosis of the legs in Behçet's syndrome. Rheumatology 2020;59(4):799–806.
48. Seyahi E, Melikoglu M, Akman C, et al. Pulmonary artery involvement and associated lung disease in Behçet disease: a series of 47 patients. Medicine (Baltim) 2012;91(1):35–48.

49. Ambrose N, Pierce IT, Gatehouse PD, et al. Magnetic resonance imaging of vein wall thickness in patients with Behçet's syndrome. Clin Exp Rheumatol 2014;32(4 Suppl 84):S99–102.

50. Alibaz-Oner F, Ergelen R, Mutis A, et al. Venous vessel wall thickness in lower extremity is increased in male patients with Behcet's disease. Clin Rheumatol 2019; 38(5):1447–51.

51. Seyahi E, Gjoni M, Durmaz EŞ, et al. Increased vein wall thickness in Behçet disease. J Vasc Surg Venous Lymphat Disord 2019;7(5):677–84.e2.

52. Aita T, Matsuo Y, Yamada Y, et al. Comment on: Femoral vein wall thickness measurement: A new diagnostic tool for Behçet's disease. Rheumatology 2021;60(9): e342–3.

53. Siva A, Saip S. The spectrum of nervous system involvement in Behçet's syndrome and its differential diagnosis. J Neurol 2009;256(4):513–29.

54. Uygunoglu U, Siva A. An uncommon disease included commonly in the differential diagnosis of neurological diseases: Neuro-Behçet's syndrome. J Neurol Sci 2021;426:117436.

55. Saip S, Siva A, Altintas A, et al. Headache in Behcet's syndrome. Headache 2005;45:911–9.

56. Kocer N, Islak C, Siva A, et al. CNS involvement in neuro-Behçet's syndrome: an MR study. Am J Neuroradiol 1999;20:1015–24.

57. Uygunoglu U, Zeydan B, Ozguler Y, et al. Myelopathy in Behçet's disease: The Bagel Sign. Ann Neurol 2017;82(2):288–98.

58. Yesilot N, Bahar S, Yilmazer S, et al. Cerebral venous thrombosis in Behçet's disease compared to those associated with other etiologies. J Neurol 2009;256(7): 1134–42.

59. Uluduz D, Midi I, Duman T, et al. Behçet's disease as a causative factor of cerebral venous sinus thrombosis: subgroup analysis of data from the VENOST study. Rheumatology 2019;58(4):600–8.

60. Borhani Haghighi A, Ittehadi H, Nikseresht AR, et al. CSF levels of cytokines in neuro-Behçet's disease. Clin Neurol Neurosurg 2009;111(6):507–10.

61. Sahin Eroglu D, Torgutalp M, Yucesan C, et al. Prognostic factors for relapse and poor outcome in neuro-Behçet's syndrome: results from a clinical long-term follow-up of a single centre. J Neurol 2022;269(4):2046–54.

62. Saruhan-Direskeneli G, Yentur SP, Mutlu M, et al. Intrathecal oligoclonal IgG bands are infrequently found in neuro-Behçet's disease. Clin Exp Rheumatol 2013;31(3 Suppl 77):25–7.

63. Hatemi I, Esatoglu SN, Hatemi G, et al. Characteristics, Treatment, and Long-Term Outcome of Gastrointestinal Involvement in Behcet's Syndrome: A Strobe-Compliant Observational Study From a Dedicated Multidisciplinary Center. Medicine (Baltim) 2016;95(16):e3348.

64. İnce B, Kibar A, Asa S, et al. 18F-Fluorodeoxyglucose Positron Emission Tomography/Magnetic Resonance Imaging Appearance of Gastrointestinal Behcet's Disease. Mol Imaging Radionucl Ther 2022;31(1):57–9.

65. Gong L, Zhang YL, Sun LX, et al. Mucosal healing in intestinal Behçet's disease: A systematic review and meta-analysis. J Dig Dis 2021;22(2):83–90.

66. Esatoglu SN, Hatemi I, Ozguler Y, et al. Faecal but not serum calprotectin levels look promising in predicting active disease in Behçet's syndrome patients with gastrointestinal involvement. Clin Exp Rheumatol 2018;36(6 Suppl 115):90–6.

67. Lawton G, Bhakta BB, Chamberlain MA, et al. The Behçet's disease activity index. Rheumatology 2004;43:73–8.

68. Forbess C, Swearingen C, Yazici Y. Behçet's Syndrome Activity Score (BSAS): a new disease activity assessment tool, composed of patient-derived measures only, is strongly correlated with The Behçet's Disease Current Activity Form (BDCAF). Ann Rheum Dis 2008;67(SII):360.
69. Mumcu G, Inanc N, Taze A, et al. A new Mucocutaneous Activity Index for Behcet's disease. Clin Exp Rheumatol 2014;32(4 Suppl 84):S80–6.
70. Senusi A, Seoudi N, Bergmeier LA, et al. Genital ulcer severity score and genital health quality of life in Behçet's disease. Orphanet J Rare Dis 2015;10:117.
71. Cheon JH, Han DS, Park JY, et al. Development, validation, and responsiveness of a novel disease activity index for intestinal Behcet's disease. Inflamm Bowel Dis 2011;17:605–13.
72. Gilworth G, Chamberlain MA, Bhakta B, et al. Development of the BD-QoL: a quality of life measure specific to Behçet's disease. J Rheumatol 2004;31:931–7.
73. Hatemi G, Mahr A, Ishigatsubo Y, et al. Trial of Apremilast for Oral Ulcers in Behçet's Syndrome. N Engl J Med 2019;381:1918–28.
74. Kural-Seyahi E, Fresko I, Seyahi N, et al. The long-term mortality and morbidity of Behçet syndrome: a 2-decade outcome survey of 387 patients followed at a dedicated center. Medicine (Baltim) 2003;82:60–76.
75. Yazici H, Pazarli H, Barnes CG, et al. A controlled trial of azathioprine in Behçet's syndrome. N Engl J Med 1990;322:281–5.
76. Ozyazgan Y, Yurdakul S, Yazici H, et al. Low dose cyclosporin A versus pulsed cyclophosphamide in Behçet's syndrome: A single masked trial. Br J Ophthalmol 1992;76:241–3.
77. Ugurlu S, Ucar D, Seyahi E, et al. Canakinumab in a patient with juvenile Behçet's syndrome with refractory eye disease. Ann Rheum Dis 2012;71(9):1589–91.
78. Bettiol A, Silvestri E, Di Scala G, et al. The right place of interleukin-1 inhibitors in the treatment of Behçet's syndrome: a systematic review. Rheumatol Int 2019; 39(6):971–90.
79. Eser Ozturk H, Oray M, Tugal-Tutkun I. Tocilizumab for the Treatment of Behçet Uveitis that Failed Interferon Alpha and Anti-Tumor Necrosis Factor-Alpha Therapy. Ocul Immunol Inflamm 2018;26(7):1005–14.
80. Ozguler Y, Leccese P, Christensen R, et al. Management of major organ involvement of Behçet's syndrome: a systematic review for update of the EULAR recommendations. Rheumatology 2018;57(12):2200–12.
81. Uygunoğlu U, Siva A. Behçet's Syndrome and Nervous System Involvement. Curr Neurol Neurosci Rep 2018;18(7):35.
82. Yoon DL, Kim YJ, Koo BS, et al. Neuro-behçet's disease in South Korea: clinical characteristics and treatment response. Int J Rheum Dis 2014;17(4):453–8.
83. Zeydan B, Uygunoglu U, Saip S, et al. Infliximab is a plausible alternative for neurologic complications of Behçet disease. Neurol Neuroimmunol Neuroinflamm 2016;3(5):e258.
84. Patocka J, Nepovimova E, Kuca K, et al. Cyclosporine A: Chemistry and Toxicity - A Review. Curr Med Chem 2021;28(20):3925–34.
85. Hatemi I, Hatemi G, Pamuk ON, et al. TNF-alpha antagonists and thalidomide for the management of gastrointestinal Behçet's syndrome refractory to the conventional treatment modalities: a case series and review of the literature. Clin Exp Rheumatol 2015;33(6 Suppl 94):S129–37.
86. Esatoglu SN, Hatemi G, Salihoglu A, et al. A reappraisal of the association between Behçet's disease, myelodysplastic syndrome and the presence of trisomy 8: a systematic literature review. Clin Exp Rheumatol 2015;33(6 Suppl 94): S145–51.

87. Soysal T, Salihoğlu A, Esatoğlu SN, et al. Bone marrow transplantation for Behçet's disease: a case report and systematic review of the literature. Rheumatology 2014;53(6):1136–41.
88. Yilmaz U, Ar MC, Esatoglu SN, et al. How to treat myelodysplastic syndrome with clinical features resembling Behçet syndrome: a case-based systematic review. Ann Hematol 2020;99(6):1193–203.

Central Nervous System Vasculitis

Primary Angiitis of the Central Nervous System and Central Nervous System Manifestations of Systemic Vasculitis

Moein Amin, MD[a], Ken Uchino, MD[b], Rula A. Hajj-Ali, MD[c],*

KEYWORDS

• PACNS • CNSV • Vasculitis • ABRA

KEY POINTS

- Central nervous system vasculitis (CNSV) is a broad group of disorders affecting central nervous system (CNS) vasculature with variable clinical presentation.
- CNSV can be divided into primary angiitis of CNS (PACNS) and secondary CNSV depending on the etiology and presence of extra-CNS involvement.
- Diagnosis of CNSV requires thorough evaluation for mimickers and commonly used testing includes serum and CSF laboratory testing, MRI, vessel imaging, and histopathological evaluation.
- Testing and evaluation of CNSV should be interpreted cautiously due to imperfect sensitivity and specificity of available testing and diagnostic criteria.

INTRODUCTION

Central nervous system vasculitis (CNSV) describes a broad category of disorders which result in intramural inflammation affecting the vasculature within the central nervous system (CNS) including the brain, spinal cord, and the meninges. In addition to categorizing the disease based on the size of the affected vessels or histopathological features, one of the most useful categorizations of CNSV is typically based on the underlying etiology.

[a] Mellen Center for Multiple Sclerosis Treatment and Research, Neurological Institute, Cleveland Clinic, Cleveland, OH, USA; [b] Cerebrovascular Center, Cleveland Clinic, Cleveland, OH, USA; [c] Cleveland Clinic Center for Vasculitis Care and Research, Cleveland Clinic, 9500 Euclid Avenue, A50, Cleveland, OH 44195, USA
* Corresponding author.
E-mail address: HAJJALR@ccf.org

Rheum Dis Clin N Am 49 (2023) 603–616
https://doi.org/10.1016/j.rdc.2023.03.011
0889-857X/23/© 2023 Elsevier Inc. All rights reserved.

rheumatic.theclinics.com

1. Primary angiitis of the central nervous system (PACNS): If vasculopathy is limited to the CNS without evidence of systemic disease.
2. Secondary CNSV: If CNS vasculopathy occurs as part of a systemic disease.

Despite being described as early as the 1950s,[1,2] the diagnosis of CNSV remains challenging due to the broad spectrum of clinical features associated with this disorder and limitations in available diagnostic modalities.

PRIMARY ANGIITIS OF THE CENTRAL NERVOUS SYSTEM
Epidemiology and Pathophysiology

Unfortunately, there is paucity of epidemiological data on the incidence and prevalence of PACNS. It is thought to be a rare disorder and its annual incidence rate is estimated to be around 2.4 cases per one million person-years with a peak incidence around the age of 50 years and a male sex predominance.[3]

The pathophysiology of this disorder remains elusive and is an area of active research possibly owing to its heterogeneous presentation. In histopathological studies, there have been three distinct common patterns of intramural pathology identified.[4]

1. Granulomatous inflammation: angiocentric infiltration of mononuclear, granulomatous, and multinucleated giant cells
2. Lymphocytic inflammation: predominantly B cell infiltration
3. Acute necrotizing: acute neutrophilic inflammation

The intramural inflammation results in damage to the vasculature and endothelial damage leading to narrowing, occlusion, or thrombosis in these vessels. Subsequently, there is CNS ischemia and injury in these affected territories which leads to the clinical findings in PACNS.

The underlying pathophysiology of PACNS is likely multifactorial and includes a combination of genetic, immunological, and environmental factors. Various immunological pathways have been implicated in the development and pathogenesis of PACNS including the significant role of expanded intrathecal Please provide the full form of cluster of differentiation 4 (CD4)+ T cells,[5] natural killer cells (NK-cells), increased interleukin-17 (IL-17), plasma cells,[6] and complements.[7] Studies evaluating the role of genetic susceptibility in the development of PACNS have shown possible involvement of certain human leukocyte antigens (HLA) haplotypes suggesting a possible genetic predisposition.[8] Furthermore, a distinct group of patients appear to develop this granulomatous inflammation in response to the deposition of amyloid beta (Aβ) peptide in the media and adventitia of CNS vessels and are referred to as Aβ-related angiitis (ABRA). Infectious (eg, human immunodeficiency virus) and systemic diseases (eg, common variable immunodeficiency) have also been associated with the development of PACNS possibly owing to their effect on the modulation of the immune system.[9]

Clinical Presentation

The clinical presenting features in PACNS are varied but most commonly include subacute onset of headache, cognitive impairment, seizures, and focal neurological deficits.[10–13] Due to the insidious nature of the symptoms, the diagnosis is often delayed[3] and a high index of suspicion is needed to consider and evaluate for this condition in the acute setting. Patients with ABRA pathology may share some clinical features with patients suffering from Alzheimer's dementia or cerebral amyloid angiopathy due to presence of common pathological Aβ protein. Although those with ABRA are usually younger than patients with Alzheimer's disease (median age of 66 years vs 71 years).[14] Less commonly, a subset of PACNS patients could have a tumor-like presentation with more acute onset of symptoms related to the mass effect.[15] Spinal cord involvement in PACNS is relatively rare (approximately 5% of cases) and most commonly affects the thoracic spine presenting with myelopathy.[10] Some of the less common presenting features include cranial neuropathies, new-onset refractory epilepsy, and anterior visual pathway involvement.[10,16,17]

PACNS should be suspected in patients with typical clinical features including multiple CNS ischemic events in different vascular territories and vasculopathy without traditional cardiovascular risk factors. In 1988, the diagnostic criteria for PACNS were set which require the presence of all of the following three criteria:[18]

1. An acquired, otherwise unexplained neurological deficit
2. Evidence of either classic angiographic or histopathologic features of angiitis within the CNS
3. No evidence of systemic vasculitis or any other condition that could elicit the angiographic or pathologic findings

Evaluation

On history and exam, presence of constitutional symptoms, peripheral nervous system involvement, or systemic inflammation argue against PACNS and alternative etiologies such as systemic infectious or inflammatory disorders should be considered.[19] Further serological testing such as antinuclear antibody panel, antineutrophil cytoplasmic antibodies (ANCA), Lyme disease serology, Syphilis testing, human immunodeficiency virus (HIV) serology, and others as clinically indicated and depending on individual risk factors, exposure, and review of symptoms should be used to exclude infectious, inflammatory, or infiltrative, causes in the appropriate setting.

Cerebrospinal fluid (CSF) analysis is an important part of the evaluation as inflammation in the CSF is one of the main features of PACNS and abnormalities are seen in the majority of patients (80%–90% based on diagnostic methods).[3,20] Currently, there are no established biomarkers in the CSF and non-specific findings such as pleocytosis (median white blood cell count 16–18 cells/mL) and mildly elevated protein (median 80–98 mg/dL) support PACNS. CSF analysis is also used for excluding alternative etiologies such as infectious causes through more advanced technologies such as metagenomic next-generation sequencing.[21]

The imaging modality of choice in PACNS is MRI which is almost always abnormal in PACNS (90%–100%).[3,11,20] Most common abnormalities include white and gray matter ischemic changes, parenchymal and leptomeningeal enhancement, micro- and macro-parenchymal hemorrhages, and brain atrophy (**Fig. 1**).

Dedicated imaging of the CNS vasculature should be obtained. PACNS is thought to have involvement of large-/medium-sized cerebral vessels (including internal carotid and proximal and second divisions of cerebral arteries) or small-sized vessels (including distal branched cerebral arteries).[22] Cerebrovascular imaging such as conventional cerebral angiogram, computer tomography angiography (CTA), or magnetic resonance angiography (MRA) is used to evaluate small to large-/medium-sized vessel involvement (**Fig. 2**). Alternating stenosis and dilatation (beading) have been reported, but irregular notched appearance might be more common.[23] Small-vessel and posterior circulation involvement could be better evaluated using conventional cerebral angiogram which has an overall sensitivity of 40% to 90% in PACNS.[24] Given the limited sensitivity of cerebral vascular imaging for small-vessel involvement, a

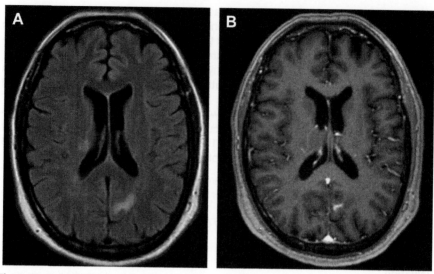

Fig. 1. Typical MRI findings in PACNS. (*A*) demonstrating multifocal areas of increased signal on FLAIR sequence involving deep or cortical/subcortical structures involving multiple vascular territories. (*B*) demonstrating gadolinium enhancement involving the affected areas and associated leptomeninges on T1-weighted post-contrast sequence.

negative study does not exclude CNSV and further workup could be considered.[25] CTA, MRA, and conventional cerebral angiogram are all imaging of the vessel lumen. Vessel wall MRI (VW-MRI) has been used to obtain more information regarding the radiographic imaging patterns of large-/medium sized cerebral arteries.[26] This technique has been used to supplement other imaging modalities to support PACNS or provide support for alternative etiologies.[27–29] Using VW-MRI imaging, possible distinction could be made between atherosclerotic plaques (eccentric non-uniform vessel wall thickening and contrast enhancement) compared to infectious or inflammatory vasculitis (usually smooth concentric uniform vessel wall enhancement likely due to increased permeability of the endothelium or vasa vasorum). In one study, using VW-MR features and concentric enhancement on VW-MR imaging, PACNS could be distinguished from other non-inflammatory vasculopathies with a sensitivity of 90.5% and specificity of 100%.[30] However, several pitfalls limit the use of vessel wall imaging including its technical limitations, incidental age-related changes, venous enhancement and contamination, and enhancement related to slow flow and vasa vasorum.[28]

The gold standard for diagnosis of PACNS is leptomeningeal and brain parenchymal biopsy for histopathological analysis which can be used to support a diagnosis of PACNS or support alternative etiologies. However, due to the multifocal involvement of PACNS biopsy is not 100% sensitive, and a negative biopsy does not exclude PACNS. With highly targeted testing, the diagnostic yield of biopsy for PACNS is around 75%.[31] Although biopsy may not confirm the diagnosis, it could yield an alternative diagnosis in CNS in approximately 30% of patients.[32] The sensitivity of biopsy with large/medium seized vessel vasculitis is likely lower due to more proximal involvement (away from site of biopsy) and biopsy can be positive in about 8% of angiogram-confirmed cases.[20] Biopsy complication rates are estimated to be around 4% to 8% and include hemorrhage and abscess formation[33,34] and the

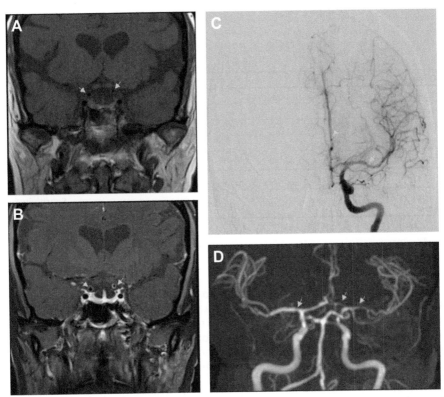

Fig. 2. Typical findings on vessel imaging in PACNS. (*A, B*) demonstrating concentric vessel wall enhancement notable on T1-weighted pre- and post-contrast sequences, respectively (*arrows*). (*C*) demonstrating diffuse multifocal stenoses noted in the left ICA, MCA, and ACA on DSA imaging (*arrows*). (*D*) demonstrating MRA findings including diffuse multifocal stenoses (*arrows*).

benefits of obtaining a biopsy must be weighed against its potential risks and complications.

Differential Diagnosis

Even after excluding secondary CNSV, the diagnosis of PACNS requires ruling out major mimics. Lack of serological, CSF, or imaging biomarkers combined with the non-specific clinical presentation of PACNS can make this process very challenging and time-consuming.

The most common vasculopathy mimicking PACNS is reversible cerebral vasoconstriction syndromes (RCVS) which is a non-inflammatory vasculopathy causing multifocal vasospasm sometimes associated with triggers such as pregnancy, posterior reversible encephalopathy syndrome, pharmaceuticals including sympathomimetics and serotonergic agents including serotonin reuptake inhibitors. Several studies have evaluated, developed, and validated a scoring system to help differentiate RCVS from PACNS (RCVS$_2$ score, **Table 1**).[35] In comparing RCVS and CNS vasculitis, arterial imaging showing "sausage on a string" or segmental dilation would be more typical of RCVS, whereas brain parenchymal imaging demonstrating deep or brainstem infarcts are specific signs of cerebral vasculitis.[23]

Table 1
Reversible cerebral vasoconstriction syndromes 2 score criteria and performance in diagnosing reversible cerebral vasoconstriction syndromes

RCVS2 Score	
Criteria	Points
Recurrent or single thunderclap headache	+5
Vasoconstrictive trigger	+3
Female sex gender	+1
Subarachnoid hemorrhage	+1
Intracranial carotid artery involvement	−2

RCVS2 Score Performance in Diagnosing RCVS	
Score	Sensitivity/ Specificity
≥5 points	86%/94%
3–4 points	11%/83%
≤2 points	77%/96%

Multifocal strokes mimicking PACNS can also be seen with recurrent embolism. The classic appearance of cerebral embolism is a wedge-shaped cortical or cerebellar infarct, but emboli may scatter or small arteries may occlude mimicking PACNS. Conditions with short-term high-risk recurrent embolism such as cardiac thrombus and valve vegetation may result in multiple acute and subacute infarcts, whereas conditions with longer-term recurrent risk such as atrial fibrillation or patent foramen ovale may be associated with acute and chronic infarcts.

Cerebral amyloid angiopathy-related inflammation (CAA-RI) is a rare disorder affecting the CNS and may mimic PACNS. The pathophysiology is thought to be similar to ABRA with inflammatory reaction to Aβ protein deposits although, on biopsy, this is limited to perivascular inflammation as opposed to intramural inflammation seen in ABRA and PACNS.[36] The clinical findings in CAA-RI include acute or subacute onset of headache, changes in behavior and consciousness, focal neurological deficits, and seizures. MRI findings in CAA-RI include unifocal or multifocal deep or subcortical white matter hyperintensities on fluid-attenuated inversion recovery (FLAIR) signal changes as well as findings consistent with cerebral amyloid angiopathy.[37]

Antiphospholipid syndrome is also associated with other neurological manifestations including cognitive impairment, headache, seizures, demyelinating events, movement disorders, and psychiatric symptoms.[38,39]

Intravascular lymphoma (IVL) is another rare mimic of PACNS causing vasculopathy with only biopsy distinguishing the two entities. It is a type of non-Hodgkin's lymphoma leading to neoplastic growth of lymphocytes within the lumen of vessels and in addition to CNS involvement, it can also lead to cutaneous involvement. Random skin biopsies containing subcutaneous tissue can be used in establishing this diagnosis but ultimately brain biopsy may be required for this diagnosis.[10]

There are several inherited disorders which can also share presenting features with PACNS and must be considered as part of the diagnostic workup. Cerebral autosomal dominant arteriopathy with subcortical infarcts and leukoencephalopathy is caused by pathological mutations in the NOTCH3 gene located on chromosome 19 and can present with migraine with aura, cognitive decline, mood changes, and epilepsy as well as FLAIR signal changes in periventricular and subcortical areas particularly affecting the anterior temporal poles and external capsules. Due to an autosomal dominant pattern with high penetrance family history should point to this diagnosis. Mitochondrial encephalomyopathy lactic acidosis (MELAS) is another inherited disorder caused by maternally inherited mitochondrial disease (most commonly m.3243 A > G pathological variation). It most commonly presents with stroke-like episodes and headaches. Cognitive impairment, seizures, lactic acidosis, and myopathy may also be present or become apparent. Involvement of brain regions is not restricted to vascular distributions and presence of hearing impairment and peripheral neuropathy might distinguish MELAS from PACNS.[40] Other rare common hereditary conditions mimicking PACNS include pathological variations in COL4A1, TREX1, and ADA2.

Treatment and Prognosis

Based on retrospective cohort studies, the treatment of PACNS is primarily immunosuppression similar to other systemic vasculitides. If not treated appropriately, it can be progressive and cause disability accumulation.[41] High-dose glucocorticoids are the mainstay of treatment of CNSV. The initial treatment of PACNS includes high-dose pulse methylprednisolone at a dose of 1 g daily over 3 to 5 days followed by oral prednisone starting at 1 mg/kg per day to a maximum of 80 mg/day followed by a taper over 6 months. The choice of steroid-sparing immunosuppressant agents in the initial induction phase depends on the severity of the disease, the pathologic pattern, and the certainty of the diagnosis. Cyclophosphamide is the preferred agent in granulomatous angiitis and necrotizing vasculitis pathologic patterns as these patterns carry a poor prognosis.[11,42,43] Mycophenolate mofetil can be considered in the induction treatment of CNSV with non-necrotizing and non-granulomatous pattern on pathology with low disease burden or when the three is lack of high diagnostic confidence despite the thorough workup.[44]

Cyclophosphamide can be administered as oral daily (1.5–2 mg/kg/day) or monthly intravenous (600–1000 mg/m^2) schedule and monitoring of white blood cell count to maintain above 3500/μL. The duration of therapy with cyclophosphamide is typically limited to 6 months due to its toxicities. Maintenance therapy, after the induction therapy, is recommended as relapses occur; mycophenolate mefetil and azathioprine are the mainstay maintenance agents. There have been reports of successful use of rituximab in CNSV although larger and additional studies evaluating the use of rituximab are needed. Methotrexate is not an ideal steroid-sparing agent in CNSV due to the low CNS penetrance. In addition, patients should be provided with prophylactic therapy for prevention of osteoporosis and opportunistic infections.

In addition to being monitored for toxicities to therapies, patients should be monitored regularly with serial neurological examinations and imaging to assess response to therapy and relapse. A recent study has shown that the enhancement of VW-MRI can be used as a marker to monitor disease activity and treatment response.[45]

PACNS is a progressive disease with more than half of patients experiencing relapses when followed for 61 months[46] and mortality rate estimated to be around 11%.[47] Prognosis in PACNS is likely influenced by initial severity of the disease, older age, and presence of strokes[48] and while no significant difference between functional outcomes and the size of involved vessel has been found, patients with small-vessel involvement are thought to have more relapses.[22]

SECONDARY CENTRAL NERVOUS SYSTEM VASCULITIS
Central Nervous System Vasculitis Secondary to Systemic Vasculitis

Although generally peripheral nervous system is more common, systemic vasculitides may also have CNS involvement. In the largest available dataset from 1368 patients with ANCA vasculitis, CNS involvement occurred in approximately 3%.[49] Granulomatosis with polyangiitis (GPA) is a systemic vasculitis with associated ANCA primarily against proteinase 3 (PR3) causing granulomatous necrotizing of small vessels predominantly involving the renal and pulmonary systems.[50] GPA can affect the CNS through involvement of the pituitary gland, the meninges, or the CNS vasculature in approximately 7%–11% of patients.[51,52] Microscopic polyangiitis (MPA) is another systemic vasculitis associated with ANCA with primary target against myeloperoxidase affecting small- to medium-sized vessels.[50] Both GPA and MPA can cause CNSV with similar presentation to PACNS although presence of systemic involvement, pachymeningitis, and pituitary involvement can help distinguish these from PACNS.[51] Although CNSV can also be seen with eosinophilic granulomatosis with polyangiitis (EGPA) and polyarteritis nodosa (PAN), in contrast to GPA and MPA, CNS involvement occurs less frequently[49] Diagnosis usually requires evaluation of different organ involvement; treatment requires treatment of the underlying systemic disease.

Behcet's disease (BD) is another chronic relapsing inflammatory disorder characterized by recurrent oral and genital ulcers associated with systemic involvement.[53] Neurological involvement termed Neuro-Behcet's disease (NBD) occurs in approximately 9% of patients involving both CNS and peripheral nervous system.[54] Typically CNS manifestations of NBD are categorized into parenchymal (affecting cerebrum, brainstem, spinal cord, and optic nerves) and non-parenchymal disease.[54] The non-parenchymal CNS NBD includes several vascular complications such as cerebral venous thrombosis, aneurysms, and dissections. The diagnosis of NBD is based on diagnostic criteria set in international consensus recommendations and given the relapsing and progressive nature of the disease treatment involves immunosuppression with steroids and steroid-sparing agents mainly with anti-tumor necrosis factor agents.[55]

Central Nervous System Vasculitis due to Infectious Vasculitis

Many infectious agents can affect the CNS vasculature including *Streptococcus pneumoniae, Neisseria meningitidis, Mycobacterium tuberculosis, Treponema pallidum,* and *Borrelia burgdorferi*. Several viruses with CNS tropism have been known to cause vasculopathy and can lead to similar presentation to PACNS. It is important to recognize these disorders as some may be treatable. The most common viruses causing CNS vasculopathy include Varicella-zoster virus (VZV),[56,57] Herpes simplex 1 and 2 (HSV 1 and 2),[58,59] and human immunodeficiency virus (HIV).[60] VZV and HSV viruses can cause a range of neurological manifestations in addition to vasculopathy including encephalitis, meningitis, cranial nerve palsies, and myelitis. Vasculopathy can be seen both in the setting of HIV infection and immune reconstitution inflammatory syndrome. Serum and CSF polymerase chain reaction (PCR) testing and consideration of metagenomic next-generation sequencing are important tools to diagnose the infectious etiologies.

Central Nervous System Vasculitis Secondary to Other Immune-Mediated Inflammatory Diseases

Several immune-mediated inflammatory diseases (IMID) have been shown to cause secondary CNSV. Systemic lupus erythematosus (SLE) can have several CNS manifestations including complications associated with antiphospholipid syndrome and neuropsychiatric manifestations associated with SLE but CNSV is estimated to be around 7% to 10%.[61] Other IMIDs can rarely cause CNSV including systemic sclerosis, mixed connective tissue disease, rheumatoid arthritis, and juvenile dermatomyositis.[48]

Sarcoidosis is a granulomatous inflammatory systemic disorder which can also have CNS involvement referred to as neurosarcoidosis (NS). Although sarcoidosis primarily affects the lung, lymph nodes, and skin, NS can be seen in about 5% of patients with sarcoidosis with common manifestations including cranial neuropathies, pachymeningitis, meningitis, parenchymal involvement, myelopathy, hypothalamic or pituitary axis involvement, peripheral neuropathy, and myopathy.[62] More recent studies have demonstrated that NS can have involvement of small, medium, or large intracranial vessels with associated enhancement on VW-MRI.[63,64] Given the broad range of possible CNS manifestations in NS, in the absence of systemic disease, it can mimic PACNS. A recent study was able to identify several features including patient's race and pattern of neurological involvement to differentiate PACNS from NS.[65]

Susac syndrome is a multisystem autoimmune endotheliopathy which can cause manifestation in the brain, inner ear, and retina. Diagnosis is typically based on the clinical presentation and findings from retinal fluorescein angiography, brain MRI (with typical "Snowball" corpus callosum lesions), and audiometry, and treatment includes immunosuppression with steroids and disease-modifying anti-rheumatic drugs.[66] Cogan syndrome is a rare vasculitis syndrome causing constitutional manifestations as well as the involvement of ocular and audio-vestibular systems. Corticosteroids are the mainstay of treatment of Cogan syndrome and disease modifying antirheumatic drugs (DMARDs).[67] Acute posterior multifocal placoid pigment epitheliopathy is a rare disorder most commonly affecting the retinal pigment epithelium characterized by acute binocular vision impairment and may be associated with cerebral vasculitis and meningoencephalitis.[68,69]

SUMMARY

CNSV is a heterogeneous group of disorders that affect the vasculature within the brain, spinal cord, and leptomeninges. Perivascular and intramural inflammation seen in CNSV can present as a primary disorder (PACNS) or secondary to another disorder (secondary CNSV). Regardless of etiology, there is vascular damage, necrosis, and tissue ischemia secondary to this process. The pathophysiology of PACNS is poorly understood but it can affect small, medium, or large vessels and the clinical presentation can vary based on the affected vessel but generally includes the insidious onset of focal neurological symptoms, headache, seizure, and cognitive impairment. There is no one test that allows diagnosis of PACNS but rather the diagnosis relies on a combination of history, physical examination, serological and CSF evaluation, MRI, vessel imaging, and in some cases, histopathological evaluation. One of the major limitations in evaluating PACNS is the lack of sensitivity and specificity in the available tests and the overlap of clinical presentations with several other mimicking conditions which need to be excluded. These include several other inflammatory and infiltrative disorders as well as secondary CNSV. Secondary CNSV could be due to systemic vasculitides, connective tissue disorders, infectious disorders, and other systemic disorders that can involve the CNS vasculature. The treatment of CNSV includes immunosuppression for PACNS or treatment of the underlying condition for secondary CNSV.

CLINICS CARE POINTS

- CNSV is divided into primary angiitis of CNS (PACNS) and secondary CNSV depending on the underlying etiology.

- CNSV affects the vasculature within the brain, spinal cord, and leptomeninges causing intramural inflammation and secondary tissue ischemia.
- Clinical manifestations of PACNS are variable, non-specific, and overlap with many other disorders which would need to be excluded in the evaluation of PACNS.
- Diagnosis of PACNS requires a thorough evaluation of serum and CSF to rule out mimickers as well as demonstrate supporting features.
- Large- and medium-sized vessel involvement can typically be evaluated using conventional vessel imaging (see **Fig. 2**) such as CT angiogram and MRA as well as VW-MRI while evaluation of small-vessel involvement typically requires digital subtraction angiography (DSA) or histopathological evaluation.
- None of the diagnostic tests in the evaluation of PACNS are 100% sensitive or specific and should be interpreted cautiously in the context of the clinical syndrome.
- PACNS is a chronic and relapsing disease and treatment of PACNS involves immunosuppression with glucocorticoids as well as steroid-sparing agents.
- Secondary CNSV could be due to various underlying disorders and the treatment usually requires treatment of the underlying disease.

DISCLOSURE

The authors have nothing to disclose.

REFERENCES

1. Newman W, Wolf A. Non-infectious granulomatous angiitis involving the central nervous system. Trans Am Neurol Assoc 1952;56(77th Meeting):114–7. Available at: http://www.ncbi.nlm.nih.gov/pubmed/13038806.
2. Cravioto H, Feigin I. Noninfectious granulomatous angiitis with a predilection for the nervous system. Neurology 1959;9:599–609. Available at: http://www.ncbi.nlm.nih.gov/pubmed/13812692.
3. Salvarani C, Brown RD, Calamia KT, et al. Primary central nervous system vasculitis: analysis of 101 patients. Ann Neurol 2007;62(5):442–51. https://doi.org/10.1002/ana.21226.
4. Miller DV, Salvarani C, Hunder GG, et al. Biopsy findings in primary angiitis of the central nervous system. Am J Surg Pathol 2009;33(1):35–43. https://doi.org/10.1097/PAS.0b013e318181e097.
5. Thom V, Schmid S, Gelderblom M, et al. IL-17 production by CSF lymphocytes as a biomarker for cerebral vasculitis. Neurol Neuroinflammation 2016;3(2):e214.
6. Strunk D, Schulte-Mecklenbeck A, Golombeck KS, et al. Immune cell profiling in the cerebrospinal fluid of patients with primary angiitis of the central nervous system reflects the heterogeneity of the disease. J Neuroimmunol 2018;321:109–16.
7. Mandel-Brehm C, Retallack H, Knudsen GM, et al. Exploratory proteomic analysis implicates the alternative complement cascade in primary CNS vasculitis. Neurology 2019;93(5):e433–44.
8. Kraemer M, Becker J, Horn PA, et al. Association of primary central nervous system vasculitis with the presence of specific human leucocyte antigen gene variant. Clin Neurol Neurosurg 2017;160:137–41.
9. Najem CE, Springer J, Prayson R, et al. Intra cranial granulomatous disease in common variable immunodeficiency: case series and review of the literature. Semin Arthritis Rheum 2018;47:890–6. Elsevier.

10. Mandal J, Chung SA. Primary angiitis of the central nervous system. Rheum Dis Clin 2017;43(4):503–18.
11. Salvarani C, Brown RD, Christianson T, et al. An update of the Mayo Clinic cohort of patients with adult primary central nervous system vasculitis: description of 163 patients. Medicine (Baltim) 2015;94(21):e738. https://doi.org/10.1097/MD.0000000000000738.
12. de Boysson H, Zuber M, Naggara O, et al. Primary angiitis of the central nervous system: description of the first fifty-two adults enrolled in the French cohort of patients with primary vasculitis of the central nervous system. Arthritis Rheumatol 2014;66(5):1315–26. https://doi.org/10.1002/art.38340.
13. Sundaram S, Menon D, Khatri P, et al. Primary angiitis of the central nervous system: Clinical profiles and outcomes of 45 patients. Neurol India 2019;67(1):105.
14. Salvarani C, Hunder GG, Morris JM, et al. Aβ-related angiitis: comparison with CAA without inflammation and primary CNS vasculitis. Neurology 2013;81(18):1596–603. https://doi.org/10.1212/WNL.0b013e3182a9f545.
15. de Boysson H, Boulouis G, Dequatre N, et al. Tumor-like presentation of primary angiitis of the central nervous system. Stroke 2016;47(9):2401–4.
16. Benson CE, Knezevic A, Lynch SC. Primary central nervous system vasculitis with optic nerve involvement. J Neuro-Ophthalmology 2016;36(2):174–7.
17. Matar RK, Alshamsan B, Alsaleh S, et al. New onset refractory status epilepticus due to primary angiitis of the central nervous system. Epilepsy Behav case reports 2017;8:100–4.
18. Calabrese LH, Mallek JA. Primary angiitis of the central nervous system. Report of 8 new cases, review of the literature, and proposal for diagnostic criteria. Medicine (Baltim) 1988;67(1):20–39. Available at: http://www.ncbi.nlm.nih.gov/pubmed/3275856.
19. Lucke M, Hajj-Ali RA. Advances in primary angiitis of the central nervous system. Curr Cardiol Rep 2014;16(10):533.
20. Beuker C, Strunk D, Rawal R, et al. Primary Angiitis of the CNS: a systematic review and meta-analysis. Neurol Neuroinflammation 2021;8(6).
21. Wilson MR, O'Donovan BD, Gelfand JM, et al. Chronic meningitis investigated via metagenomic next-generation sequencing. JAMA Neurol 2018;75(8):947–55.
22. de Boysson H, Boulouis G, Aouba A, et al. Adult primary angiitis of the central nervous system: isolated small-vessel vasculitis represents distinct disease pattern. Rheumatology 2017;56(3):439–44. https://doi.org/10.1093/rheumatology/kew434.
23. Singhal AB, Topcuoglu MA, Fok JW, et al. Reversible cerebral vasoconstriction syndromes and primary angiitis of the central nervous system: clinical, imaging, and angiographic comparison. Ann Neurol 2016;79(6):882–94.
24. Deb-Chatterji M, Schuster S, Haeussler V, et al. Primary angiitis of the central nervous system: new potential imaging techniques and biomarkers in blood and cerebrospinal fluid. Front Neurol 2019;10:568.
25. Schuster S, Bachmann H, Thom V, et al. Subtypes of primary angiitis of the CNS identified by MRI patterns reflect the size of affected vessels. J Neurol Neurosurg Psychiatry 2017;88(9):749–55.
26. Kesav P, Krishnavadana B, Kesavadas C, et al. Utility of intracranial high-resolution vessel wall magnetic resonance imaging in differentiating intracranial vasculopathic diseases causing ischemic stroke. Neuroradiology 2019;61(4):389–96.
27. Eiden S, Beck C, Venhoff N, et al. High-resolution contrast-enhanced vessel wall imaging in patients with suspected cerebral vasculitis: Prospective comparison

of whole-brain 3D T1 SPACE versus 2D T1 black blood MRI at 3 Tesla. PLoS One 2019;14(3):e0213514.

28. Mandell DM, Mossa-Basha M, Qiao Y, et al. Intracranial vessel wall MRI: principles and expert consensus recommendations of the American Society of Neuroradiology. Am J Neuroradiol 2017;38(2):218–29.

29. Obusez EC, Hui F, Hajj-Ali RA, et al. High-resolution MRI vessel wall imaging: spatial and temporal patterns of reversible cerebral vasoconstriction syndrome and central nervous system vasculitis. Am J Neuroradiol 2014;35(8):1527–32.

30. Karaman AK, Korkmazer B, Arslan S, et al. The diagnostic contribution of intracranial vessel wall imaging in the differentiation of primary angiitis of the central nervous system from other intracranial vasculopathies. Neuroradiology 2021; 63(10):1635–44.

31. Bai HX, Zou Y, Lee AM, et al. Diagnostic value and safety of brain biopsy in patients with cryptogenic neurological disease: a systematic review and meta-analysis of 831 cases. Neurosurgery 2015;77(2):283–95.

32. Torres J, Loomis C, Cucchiara B, et al. Diagnostic yield and safety of brain biopsy for suspected primary central nervous system angiitis. Stroke 2016;47(8):2127–9.

33. Schuette AJ, Taub JS, Hadjipanayis CG, et al. Open biopsy in patients with acute progressive neurologic decline and absence of mass lesion. Neurology 2010; 75(5):419–24.

34. Magaki S, Gardner T, Khanlou N, et al. Brain biopsy in neurologic decline of unknown etiology. Hum Pathol 2015;46(4):499–506.

35. Rocha EA, Topcuoglu MA, Silva GS, et al. RCVS 2 score and diagnostic approach for reversible cerebral vasoconstriction syndrome. Neurology 2019; 92(7). https://doi.org/10.1212/WNL.0000000000006917.

36. Salvarani C, Morris JM, Giannini C, et al. Imaging findings of cerebral amyloid angiopathy, Aβ-Related Angiitis (ABRA), and cerebral amyloid angiopathy–related inflammation: a single-institution 25-year experience. Medicine (Baltim) 2016; 95(20).

37. Auriel E, Charidimou A, Gurol ME, et al. Validation of clinicoradiological criteria for the diagnosis of cerebral amyloid angiopathy–related inflammation. JAMA Neurol 2016;73(2):197–202.

38. Yelnik CM, Kozora E, Appenzeller S. Non-stroke central neurologic manifestations in antiphospholipid syndrome. Curr Rheumatol Rep 2016;18(2):11.

39. D'Angelo C, Franch O, Fernández Paredes L, et al. Antiphospholipid Antibodies overlapping in Isolated Neurological Syndrome and Multiple Sclerosis: Neurobiological Insights and Diagnostic Challenges. Front Cell Neurosci 2019;13:107.

40. El-Hattab AW, Adesina AM, Jones J, et al. MELAS syndrome: clinical manifestations, pathogenesis, and treatment options. Mol Genet Metab 2015; 116(1–2):4–12.

41. Byram K, Hajj-Ali RA, Calabrese L. CNS vasculitis: An approach to differential diagnosis and management. Curr Rheumatol Rep 2018;20(7):37.

42. Salvarani C, Brown RD Jr, Calamia KT, et al. Rapidly progressive primary central nervous system vasculitis. Rheumatology 2011;50(2):349–58.

43. Salvarani C, Brown RD Jr, Christianson TJH, et al. Long-term remission, relapses and maintenance therapy in adult primary central nervous system vasculitis: A single-center 35-year experience. Autoimmun Rev 2020;19(4):102497.

44. Salvarani C, Brown RD Jr, Christianson TJH, et al. Mycophenolate mofetil in primary central nervous system vasculitis. Semin Arthritis Rheum 2015;45:55–9. Elsevier.

45. Shimoyama T, Uchino K, Calabrese LH, et al. Serial vessel wall enhancement pattern on high-resolution vessel wall magnetic resonance imaging and clinical implications in patients with central nervous system vasculitis. Clin Exp Rheumatol 2022;40(4):811–8.
46. Schuster S, Ozga A-K, Stellmann J-P, et al. Relapse rates and long-term outcome in primary angiitis of the central nervous system. J Neurol 2019;266(6):1481–9.
47. Hajj-Ali RA, Saygin D, Ray E, et al. Long-term outcomes of patients with primary angiitis of the central nervous system. Clin Exp Rheumatol 2019;37(117):S45–51.
48. Dutra LA, de Souza AWS, Grinberg-Dias G, et al. Central nervous system vasculitis in adults: An update. Autoimmun Rev 2017;16(2). https://doi.org/10.1016/j.autrev.2016.12.001.
49. Hajj-Ali R, Butler R, Langford C, et al. Neurologic Involvement in ANCA-associated Vasculitis: Data from Multicenter Longitudinal Observational Study. Arthritis Rheumatol 2021. Available at: https://acrabstracts.org/abstract/neurologic-involvement-in-anca-associated-vasculitis-data-from-multicenter-longitudinal-observational-study/. Accessed August 2, 2022.
50. Imboden JB, Hellmann DB, Stone JA. Current diagnosis & treatment in rheumatology. New York, NY: McGraw Hill Professional; 2020.
51. Ghinoi A, Zuccoli G, Pipitone N, et al. Anti-neutrophil cytoplasmic antibody (ANCA)-associated vasculitis involving the central nervous system: case report and review of the literature. Clin Exp Rheumatol 2010;28(5):759–66.
52. Seror R, Mahr A, Ramanoelina J, et al. Central nervous system involvement in Wegener granulomatosis. Medicine (Baltim) 2006;85(1):53–65.
53. Bulur I, Onder M. Behçet disease: new aspects. Clin Dermatol 2017;35(5):421–34.
54. Borhani-Haghighi A, Kardeh B, Banerjee S, et al. Neuro-Behcet's disease: An update on diagnosis, differential diagnoses, and treatment. Mult Scler Relat Disord 2020;39:101906.
55. Kalra S, Silman A, Akman-Demir G, et al. Diagnosis and management of Neuro-Behçet's disease: international consensus recommendations. J Neurol 2014;261(9):1662–76.
56. Carod Artal FJ. Clinical management of infectious cerebral vasculitides. Expert Rev Neurother 2016;16(2):205–21.
57. Nagel MA, Cohrs RJ, Mahalingam R, et al. The varicella zoster virus vasculopathies: clinical, CSF, imaging, and virologic features. Neurology 2008;70(11):853–60.
58. Guerrero WR, Dababneh H, Hedna S, et al. Vessel wall enhancement in herpes simplex virus central nervous system vasculitis. J Clin Neurosci 2013;20(9):1318–9.
59. Fan TH, Khoury J, Cho S-M, et al. Cerebrovascular complications and vasculopathy in patients with herpes simplex virus central nervous system infection. J Neurol Sci 2020;419:117200.
60. Gutierrez J, Ortiz G. HIV/AIDS patients with HIV vasculopathy and VZV vasculitis. Clin Neuroradiol 2011;21(3):145.
61. Barile-Fabris L, Hernández-Cabrera MF, Barragan-Garfias JA. Vasculitis in systemic lupus erythematosus. Curr Rheumatol Rep 2014;16(9):1–6.
62. Bradshaw MJ, Pawate S, Koth LL, et al. Neurosarcoidosis: pathophysiology, diagnosis, and treatment. Neurol Neuroinflammation 2021;8(6).
63. Bathla G, Watal P, Gupta S, et al. Cerebrovascular manifestations of neurosarcoidosis: an underrecognized aspect of the imaging spectrum. Am J Neuroradiol 2018;39(7):1194–200.

64. Bathla G, Abdel-Wahed L, Agarwal A, et al. Vascular involvement in neurosarcoidosis: early experiences from intracranial vessel wall imaging. Neurol Neuroinflammation 2021;8(6).

65. Saygin D, Jones S, Sundaram P, et al. Differentiation between neurosarcoidosis and primary central nervous system vasculitis based on demographic, cerebrospinal and imaging features. Clin Exp Rheumatol 2020;124(2):135–8.

66. Pereira S, Vieira B, Maio T, et al. Susac's syndrome: an updated review. Neuro Ophthalmol 2020;44(6):355–60.

67. Espinoza GM, Wheeler J, Temprano KK, et al. Cogan's syndrome: Clinical presentations and update on treatment. Curr Allergy Asthma Rep 2020;20(9):1–6.

68. Matamala JM, Feuerhake W, Verdugo R. Delayed recurrent stroke in a young patient with acute posterior multifocal placoid pigment epitheliopathy. J Stroke Cerebrovasc Dis 2013;22(8):e630–4.

69. de Vries JJ, den Dunnen WFA, Timmerman EA, et al. Acute posterior multifocal placoid pigment epitheliopathy with cerebral vasculitis: a multisystem granulomatous disease. Arch Ophthalmol 2006;124(6):910–3.

Vasculitis Mimics and Other Related Conditions

Jason M. Springer, MD, MS[a],*, Alexandra Villa-Forte, MD, MPH[b]

KEYWORDS

- Large vessel vasculitis • Medium vessel vasculitis • Small vessel vasculitis
- Vasculitis mimics

KEY POINTS

- Vasculitis should be considered in the context of a systemic inflammatory diease of multiple organs or unexplained ischemia.
- The differential for primary forms of vasculitis should include non-autoimmune vasculopathies and inflammatory disorders causing secondary vasculitis or vasculitis-like inflammation.
- The differential for cutaneous vasculitis is broad. A skin biopsy is the gold standard for diagnosis. Secondary causes of cutaneous vasculitis should be considered.
- Atherosclerosis and reversible cerebral vasoconstriction syndrome (RCVS) are common mimics of primary angiitis of the central nervous system (PACNS).

INTRODUCTION

The 2012 Chapel Hill Consensus Conference classifies different forms of vasculitis by the size of the vessel predominantly affected, most commonly arteries.[1] Large vessel disease typically involves the aorta and proximal branches of the aorta, but may also affect other vessel sizes, including the extracranial arteries in the head. Medium vessel disease includes arteries that are smaller but still have a muscular layer, whereas small vessel disease typically involves microscopic arterioles, capillaries, and post-capillary venules. This classification is not perfect, with overlapping vessels affected between groups. In addition, some forms of primary vasculitis do not fit neatly into this paradigm, such as Behçet's disease which can manifest in any sized vessel. However, this nomenclature forms a useful framework for guiding the clinician in identifying mimics (**Table 1**).

WHEN TO SUSPECT VASCULITIS

There are two main clinical presentations when vasculitis should always be considered and excluded: (1) a systemic inflammatory disease affecting multiple organs, and (2)

a Vanderbilt University Medical Center, 1161 21st Avenue South, T-3113 Medical Center North, Nashville, TN 37232-2681, USA; b Cleveland Clinic, 9500 Euclid Avenue, A50, Cleveland, OH 44195, USA
* Corresponding author.
E-mail address: jason.springer@vumc.org

Rheum Dis Clin N Am 49 (2023) 617–631
https://doi.org/10.1016/j.rdc.2023.03.008
0889-857X/23/Published by Elsevier Inc.

rheumatic.theclinics.com

Table 1
Mimics of primary forms of vasculitis[a]

Cutaneous Vasculitis/LCV Mimics	SVV Mimics	MVV Mimics	LVV Mimics	PACNS Mimics
Arthropod bites	Infective endocarditis	Atherosclerosis	Atherosclerosis	RCVS
Pigmented purpuric dermatoses	COVID-19	Thromboembolic disease	NAION	Atherosclerosis
Macular purpura	Cocaine/Levamisole	vEDS	Infections	Thromboembolic disease
Hypercoagulable/thrombotic disease	Infectious vasculopathy	Loeys-Dietz syndrome	Marfan syndrome	Infections
Pyoderma gangrenosum	HBV, HCV, HIV, etc.	FMD	Loeys-Dietz syndrome	HSV, VZV, HIV, etc.
Cholesterol crystal embolization	Anti-GBM disease	SAM	Turner syndrome	Intravascular lymphoma/paraneoplastic
Calciphylaxis	SLE	IE	IgG4-related disease	SLE
Livedoid vasculopathy	Sarcoidosis	Infectious vasculopathy	Erdheim-Chester disease	Sarcoidosis
Drugs/toxins vasculopathy	Malignancy/paraneoplastic	HBV, HCV, HIV, etc.	VEXAS syndrome	APLS
Cocaine, Minocycline, etc.	Eosinophilic diseases	Ergotism		Susac syndrome
Infectious vasculopathy	HES, ABPA, etc.	Radiation fibrosis		CADASIL
RMSF, COVID-19, etc.		Malignant atrophic papulosis (Degos disease)		MELAS
Purpura fulminans		Thromboangiitis obliterans (Buerger's disease)		Cerebroretinal vasculopathy syndrome
Systemic amyloidosis				Moyamoya disease
Septic emboli				Amyloid angiopathy
Pernio				
Scurvy				

Abbreviations: ABPA, allergic bronchopulmonary aspergillosis; APLS, antiphospholipid syndrome; CADASIL, cerebral autosomal dominant arteriopathy with subcortical infarcts and leukoencephalopathy; GBM, glomerular basement disease; HBV, hepatitis B virus; HCV, hepatitis C virus; HES, hypereosinophilic syndrome; HIV, human immunodeficiency virus; HSV, herpes simplex virus; LCV, leukocytoclastic vasculitis; LVV, large vessel vasculitis; MELAS, mitochondrial encephalomyopathy lactic acidosis and stroke syndrome; MVV, medium vessel vasculitis; NAION, nonarteritic ischemic optic neuropathy; PACNS, primary angiitis of central nervous system; RCVS, reversible cerebral vasoconstrictive syndrome; RMSF, rocky mountain spotted fever; SAM, segmental arterial mediolysis; SLE, systemic lupus erythematosus; SVV, small vessel vasculitis; vEDS, vascular Ehlers-Danlos syndrome; VEXAS, vacuoles E1 enzymes X-linked enzyme autoinflammatory somatic; VZV, varicella zoster virus.

[a] Secondary forms of vasculitis have been excluded from this list; but many mimics can also cause secondary vasculitis (eg, drugs and infections).

unexplained ischemia. In the first group, patients commonly present with non-specific symptoms of fever, weight loss, fatigue, joint and muscle pain, in addition to symptoms related to specific organ involvement, for example, palpable purpura and mononeuritis multiplex. The suspicion for vasculitis should be high in the presence of a robust systemic inflammatory response and a high number of involved organs. However, patients with single-organ vasculitis may be asymptomatic or display specific manifestations related to the affected organ. Sometimes, vasculitis is an incidental finding following surgery (eg, hysterectomy) in asymptomatic patients. In that situation, it cannot be clinically suspected. Depending on the stage of the disease, symptoms vary from a few, at onset, to many, with disease progression. In the second group, patients present with organ ischemia or infarction in the absence of risk factors or typical vessel distribution for atherosclerosis. Patients may also be younger than expected for significant vessel damage from atherosclerosis. Manifestations of ischemia may be apparent when symptoms of claudication are present or may be subtle when the only abnormal findings are related to the physical exam (eg, discrepancy in blood pressure and/or pulses, or vascular bruits). Another challenging clinical presentation of vasculitis consists of a non-specific illness of low-grade fever, unintentional weight loss, fatigue, anemia, and high laboratorial markers of inflammation. Patients may lack localizing symptoms making the diagnosis very difficult. This can happen in large vessel vasculitis.

MEDIUM AND LARGE VESSEL VASCULITIS MIMICS
Atherosclerosis and Thromboembolic Diseases

Atherosclerosis is a common mimic of forms of vasculitis affecting the elderly, such as giant cell arteritis. However, familial forms of atherosclerosis may be potential mimics of Takayasu's arteritis, which generally presents before the age of 40 (**Fig. 1**). The pattern of large vessel involvement can help distinguish atherosclerosis from primary large vessel vasculitis, with the latter more commonly involving the thoracic aorta and major thoracic branches, particularly the subclavian arteries.[2] Extensive vessel calcification can be seen in atherosclerosis as well as late stages of large vessel vasculitis, however, coronary artery calcification is more commonly found in atherosclerosis[3]

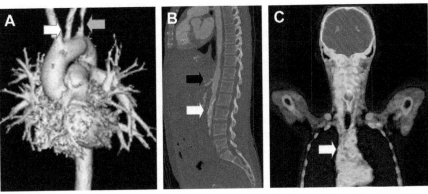

Fig. 1. A 35-year-old woman with familial hypercholesterolemia. Atherosclerosis is noted diffusely in a distribution similar to large vessel vasculitis. (A) CTA reconstruction is notable for left subclavian artery stenosis (*gray arrow*) and left common carotid stenosis (*white arrow*). (B) CTA demonstrates calcification of the abdominal aorta (*white arrow*) as well as marked narrowing of the superior mesenteric artery (*black arrow*). (C) PET demonstrates uptake within the ascending aorta as well as the aortic arch (*white arrow*).

(see **Fig. 1**B). In addition, atherosclerosis can involve medium-sized arteries such as the visceral, carotid, vertebral, and intracranial arteries. Generally, atherosclerosis affects branch points or curving portions of the artery. Atherosclerosis should be considered in patients with risk factors (eg, diabetes, smoking, hypertension) in the setting of extensive arterial irregularities involving both large- and medium-sized arteries. Atherosclerosis can cause vascular enhancement on PET imaging, which can have a similar pattern to that seen in large vessel vasculitis (see **Fig. 1**C). Clues favoring a diagnosis of vasculitis over atherosclerosis on non-invasive vascular imaging include perivascular contrast enhancement, concentric wall thickening (vs eccentric thickening), and involvement of long segments of blood vessels (vs focal disease). The thromboembolic disease can result in end-organ ischemia of medium to small arteries. Coagulopathies, such as antiphospholipid syndrome, should be considered in cases presenting as multiorgan ischemia.

Nonarteritic Ischemic Optic Neuropathy

Sudden vision loss in patients over the age of 50 should prompt consideration of ischemic optic neuropathy (ION) related to giant cell arteritis. ION can be either anterior (ie, affecting the optic disk) or posterior (ie, retrobulbar). Nonarteritic ischemic optic neuropathy (NAION) can be difficult to differentiate from arteritic causes, the latter usually from giant cell arteritis. Potential causes of NAION can include thromboembolic diseases or hypotensive episodes. In the absence of recent surgery or hypotensive episode, posterior ION should prompt a high suspicion for giant cell arteritis.[4–6] Bilateral ION occurring in rapid succession should raise suspicion for arteritic ischemic optic neuropathy. A careful history must be obtained to evaluate for extra-ocular manifestations of giant cell arteritis.

Infections

Arterial infections can result in aneurysms of medium or large arteries, mimicking primary forms of vasculitis. Compared to noninfectious causes of aortitis, infectious aortitis was more frequently associated with aortic aneurysms (78% vs 18%), especially in the abdominal aorta.[7] Infections of the arterial wall can develop from either direct inoculation related to vascular damage, arterial seeding to vulnerable areas (eg, pre-existing aneurysms or atherosclerotic plaques), spread from proximal infections or septic emboli from the heart. The most common infections include *Staphylococcus aureus* (28%–71% of reported cases),[8–10] and *Salmonella* spp (15%–24% of case),[8,10] with the diseased aorta (eg, atherosclerosis) particularly more susceptible to the latter. Other, less common, infections include *Streptococcus pneumonia*, *Treponema pallidum*, *Mycobacterium* spp (*bovis* and *tuberculosis*), *Coxiella burnetii,* and fungal organisms. The femoral artery and abdominal aorta are more common sites of infectious aneurysms.[8] A heightened suspicion is appropriate in at-risk populations including a history of a prior vascular injury, intravenous drug use, pre-existing aneurysm, antecedent infection, extensive atherosclerosis, or impaired immunity. Blood cultures (anaerobic, aerobic, and fungal) should be sent of any patient with suspected infectious arteritis. Given the high mortality rate associated with infective aortitis,[7] initiation of antibiotics should be considered before the results of blood cultures in cases in which there is a high level of suspicion.

Genetic Connective Tissue Diseases

Syndromic connective tissue diseases can cause vascular aneurysms, mimicking medium to large vessel vasculitis. These diseases typically lack the systemic symptoms and serologic markers of inflammation typically seen with primary vasculitis.

Marfan syndrome

Marfan syndrome is an autosomal dominant disorder caused by mutation in the FBN-1 gene in most cases, causing a deficiency of fibrillin-1, a component of the extracellular microfibrils.[11] Aortic aneurysms can form, typically at the root, and be associated with a high mortality rate if not identified early.[12] Other manifestations include tall stature, characteristic facial features (eg, small jaw, down-slanting palpebral fissures, dolichocephaly, enophthalmos), high-arched palate, kyphoscoliosis, arachnodactyly, pectus excavatum, flat feet, hypermobility, lens dislocations, emphysematous changes of the lungs and/or history of spontaneous pneumothorax, striae distention, or inguinal/incisional hernias.[13]

Vascular Ehlers-Danlos

Vascular Ehlers-Danlos syndrome is an autosomal dominant condition resulting, most commonly, from mutations in the COL3A1 gene, causing altered type III procollagen.[14] The commonly affected arteries include the mesenteric (32%), cerebrovascular (17%), iliac (17%), and renal (12%), but the aorta can also be affected. Arterial complications can be life-threatening and include arterial aneurysms (54%), dissections (35%), rupture (10%), pseudoaneurysm (3%), thrombosis (3%), and carotid cavernous fistulae (4%).[15] The skin may appear translucent, with prominent veins. Patients can easily get surgical wound complications or easy bruising. Musculoskeletal features may include acrogeria (loss of subcutaneous fat in the distal extremities), characteristic facial features (ie, prominent eyes, thin face/nose, and lobeless ears), clubfoot, and congenital hip dislocation.[16] Other manifestations include gingival recession, uterine rupture, spontaneous colon perforation, and emphysema.[14,16] Unlike classic Ehlers-Danlos syndrome, hypermobility is not a common feature of the vascular subtype.

Loeys-Dietz syndrome

Loeys-Dietz syndrome affects the genes for either type I or type II transforming growth factor beta receptor (TGFBR1 or TGFBR2 genes, respectively) in an autosomal dominant inheritance pattern.[17] Loeys-Dietz syndrome can cause isolated ascending aortic aneurysms or dissections, but a generalized arterial vasculopathy can also occur.[18] Other findings include widely spaced eyes (hypertelorism), bifid uvula, cleft palate, early fusion of the skull (ie, craniosynostosis), structural brain abnormalities, mental retardation, or congenital heart disease.[17]

Turner syndrome. Turner syndrome is caused by loss of part or all the X chromosomes, estimated to affect 1 in 2500 live female individuals births.[19] Milder phenotypes may not be diagnosed until late adulthood.[20] Patients can present with thoracic aortic dilations or dissections, typically of the ascending aorta. However, in most cases (90%), there is an associated cardiovascular malformation, such as coarctation or bicuspid aortic valve.[21] Other typical manifestations of Turner syndrome include short stature, "shield" chest with wide spaced nipples, webbed neck, pronounced radial angle of forearms with arm extended (cubitus valgus), underdeveloped jaw (micrognathia), high-arched palate, and genu valgum.

Fibromuscular Dysplasia

Fibromuscular dysplasia (FMD) is a non-inflammatory vasculopathy notable for a characteristic "string of beads" appearance on angiography. The true prevalence of FMD in the general population is not known, as incidental cases of FMD have been found in up to 6% of asymptomatic individuals,[22] suggesting FMD may be underdiagnosed. Although approximately 90% of adult patients are women,[23] this gender bias is not seen in pediatric patients with FMD.[24] The most common presenting symptoms include headaches, renovascular hypertension, and pulsatile tinnitus.[23] The commonly involved arteries include the renal (80%), extracranial carotid (74%), vertebral (37%), mesenteric (26%) and intracranial carotids (16%),[23] however arterial changes have been reported in virtually every arterial bed. Aortic aneurysms of both the thoracic and abdominal aorta have been reported in 3% of patients.[23] Vascular events can include transient ischemic strokes (19%), dissections (20%), and aneurysms (17%).[23] Current classification of FMD is based on angiographic appearance.[25] Multifocal FMD is characterized by the typical alternating stenotic and post-stenotic dilation (ie, "string of bead" appearance), most commonly caused by medial or peri-medial fibroplasia. Focal FMD is characterized by circumferential stenosis, most caused by intimal fibroplasia.

Immunoglobulin G(IgG)-Related Disease

IgG4-related disease, an immune-mediated multisystem disease, was first recognized as a distinct clinical entity in 2003.[26] Although several distinct phenotypes of the disease may mimic certain vasculitis syndromes, the retroperitoneal fibrosis and aortitis/peri-aortitis phenotype is most associated with the presence of true vasculitis. IgG4-related disease is a frequent cause of inflammatory abdominal aortic aneurysms[27] and retroperitoneal fibrosis may accompany the aortitis.[28] The most common site of aortic involvement is the infrarenal aorta with extension into the iliac arteries, estimated to occur in 45% of those with IgG4-related aortitis.[29] Other common manifestations of IgG4-related disease can include lymphadenopathy, autoimmune pancreatitis, sclerosing cholangitis, salivary/lacrimal gland involvement, ocular/orbital inflammatory disease, thyroiditis, lung/pleural involvement, and renal involvement. IgG4-related disease is primarily a histopathologic diagnosis notable for a lymphoplasmacytic infiltrate with a predominance of IgG4+ plasma cells, storiform fibrosis, obliterative phlebitis, and an increased number of eosinophils.[30] Although an elevated serum IgG4 level is suggestive of the disease, it can be normal in up to 50% of cases during active disease[31] and also has poor specificity.[32]

Erdheim-Chester Disease

Erdheim-Chester disease is a rare non-Langerhans histiocytic disorder characterized by somatic mutations of myeloid progenitor cells. Circumferential soft tissue sheathing of the thoracic and abdominal aorta ("coated aorta") can occur, with potential complications including renal artery hypertension or myocardial infarction.[33,34] Erdheim-Chester disease is more commonly seen in men (3:1 ratio of males to females) with a mean age of diagnosis between 50 and 60 years old.[35] Although most patients (>90%) have bone involvement, only about 50% will report bone pain, typically presenting as juxta-articular bone pain, especially in the lower extremities.[36] Typical radiographic changes include cortical osteosclerosis of the diaphyseal and metaphyseal regions of long bones.[36] Other manifestations include cardiac conduction abnormalities, cardiac valve abnormalities, lung parenchymal/pleural changes, central nervous system infiltration, pituitary disease (commonly manifesting as central diabetes insipidus), xanthelasma, retro-orbital infiltration, and/or infiltration of perinephric tissue ("hairy kidney").

SMALL VESSEL VASCULITIS MIMICS
Infections

Infections are well-known causes of secondary vasculitis but are also important vasculitis mimics, in the absence of vessel inflammation. Although infections may mimic vasculitides of any vessel size, they are associated with clinical manifestations that frequently mimic systemic small vessel vasculitis. Most infections present with constitutional symptoms, multiorgan involvement causing a variety of symptoms, laboratory abnormalities suggesting the presence of inflammation such as elevated erythrocyte sedimentation rate (ESR) and c-reactive protein (CRP), and other radiographic abnormalities (eg, lung ground-glass opacities or mass on chest imaging) that may be indistinguishable from systemic small vessel vasculitis. Antineutrophil cytoplasmic antibodies (ANCA) directed against proteinase 3 (PR3) and myeloperoxidase (MPO) are strongly associated with the group of systemic small vessel vasculitis known as ANCA-associated vasculitis (AAV), which includes granulomatosis with polyangiitis (GPA), microscopic polyangiitis (MPA), and eosinophilic granulomatosis with polyangiitis (EGPA).[1] ANCA is commonly used in the diagnosis of these conditions but can also be present in non-vasculitic disorders, particularly infections. ANCA has been reported in various infections, such as chronic viral hepatitis, parvovirus B19, human immunodeficiency virus, bacterial, fungal (eg, *Aspergillus* and *Histoplasma*), and parasitic (eg, *Entamoeba histolytica*).[37] Although any ANCA pattern can be seen with infections, discordance between the immunofluorescence (ie, c-ANCA and p-ANCA) and the enzyme immunoassay (ie, PR3-ANCA and MPO-ANCA), can be a clue to an infectious cause. Some of these infectious agents can cause lung nodules, cavitary lesions, or masses, which in the presence of a positive ANCA test may pose a challenge to distinguish from GPA. Many cases require a positive tissue culture to confirm the diagnosis. Lung cavitary lesions can be caused by many infectious agents such as *Mycobacterium tuberculosis*, atypical mycobacteria (*Mycobacterium avium-intracellulare* and *Mycobacterium kansaii*), *Streptococcus pneumoniae, S aureus, Klebsiella pneumoniae, Aspergillus fumigatus, and Pneumocystis jirovecii,* among others.[38] Malignancies should also be considered in the differential diagnosis of a cavitary lesion. A wall thickness greater than 24 mm and the lack of perilesional centrilobular nodules are highly suggestive of malignancy.[39]

Infective Endocarditis

Infective endocarditis (IE) is one of the most important and elusive mimics of systemic small vessel vasculitis at many different levels: clinical manifestations, laboratory abnormalities, and even at the histopathological level. Skin manifestations of IE may be a true mimic (without vessel wall inflammation) or a secondary vasculitis (leukocytoclastic vasculitis). Patients may present with fever, weight loss, constitutional symptoms, polyarthritis, skin rashes, extremity infarcts, cerebral lesions from the embolic phenomenon, and glomerulonephritis. Gram-positive organisms (*S aureus, S viridans,* or *bovis*) and *Bartonella* species have been associated with ANCA-positive IE. *Bartonella* species is particularly important as it is one of the most frequent causes of culture-negative IE in the United States.[40] IE may be preceded by other sites of infection such as recurrent sinusitis, raising suspicion for GPA, especially in the presence of a positive ANCA test. ANCA positivity is seen in up to 33% of patients with IE, with available ANCA results.[41–43] Many case reports or series have reported that the combination of the indirect immunofluorescence testing for c-ANCA and p-ANCA with the antigen-specific enzyme-linked immunosorbent assay tests for anti-PR3 and anti-MPO may improve the specificity of ANCA testing. Nevertheless, patients with IE have more frequent c-ANCA than p-ANCA (84% vs 14%); and PR3-ANCA compared with MPO-ANCA and dual PR3 and MPO-ANCA (63% vs 17% vs 10%).[42] Other laboratory test abnormalities, such as anemia, high ESR, and CRP are indistinguishable from vasculitis. Rheumatoid factor may be elevated in IE, as well as in up to 70% of patients with GPA. Differentiating between AAV and IE may be challenging and important features that may help establish the diagnosis of IE include the presence of positive blood cultures, thrombocytopenia, low complement levels, the onset of a new heart murmur, and the presence of valve vegetation in the echocardiogram; all of these are either absent or rarely seen in AAV.[43] The renal histology may also help distinguish between AAV and IE. Different histological types may be seen in infectious endocarditis such as endocapillary proliferative, membranoproliferative, and crescentic glomerulonephritis. Immunofluorescence may show an immune complex-mediated or pauci-immune immunologic mechanism. Most cases show positive immunofluorescence of the mesangial area, and some also show deposition in the basement membrane.[44,45] Even in the cases of pauci-immune glomerulonephritis on immunofluorescence, mesangial subepithelial deposits can sometimes be seen on electron microscopy, which could help differentiate from AAV. Patients with AAV more frequently have pulmonary and peripheral nerve system involvement. Interestingly, patients with IE and positive ANCA were noted to have more frequently documented vegetations on the echocardiogram in one study, and more ischemic lesions on cerebral MRI in another report.[43] Renal impairment also tended to be more frequent in patients with positive ANCA.[42] These associations, however, were not observed across all studies. A case of culture-negative, positive PR3-ANCA, and pauci-immune glomerulonephritis IE can be very difficult to distinguish from AAV, however, this distinction is critical because of the severe negative consequences of immunosuppressive therapy in the setting of an infection.

Coronavirus Disease 2019 (COVID-19)

A thrombogenic vasculopathy with different clinical manifestations has been linked to COVID-19. Vascular dysfunction in COVID-19 may result in alveolar hemorrhage, pulmonary thrombosis, deep vein thrombosis, and multiorgan venous and arterial thromboses with a high risk of mortality.[46] Some cases have been associated with findings of true secondary vasculitis affecting many different organs, primarily the skin. Herein, we highlight the COVID-19-associated non-vasculitic skin and brain lesions, that mimic vasculitis. Many case reports or series have described necrotic skin lesions in up to 6% of patients, mostly associated with older age, severe disease, and a higher risk of mortality.[47] These lesions have been characterized by a pauci-immune thrombogenic vasculopathy with terminal complement activation in the vessel walls, and occasional Severe Acute Respiratory Syndrome Coronavirus 2 (SARS-CoV-2) spike protein deposition.[47–49] Some cases have shown extensive cutaneous vascular thrombosis in the absence of inflammatory cells. Another situation where COVID-19 may mimic vasculitis includes disseminated intravascular coagulation in critically ill patients with clinical manifestations of ischemia in the fingers and toes (cyanosis and gangrene). Single or multifocal central nervous system (CNS) lesions have been reported in association with COVID-19 and raised the question of possible CNS vasculitis. However, brain neuropathological studies have reported findings of ischemia without evidence of vasculitis. Mechanisms of thromboembolism are favored over vasculitis.[48]

Cocaine-Induced Midline Destructive Lesions

Inhalation of nasal cocaine is well-known to cause nasal ischemia and necrosis with the destruction of the nasal septum. Early nasal lesions consist of nasal mucosa congestion, crusting, and bleeding. The continuous use of cocaine can cause more extensive destructive lesions affecting the septum, inferior, middle, and superior turbinates, lateral nasal wall, sinonasal walls, and the floor of the nasal cavity.[50] Clinical distinction between cocaine-induced midline destructive lesions (CIMDL) and GPA may be very difficult, particularly in patients with upper airway-limited GPA presentations and because of the high frequency of ANCA positivity associated with CIMDL (up to 72%),[50] and lower frequency of ANCA positivity in GPA without renal involvement (~60%). Histopathology in CIMDL shows more often non-specific findings of inflammation, necrosis, and fibrosis. When compared to GPA, extravascular necrosis, microabscesses, granulomas, and giant cells were not seen with cocaine use and these may be helpful in the diagnosis of GPA when present.[51] Some studies comparing GPA with CIMDL could not find a distinguishing factor in the immunofluorescence ANCA test between the two groups. However, it has been reported that ANCA reacting to human neutrophil elastase was found in a higher-than-expected frequency in CIMDL, and not present in GPA.[52] Routine immunofluorescence ANCA testing alone may not allow for the differentiation between GPA and CIMDL but detailed analysis of antigen specificity is important in diagnostic confirmation. Another factor that may be helpful in distinguishing the two conditions is the frequent lack of systemic inflammation, despite extensive midline destructive lesions in CIMDL.

CUTANEOUS VASCULITIS MIMICS

Many non-vasculitic cutaneous disorders cause lesions that may be clinically indistinguishable from vasculitic skin lesions. Lesions may present in different stages and include a great variety of manifestations such as urticaria, petechiae, purpura, papules, hemorrhagic vesicles and bullae, subcutaneous nodules, livedo, ulcers, and gangrene. Skin biopsy is the gold standard for the diagnosis of cutaneous vasculitis but is not always definitive.

Pyoderma Gangrenosum

Pyoderma gangrenosum is a rare inflammatory disorder, classified as a neutrophilic dermatosis, and characterized by chronic and recurrent painful skin ulcers (see **Fig. 2C**). There are several distinct clinical variations of pyoderma gangrenosum with classic (or ulcerative) pyoderma gangrenosum being characterized by erythematous or violaceous papules or pustules, evolving into ulcers or necrotic plaques, usually in the legs.[53,54] Mucosal lesions (oropharynx or genital) may need to be differentiated from Behçet disease. Pathergy phenomenon resulting in the development of skin lesions at sites of injury is very common in pyoderma gangrenosum.[54] Disorders most associated with classic pyoderma gangrenosum are inflammatory bowel disease and rheumatoid arthritis. The diagnosis of pyoderma gangrenosum is very difficult as histopathological features are not specific and biopsies are non-diagnostic. Exclusion of other causes of skin ulcers, such as vasculitis, is essential.

Cholesterol Crystal Embolization

Embolization of cholesterol crystals from atheromatous plaques in the major vessel walls results in a variety of clinical manifestations. Microemboli of cholesterol crystals may lodge in small and medium arteries, affecting multiple organs, especially the kidneys, skin, gastrointestinal system, and brain. Risk factors for atherosclerosis, male sex, older age, and anticoagulation are major risk factors for cholesterol crystal embolization.[55] Clinical manifestations depend on the anatomic location and extent of organ involvement. Common symptoms are non-specific including constitutional symptoms, weight loss, fever, and myalgias. Patients may also develop acute neurologic deficits, amaurosis fugax, polyneuropathies, acute renal failure, and skin changes, primarily livedo reticularis.[56] Laboratory test results overlap with systemic small vessel vasculitis with elevated ESR and CRP, anemia, and hypereosinophilia. In contrast to the systemic small vessel vasculitides, patients with cholesterol crystal embolization may

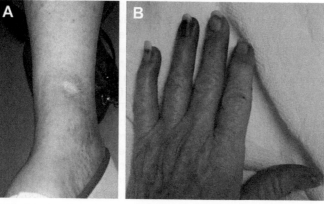

Fig. 2. Mimics of cutaneous vasculitis. (*A*) Livedoid vasculopathy with atrophie blanche, (*B*) cholesterol crystal embolization, and (*C*) pyoderma gangrenosum.

have thrombocytopenia. Cutaneous manifestations also vary and closely mimic vasculitis with livedo of limbs, cyanosis (**Fig. 2**B), ulcers, and gangrene of extremities. Cholesterol crystal embolization skin lesions are more common in the feet and toes, generally bilaterally. Clinical diagnosis requires a high degree of suspicion. Early diagnosis is often missed but remains crucial given the poor prognosis associated with multisystem cholesterol crystal embolization. The histopathologic hallmark of cholesterol crystal embolization is the finding of cholesterol clefts (intravascular cholesterol crystals).[57]

Calciphylaxis

Calciphylaxis is a rare, non-inflammatory, cutaneous vasculopathy that causes painful ischemic skin lesions. Skin manifestations are the result of micro-vessel calcification, intimal fibrosis, hyperplasia, and thrombosis in the subcutaneous tissue and dermis.[58] Vessel occlusion results in ischemia and necrosis of epidermal and adipose tissue. Initial skin lesions may appear as induration, plaques, nodules, livedo, or purpura. Extravascular calcification is common.[58,59] The disease has been described in association with hemodialysis or peritoneal dialysis, hence the alternative term, calcific uremic arteriolopathy. It occurs in up to 4% of hemodialysis patients but can occur in nonuremic patients as well. Other risk factors include elevated calcium and phosphate levels, obesity, and diabetes mellitus. Although skin biopsy is considered the best tool to confirm a clinically suspected diagnosis, it carries the risk of provoking a new ulcer and infection. Therefore, the diagnosis of calciphylaxis in the presence of a typical painful necrotic ulcer in a patient with end-stage renal disease (ESRD) may be established without histologic confirmation. Conversely, early or atypical skin lesions, in the absence of ESRD, may require biopsy to exclude other causes, including necrotizing small vessel vasculitis.[59] The presence of extravascular subcutaneous net-like calcification on plain radiographs may offer strong suspicion for calciphylaxis when the biopsy is inconclusive.

Livedoid Vasculopathy

Livedoid vasculopathy is a thrombo-occlusive condition that causes chronic painful recurrent ulcers of the legs, mainly in the ankles.[60] It is more common in women. The ulcers are very slow to heal and frequently recur. Early lesions may consist of painful erythematous nodules, purpuric papules or plaques, that rapidly evolve into ulcerations. The typical appearance of the star-shaped white atrophic scars has led to the synonymous use of the term "atrophie blanche" (**Fig. 2**A). However, not all cases of atrophie blanche are due to livedoid vasculopathy and a distinction has been suggested: (1) atrophie blanche associated with livedoid vasculopathy, and (2) atrophie blanche in chronic venous insufficiency.[61] The histopathology of livedoid vasculopathy is characterized by intraluminal thrombosis (occlusion of dermal vessels by fibrin thrombi), endothelial proliferation, and subintimal hyaline degeneration. Although a sparse perivascular lymphocytic infiltration may be seen and immunofluorescence may demonstrate immunoglobulin (IgG and IgM) and complement (C3) in the vessel walls; vasculitis is not present in livedoid vasculopathy.[62] Increased coagulation and/or impaired fibrinolysis likely play a central role in pathogenesis. At least half of the patients have a hypercoagulable risk factor such as antiphospholipid antibodies or factor V Leiden mutation.[62] Livedoid vasculopathy ulcers may mimic both small and medium vessel cutaneous vasculitis. The diagnosis is based on clinical, laboratory (hypercoagulability studies if clinically indicated), and histopathology abnormalities. The appearance and location of the ulcers or scars (eg, atrophie blanche) may be highly suggestive in some patients; however, a biopsy may be necessary to confirm the diagnosis and exclude mimicking conditions.

CENTRAL NERVOUS SYSTEM VASCULITIS MIMICS
Reversible Cerebral Vasoconstriction Syndrome

Reversible cerebral vasoconstriction syndrome (RCVS) is a heterogenous disorder caused by non-inflammatory vasoconstriction of intracerebral arteries. The diffuse intracerebral vessel spasm may be triggered by vasoactive medications (eg, pseudoephedrine), exertion, or may occur during the postpartum period. It is more common in young women and people with a history of migraine. RCVS is the most frequent and challenging mimicker of primary angiitis of the CNS (PACNS), as both conditions are characterized by a diffuse vessel involvement pattern. Patients with RCVS typically present with a sudden severe headache, often referred to as thunderclap headache, that can recur over a short time, and may result in stroke, neurologic deficits, or hemorrhage.[63] Initial brain MRI may be normal or shows cortical-only infarctions or vasogenic edema in RCVS, as opposed to PACNS when nearly all patients have an initial abnormal brain MRI.[64] In PACNS, the headache is usually subacute and less severe. Cerebral arteriogram is characterized by alternating areas of stenosis and ectasia in multiple vessel beds, similar in both conditions. The arteriogram is suggestive of RCVS if the abnormalities show reversibility within a short period.[65] The spinal fluid is helpful in differentiating the two conditions as it is usually normal in RCVS and shows increased cells and/or protein levels in nearly all patients with PACNS. The distinction between RCVS and PACNS may be challenging but it is crucial as immunosuppressive medications have no role in the treatment of RCVS.

DISCUSSION

The 2012 Chapel Hill Consensus Conference definitions of the primary vasculitides provide a good framework for the clinician to structure a differential diagnosis. The differential includes not only diseases that can cause secondary vasculitis, such as infections or drugs; but also, non-inflammatory diseases causing a vasculopathy in the same vascular beds. Although there can be some overlap in the size of affected blood vessels in primary vasculitis, odd patterns of vessel involvement, such as concomitant small and larger vessels or intracranial and extracranial involvement, should prompt one to consider mimics more strongly. In addition, the presence of blood cell line cytopenia would be atypical for primary forms of vasculitis.

SUMMARY

The differential diagnosis for primary forms of systemic vasculitis can be broad including secondary vasculitis and non-inflammatory mimics. Increased awareness of the vasculitis mimics is crucial to prevent toxicities from unnecessary immunosuppressive treatment. The pattern of vascular involvement, extravascular manifestations, and histopathology can help to differentiate between them.

CLINICS CARE POINTS

- Vasculitis should be considered in any patient presenting with systemic inflammatory disease affecting multiple organs or patients with unexplained ischemia, however, it is always important to exclude the vasculitis mimics.
- Mimics of vasculitis consist of non-inflammatory vasculopathies with a similar vessel distribution as primary forms of vasculitis, and include diseases that, at times, can also cause secondary vasculitis (eg, infections, drugs).
- Cutaneous small vessel vasculitis can have a long list of mimics to consider, including pyoderma gangrenosum, cholesterol crystal embolization, calciphylaxis, and livedoid vasculopathy

DISCLOSURE

J.M. Springer has served as a consultant for Chemocentryx. A. Villa-Forte has served as consultant for Chemocentryx and Amgen.

REFERENCES

1. Jennette JC, Falk RJ, Bacon PA, et al. 2012 revised International Chapel Hill Consensus Conference Nomenclature of Vasculitides. Arthritis Rheum 2013; 65:1–11.
2. Grayson PC, Maksimowicz-McKinnon K, Clark TM, et al. Distribution of arterial lesions in Takayasu's arteritis and giant cell arteritis. Ann Rheum Dis 2012;71: 1329–34.
3. Banerjee S, Bagheri M, Sandfort V, et al. Vascular calcification in patients with large-vessel vasculitis compared to patients with hyperlipidemia. Semin Arthritis Rheum 2019;48:1068–73.
4. Sadda SR, Nee M, Miller NR, et al. Clinical spectrum of posterior ischemic optic neuropathy. Am J Ophthalmol 2001;132:743–50.
5. Dunker S, Hsu HY, Sebag J, et al. Perioperative risk factors for posterior ischemic optic neuropathy. J Am Coll Surg 2002;194:705–10.
6. Hayreh SS. Posterior ischaemic optic neuropathy: clinical features, pathogenesis, and management. Eye (Lond) 2004;18:1188–206.
7. Carrer M, Vignals C, Berard X, et al. Retrospective multicentric study comparing infectious and non-infectious aortitis. Clin Infect Dis 2022;76(3):e1369–78.
8. Brown SL, Busuttil RW, Baker JD, et al. Bacteriologic and surgical determinants of survival in patients with mycotic aneurysms. J Vasc Surg 1984;1:541–7.
9. Johnson JR, Ledgerwood AM, Lucas CE. Mycotic aneurysm. New concepts in therapy. Arch Surg 1983;118:577–82.

10. Moneta GL, Taylor LM Jr, Yeager RA, et al. Surgical treatment of infected aortic aneurysm. Am J Surg 1998;175:396–9.
11. Neptune ER, Frischmeyer PA, Arking DE, et al. Dysregulation of TGF-beta activation contributes to pathogenesis in Marfan syndrome. Nat Genet 2003;33:407–11.
12. Gott VL, Greene PS, Alejo DE, et al. Replacement of the aortic root in patients with Marfan's syndrome. N Engl J Med 1999;340:1307–13.
13. Judge DP, Dietz HC. Marfan's syndrome. Lancet 2005;366:1965–76.
14. Pepin M, Schwarze U, Superti-Furga A, et al. Clinical and genetic features of Ehlers-Danlos syndrome type IV, the vascular type. N Engl J Med 2000;342:673–80.
15. Shalhub S, Byers PH, Hicks KL, et al. A multi-institutional experience in the aortic and arterial pathology in individuals with genetically confirmed vascular Ehlers-Danlos syndrome. J Vasc Surg 2019;70:1543–54.
16. Malfait F, Francomano C, Byers P, et al. The 2017 international classification of the Ehlers-Danlos syndromes. Am J Med Genet C Semin Med Genet 2017;175:8–26.
17. Loeys BL, Chen J, Neptune ER, et al. A syndrome of altered cardiovascular, craniofacial, neurocognitive and skeletal development caused by mutations in TGFBR1 or TGFBR2. Nat Genet 2005;37:275–81.
18. Loeys BL, Schwarze U, Holm T, et al. Aneurysm syndromes caused by mutations in the TGF-beta receptor. N Engl J Med 2006;355:788–98.
19. Bondy CA, Turner Syndrome Study G. Care of girls and women with Turner syndrome: a guideline of the Turner Syndrome Study Group. J Clin Endocrinol Metab 2007;92:10–25.
20. Gunther DF, Eugster E, Zagar AJ, et al. Ascertainment bias in Turner syndrome: new insights from girls who were diagnosed incidentally in prenatal life. Pediatrics 2004;114:640–4.
21. Lin AE, Lippe B, Rosenfeld RG. Further delineation of aortic dilation, dissection, and rupture in patients with Turner syndrome. Pediatrics 1998;102:e12.
22. Hendricks NJ, Matsumoto AH, Angle JF, et al. Is fibromuscular dysplasia underdiagnosed? A comparison of the prevalence of FMD seen in CORAL trial participants versus a single institution population of renal donor candidates. Vasc Med 2014;19:363–7.
23. Olin JW, Froehlich J, Gu X, et al. The United States Registry for Fibromuscular Dysplasia: results in the first 447 patients. Circulation 2012;125:3182–90.
24. Green R, Gu X, Kline-Rogers E, et al. Differences between the pediatric and adult presentation of fibromuscular dysplasia: results from the US Registry. Pediatr Nephrol 2016;31:641–50.
25. Olin JW, Gornik HL, Bacharach JM, et al. Fibromuscular dysplasia: state of the science and critical unanswered questions: a scientific statement from the American Heart Association. Circulation 2014;129:1048–78.
26. Kamisawa T, Funata N, Hayashi Y, et al. A new clinicopathological entity of IgG4-related autoimmune disease. J Gastroenterol 2003;38:982–4.
27. Kasashima S, Zen Y, Kawashima A, et al. Inflammatory abdominal aortic aneurysm: close relationship to IgG4-related periaortitis. Am J Surg Pathol 2008;32:197–204.
28. Stone JR. Aortitis, periaortitis, and retroperitoneal fibrosis, as manifestations of IgG4-related systemic disease. Curr Opin Rheumatol 2011;23:88–94.
29. Ozawa M, Fujinaga Y, Asano J, et al. Clinical features of IgG4-related periaortitis/periarteritis based on the analysis of 179 patients with IgG4-related disease: a case-control study. Arthritis Res Ther 2017;19:223.
30. Smyrk TC. Pathological features of IgG4-related sclerosing disease. Curr Opin Rheumatol 2011;23:74–9.

31. Wallace ZS, Deshpande V, Mattoo H, et al. IgG4-related disease: clinical and laboratory features in one hundred twenty-five patients. Arthritis Rheumatol 2015;67: 2466–75.

32. Carruthers MN, Khosroshahi A, Augustin T, et al. The diagnostic utility of serum IgG4 concentrations in IgG4-related disease. Ann Rheum Dis 2015;74:14–8.

33. Haroche J, Amoura Z, Dion E, et al. Cardiovascular involvement, an overlooked feature of Erdheim-Chester disease: report of 6 new cases and a literature review. Medicine (Baltimore) 2004;83:371–92.

34. Serratrice J, Granel B, De Roux C, et al. "Coated aorta": a new sign of Erdheim-Chester disease. J Rheumatol 2000;27:1550–3.

35. Cavalli G, Guglielmi B, Berti A, et al. The multifaceted clinical presentations and manifestations of Erdheim-Chester disease: comprehensive review of the literature and of 10 new cases. Ann Rheum Dis 2013;72:1691–5.

36. Haroche J, Arnaud L, Amoura Z. Erdheim-Chester disease. Curr Opin Rheumatol 2012;24:53–9.

37. Konstantinov KN, Ulff-Moller CJ, Tzamaloukas AH. Infections and antineutrophil cytoplasmic antibodies: triggering mechanisms. Autoimmun Rev 2015;14:201–3.

38. Gadkowski LB, Stout JE. Cavitary pulmonary disease. Clin Microbiol Rev 2008; 21:305–33, table of contents.

39. Nin CS, de Souza VV, Alves GR, et al. Solitary lung cavities: CT findings in malignant and non-malignant disease. Clin Radiol 2016;71:1132–6.

40. Houpikian P, Raoult D. Blood culture-negative endocarditis in a reference center: etiologic diagnosis of 348 cases. Medicine (Baltimore) 2005;84:162–73.

41. Ying CM, Yao DT, Ding HH, et al. Infective endocarditis with antineutrophil cytoplasmic antibody: report of 13 cases and literature review. PLoS One 2014;9: e89777.

42. Langlois V, Lesourd A, Girszyn N, et al. Antineutrophil cytoplasmic antibodies associated with infective endocarditis. Medicine (Baltimore) 2016;95:e2564.

43. Mahr A, Batteux F, Tubiana S, et al. Brief report: prevalence of antineutrophil cytoplasmic antibodies in infective endocarditis. Arthritis Rheumatol 2014;66:1672–7.

44. Majumdar A, Chowdhary S, Ferreira MA, et al. Renal pathological findings in infective endocarditis. Nephrol Dial Transplant 2000;15:1782–7.

45. Raybould JE, Raybould AL, Morales MK, et al. Bartonella endocarditis and pauci-immune glomerulonephritis: a case report and review of the literature. Infect Dis Clin Pract (Baltim Md) 2016;24:254–60.

46. Menter T, Haslbauer JD, Nienhold R, et al. Postmortem examination of COVID-19 patients reveals diffuse alveolar damage with severe capillary congestion and variegated findings in lungs and other organs suggesting vascular dysfunction. Histopathology 2020;77:198–209.

47. McGonagle D, Bridgewood C, Ramanan AV, et al. COVID-19 vasculitis and novel vasculitis mimics. Lancet Rheumatol 2021;3:e224–33.

48. Llamas-Velasco M, Munoz-Hernandez P, Lazaro-Gonzalez J, et al. Thrombotic occlusive vasculopathy in a skin biopsy from a livedoid lesion of a patient with COVID-19. Br J Dermatol 2020;183:591–3.

49. Magro C, Mulvey JJ, Berlin D, et al. Complement associated microvascular injury and thrombosis in the pathogenesis of severe COVID-19 infection: a report of five cases. Transl Res 2020;220:1–13.

50. Trimarchi M, Gregorini G, Facchetti F, et al. Cocaine-induced midline destructive lesions: clinical, radiographic, histopathologic, and serologic features and their differentiation from Wegener granulomatosis. Medicine (Baltimore) 2001;80: 391–404.

51. Rachapalli SM, Kiely PD. Cocaine-induced midline destructive lesions mimicking ENT-limited Wegener's granulomatosis. Scand J Rheumatol 2008;37:477–80.
52. Wiesner O, Russell KA, Lee AS, et al. Antineutrophil cytoplasmic antibodies reacting with human neutrophil elastase as a diagnostic marker for cocaine-induced midline destructive lesions but not autoimmune vasculitis. Arthritis Rheum 2004;50:2954–65.
53. Callen JP, Jackson JM. Pyoderma gangrenosum: an update. Rheum Dis Clin North Am 2007;33:787–802, vi.
54. Ahn C, Negus D, Huang W. Pyoderma gangrenosum: a review of pathogenesis and treatment. Expert Rev Clin Immunol 2018;14:225–33.
55. Agrawal A, Ziccardi MR, Witzke C, et al. Cholesterol embolization syndrome: an under-recognized entity in cardiovascular interventions. J Interv Cardiol 2018;31:407–15.
56. Ghanem F, Vodnala D, Kalanakunta JK, et al. Cholesterol crystal embolization following plaque rupture: a systemic disease with unusual features. J Biomed Res 2017;31:82–94.
57. Falanga V, Fine MJ, Kapoor WN. The cutaneous manifestations of cholesterol crystal embolization. Arch Dermatol 1986;122:1194–8.
58. Nigwekar SU, Kroshinsky D, Nazarian RM, et al. Calciphylaxis: risk factors, diagnosis, and treatment. Am J Kidney Dis 2015;66:133–46.
59. Ghosh T, Winchester DS, Davis MDP, et al. Early clinical presentations and progression of calciphylaxis. Int J Dermatol 2017;56:856–61.
60. Callen JP. Livedoid vasculopathy: what it is and how the patient should be evaluated and treated. Arch Dermatol 2006;142:1481–2.
61. Alavi A, Hafner J, Dutz JP, et al. Livedoid vasculopathy: an in-depth analysis using a modified Delphi approach. J Am Acad Dermatol 2013;69:1033–42.e1.
62. Hairston BR, Davis MD, Pittelkow MR, et al. Livedoid vasculopathy: further evidence for procoagulant pathogenesis. Arch Dermatol 2006;142:1413–8.
63. de Boysson H, Parienti JJ, Mawet J, et al. Primary angiitis of the CNS and reversible cerebral vasoconstriction syndrome: a comparative study. Neurology 2018;91:e1468–78.
64. Singhal AB, Topcuoglu MA, Fok JW, et al. Reversible cerebral vasoconstriction syndromes and primary angiitis of the central nervous system: clinical, imaging, and angiographic comparison. Ann Neurol 2016;79:882–94.
65. Calabrese LH, Dodick DW, Schwedt TJ, et al. Narrative review: reversible cerebral vasoconstriction syndromes. Ann Intern Med 2007;146:34–44.

Ear, Nose, and Throat Manifestations of Vasculitis and Other Systemic Autoimmune Diseases: Otologic, Sinus, and Airway

Isaac Wasserman, MD[a], Divya A. Chari, MD[a,b],
Stacey T. Gray, MD[a], Matthew R. Naunheim, MD[a],
Eli M. Miloslavsky, MD[c,*]

KEYWORDS

- Otology • SINUS • Otolaryngology • Vasculitis

KEY POINTS

- Otologic, sinus, and airway involvement can be the presenting manifestation of vasculitis and other systemic rheumatic diseases.
- Ear, nose, and throat (ENT) involvement of rheumatic diseases can be difficult to distinguish from other more common etiologies, therefore, a high index of suspicion is required.
- Interpretation of audiology, endoscopic, and imaging findings as well as pathology is important in the diagnosis of ENT manifestations.
- Treatment of the underlying systemic disease is often effective for controlling ENT manifestations, however, both topical and surgical therapies are important aspects of therapy.

INTRODUCTION

Auricular, nasal, and laryngeal manifestations occur frequently in rheumatic diseases. Inflammatory ear, nose, and throat (ENT) processes often result in organ damage and have profound effects on quality of life. However, patients may experience delays in diagnosis and treatment due to non-specific symptoms, limited specificity of currently available testing, and a relative lack of data on treatment efficacy. Herein, we review the otologic, nasal, and laryngeal involvement of rheumatic diseases, focusing on their clinical presentation and diagnosis. ENT manifestations generally respond to

[a] Department of Otolaryngology, Massachusetts Eye and Ear Infirmary, Harvard Medical School, Boston, MA, USA; [b] Department of Otolaryngology, University of Massachusetts Memorial Health Center, Worcester, MA, USA; [c] Division of Rheumatology, Allergy and Immunology, Department of Medicine, Massachusetts General Hospital, Harvard Medical School, Boston, MA, USA
* Corresponding author. Massachusetts General Hospital, 55 Fruit Street, Yawkey 2B, Boston, MA 02114.
E-mail address: emiloslavsky@mgh.harvard.edu

Rheum Dis Clin N Am 49 (2023) 633–645
https://doi.org/10.1016/j.rdc.2023.03.012
0889-857X/23/© 2023 Elsevier Inc. All rights reserved.

treatment of the systemic disease, which is outside the scope of this review; however, adjunctive topical and surgical treatment approaches, as well as treatment of idiopathic inflammatory ENT manifestations will be reviewed.

OTOLOGY

Rheumatic diseases can involve the organs of hearing and balance, occasionally presenting first with clinical symptoms isolated to the ear. Symptoms include hearing loss (conductive, sensorineural, or mixed), tinnitus, vertigo/impaired vestibular function, or inflammatory ear symptoms (including otorrhea and aural fullness). These features are non-specific, however, and can be found in a variety of different etiologies. Therefore, a high index of suspicion combined with other systemic findings are required to identify a rheumatic disease process. An otologic-focused history and exam should be performed that includes an otoscopic examination, assessment of cranial nerve function, tuning fork exam, and, when appropriate, vestibular testing. In addition, a comprehensive audiologic evaluation including measurement of pure tone thresholds, word recognition score, tympanometry, and acoustic reflex testing is strongly recommended.

A conventional audiogram includes pure tone thresholds (the lowest decibel required to register a sound at least half of the time) of air and bone conduction across a wide range of frequencies (250–8 kHz). Examining various pure tone thresholds allows one to assess the severity of hearing loss and categorize it as (1) sensorineural (SNHL), where air and bone conduction thresholds will overlap, (2) conductive (CHL), which appears as an air-bone gap in the conduction thresholds, or (3) mixed (MHL), which has both an air-bone gap and overall decrease in the bone thresholds.

Autoimmune Inner Ear Disease

Primary autoimmune inner ear disease (AIED) is a rapidly progressive, bilateral hearing loss that occurs over a period of weeks to months.[1] The annual incidence of AIED is estimated at fewer than five cases per 100,000, with a prevalence of 15/100,000 and a female sex predominance in women in the third and sixth decades of life.[2] Although typically AIED occurs bilaterally, some patients present with unilateral disease initially. Over half of the patients will have concomitant vestibular disturbances.[3,4] A hallmark of primary AIED is responsiveness to high-dose steroid treatment, and it must be differentiated from secondary AIED that occurs in the setting of systemic autoimmune diseases. Unlike secondary AIED, cartilage destruction or middle ear disease is absent in AIED (**Fig. 1**).

Responsiveness to glucocorticoids with improvement in pure tone thresholds is expected, but the challenge is that most patients will experience a recurrent decline in hearing once the steroid treatment is discontinued. Intratympanic corticosteroids can be used, particularly in patients presenting with sudden or rapidly progressive sensorineural hearing loss. Risks of intratympanic injection include otorrhea, persistent tympanic membrane perforation, temporary altered taste disturbance, and vestibular symptoms. A variety of steroid-sparing agents has been studied in patients with AIED, including methotrexate, mycophenolate, azathioprine, cyclophosphamide, tumor necrosis alpha inhibitors (TNF)-inhibitors, intravenous immunoglobulin (IVIG), and anakinra among others.[4–6] Methotrexate was the most common steroid-sparing agent used before a negative randomized trial in autoimmune hearing loss published in 2003.[5] Our current approach is to start with mycophenolate mofetil and consider a TNF-inhibitor as second-line therapy; however, no high-quality data currently exist with the use of either agent. The natural history of AIED typically results in severe to profound sensorineural hearing loss in one or both ears.

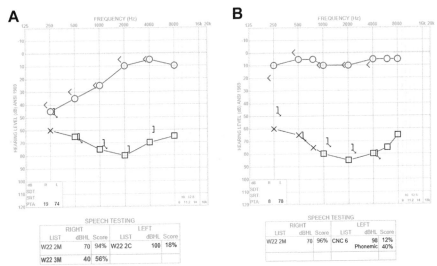

Fig. 1. (A) Pre-treatment audiogram of a 30-year-old woman with bilateral AIED. The audiogram shows asymmetric sensorineural hearing loss, left worse than right, with poor word recognition score on the left (18% at 100 dB hearing level [dBHL]) and excellent word recognition score on the right (94% at 70 dBHL). (B) Post-treatment audiogram after a 4-week course of high-dose oral steroids. Audiogram shows improvement in the pure tone thresholds on the right to the normal range in all frequencies with excellent word recognition score and no change in pure tone thresholds on the left with poor word recognition score (12% at 98 dBHL).

Cogan's Syndrome

Presenting with non-syphilitic ocular keratitis and audio-vestibular disruption, Cogan's syndrome can result in sensorineural hearing loss, tinnitus, and vertigo. The otologic manifestation may be separated from the ocular presentation by 6 months, but 85% of patients will demonstrate ocular and vestibulocochlear symptoms within 2 years.[7] Hearing loss is bilateral and, although fluctuating, is often progressive and occurs in 44% to 60% of patients with Cogan's.[8,9] The vestibular manifestations can be bilateral and include vertigo with resulting nausea and vomiting.

Antineutrophil Cytoplasmic Antibody -Associated Vasculitides

Granulomatosis with polyangiitis (GPA) is a necrotizing vasculitis of small- and medium-sized vessels. Of patients with GPA, 20% to 40% have otologic involvement,[10] commonly affecting the middle ear and mastoid.[11,12] Involvement of these structures may result in Eustachian tube obstruction with secondary serous otitis media and resulting conductive hearing loss. Less commonly, some patients may experience purulent otitis media or granulomatous involvement of the middle ear and mastoid. Progressive cases can extend to involve the inner ear, resulting in a sensorineural component of hearing loss, as well as vestibular symptoms.

Sarcoidosis

Characterized by noncaseating granulomas, sarcoidosis classically targets the lungs, although it can affect myriad organ systems. Otologic involvement is rare, and consistent estimates of prevalence are unavailable. Because of its predilection for neurologic involvement presenting symptoms typically include sensorineural hearing loss and vestibular dysfunction.[13]

Relapsing Polychondritis

Affecting hyaline elastic and fibrous cartilaginous tissues, relapsing polychondritis (RP) is episodic and generally progressive.[14] The most common feature (in nearly 90% of patients) is auricular chondritis that presents with acute swelling, erythema, and tenderness of the ear, sparing the lobule.[15] This inflammation may result in conductive hearing loss (secondary to chondritis of the auditory tubal cartilage). There may also be involvement of the inner ear (reported in a smaller proportion of cases), which may result in sensorineural hearing loss (thought to be secondary to vasculitis of the labyrinthine artery or its cochlear branch).

Systemic Lupus Erythematosus

Sensorineural hearing loss can be associated with systemic lupus erythematosus (SLE), but reports range from 15% to 66%, in part secondary to the asymptomatic severity of the hearing loss.[16,17] This hearing loss is typically bilateral and high frequency without correlation to the severity of the underlying disease or treatment. Vestibular symptoms are variable, with reports documenting incidence between 5% and 70% of patients with SLE.[18]

Idiopathic Sudden Sensorineural Hearing Loss

Unlike the hearing loss associated with primary AIED, the sensorineural hearing loss in idiopathic sudden sensorineural hearing loss (iSSNHL) occurs either all at once or over a few days (instead of over weeks to months). Another differentiation is the typical unilateral nature. Idiopathic sudden SNHL occurs annually in 5 to 20 people per 100,000.[19] Diagnosis is confirmed with an audiogram. Treatment consists of oral or intratympanic steroids, with a consideration of hyperbaric oxygen. Recurrence is reported in 5% to 10% of patients.[20]

Summary

The ear—its external pinna, middle ear, as well as inner ear—is vulnerable to rheumatic disorders. Elucidating the underlying cause is important for determining both the duration of treatment (eg, short-course steroids in iSSNHL) and the need for steroid-sparing agents (eg, secondary AIED and relapsing primary AIED). Surgical implantation of a cochlear implant for severe/profound sensorineural hearing loss may be necessary in refractory cases.

RHINOLOGY

"Congestion, facial pressure, and nasal discharge." These symptoms are common and present in myriad sinonasal disease processes including rheumatologic disorders. Generally, systemic signs of underlying inflammation serve as the clue, but, rarely, sinonasal manifestations can be the presenting symptom of a rheumatologic disorder. Additionally, epistaxis and anosmia are other symptoms observed. Persistent nasal crusting should raise suspicion of an underlying inflammatory process. To complement the sinonasal history including prior sinus and upper respiratory tract infections, surgeries, asthma, and allergies, direct visualization of the nasal cavity with an endoscope is often necessary. In addition, non-contrast axial imaging is typically employed to determine the degree of sinonasal disease.

Antineutrophil Cytoplasmic Antibody -Associated Vasculitides

Sinonasal involvement has been documented in up to 90% of GPA cases.[21] Lesions in the nasal and paranasal mucosa result in nasal obstruction, crusting, rhinorrhea, hyposmia, as well as epiphora secondary to nasolacrimal duct obstruction. Involvement of the turbinates, nasal bones, and septum are also seen. Physical exam, including endoscopy, demonstrates inflamed, ulcerated, and often "cobblestone-appearing" mucosa. Computed tomography can demonstrate mucosal thickening (in up to 88% of patients with GPA), along with bony erosion (up to 60%; **Fig. 2**).[22,23] Biopsy is often undertaken, but the yield is low, with one study demonstrating only 24% of biopsies consistent with GPA in the setting of GPA.[24]

Eosinophilic granulomatosis with polyangiitis (EGPA) can also result in sinonasal symptoms. Presentation is more similar to allergic rhinitis, with obstruction, sinusitis, and nasal polyps found in nearly 60% of affected patients.[25]

Sarcoidosis

Involvement of the sinonasal tract in sarcoidosis has been reported in 1% to 30% of patients affected.[26,27] Nasal symptoms include obstruction, congestion, rhinorrhea, anosmia, crusting, and septal perforation. Endoscopy may demonstrate small nodules or granulation, crusts, or synechiae of the mucosa. Biopsy of affected mucosa should reveal non-caseating epithelioid giant cell granulomas.

Cocaine-Induced Midline Destructive Lesion

Positive antineutrophil cytoplasmic antibody (ANCA) can also be seen in cocaine-induced midline destructive lesions (CIMDL), with corresponding radiographic and histopathologic abnormalities of nasal structures. Septal perforation and crusting are hallmarks of CIMDL.[28] Cutaneous ulcers along the nasal tip, sub-nasal sulcus, and philtrum may also be present. Among users of cocaine, there is an approximately 5% prevalence of this complication.[29] There are no disease-specific histopathologic

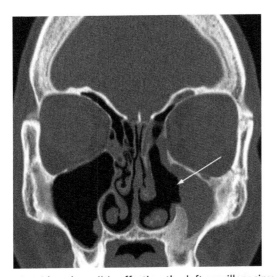

Fig. 2. Granulomatosis with polyangiitis affecting the left maxillary sinus with significant sclerosis of the maxillary sinus walls and absence of the medial maxillary wall (*arrow;* without prior surgery).

features of CIMDL as there is an overlap with GPA. Cocaine metabolites and human neutrophil elastase (HNE) ANCA are two systemic tests that can help differentiate CIMDL from GPA. Cocaine can also induce a double positive ANCA, which can serve as a clue to this etiology.[30] The role of immunosuppression is limited, with the mainstay of treatment being the cessation of cocaine use.

Relapsing Polychondritis

Nasal symptoms of RP include pain, erythema, crusting, and congestion. As the disease progresses, a saddle nose deformity may develop (nearly one-quarter of patients at the time of diagnosis), although over 50% of patients with polychondritis will have nasal cartilage involvement.[31] Biopsy demonstrates chondrolysis, chondritis, and perichondritis.

Immunoglobin G4-Related Disease

Immunoglobin G4-related disease (IgG4-RD) is a chronic fibro-inflammatory disease that can have manifestations throughout the body.[32] There are no good estimates of sinonasal involvement in this disease. The most common sinonasal structures involved are the maxillary sinus, ethmoid sinus, nasal cavity/septum, and sphenoid sinus (in decreasing frequency).[33] Symptoms include nasal obstruction/congestion, facial swelling, headache, and epistaxis. Serum IgG4 levels generally lack sensitivity and specificity for diagnosis, making a histopathologic examination of biopsies an integral part of the diagnosis.

Summary

Sinonasal manifestations of GPA, sarcoid, IgG4RD, RP, and cocaine use can be indistinguishable from one another. Therefore, diagnosis relies on serologic testing, identifying manifestations outside of the nose and ruling out a history of cocaine use. In isolated sinus disease with negative or equivocal serologies, biopsy is important to exclude other mimickers such as infection and malignancy. In a minority of patients, biopsy can be diagnostic of a systemic rheumatic process. The mainstay of treatment of most sinonasal manifestations of rheumatologic disorders is systemic (immunosuppressive) treatment. Surgical intervention is sometimes necessary to address an impending complication of sinus disease due to obstruction affecting the orbit or intracranial cavity. In select cases, especially EGPA, surgical intervention to address nasal polyps can also be utilized. Topical therapy with steroid sprays, irrigations, and emollients can often help improve patient symptomatology. Frequent endoscopic evaluation and repeat imaging are necessary to evaluate for disease progression and assessment of nasal disease.

LARYNGOLOGY

Although rare, manifestations of rheumatologic disorders in the larynx may result in dysphonia, dysphagia, or dyspnea.[34,35] Many conditions affecting the larynx result in similar, non-specific symptoms secondary to inflammation, including globus, dysphonia, dyspnea, and pain. On the other hand, given the exquisite sensitivity to inflammation of the vocal cords, dysphonia can sometimes be the presenting symptom of a rheumatologic disorder.[36]

Guidelines suggest indirect visualization of the larynx with laryngoscope with or without stroboscopy if voice changes persist for greater than 4 weeks.[37] If there is a known disease process, however, that can affect the airway, we recommended visualization of the larynx earlier than 4 weeks given the risk for airway compromise.

Stridor in a patient with known rheumatologic disease warrants an urgent airway evaluation by laryngology. Finally, routine radiologic imaging is generally unhelpful in clarifying the etiology of mucosal disease and inflammation.

Granulomatosis with Polyangiitis

Granulomatosis with polyangiitis (GPA) can lead to subglottic stenosis (SGS) in approximately 16% to 23% of patients,[38] while EGPA is a rarer cause of this complication.[39] Narrowing may be asymptomatic until an additional upper respiratory tract infection results in even more narrowing, leading to evaluation. Classically, narrowing in the subglottis (as opposed to the supraglottis) will lead to biphasic (inspiratory and expiratory) stridor **(Fig. 3)**. Of note, subglottic stenosis can progress despite seemingly quiescent systemic vasculitis.[40]

Both medical and surgical options are important for treating SGS because medical management alone is unlikely to resolve the stenosis. Various surgical options can help dilate the airway, including endoscopic balloon dilation, laser resection, and intra-lesional steroid injections. Open airway surgery to resect and reconstruct is typically reserved for late-stage or refractory cases. Often, multiple, repeat procedures

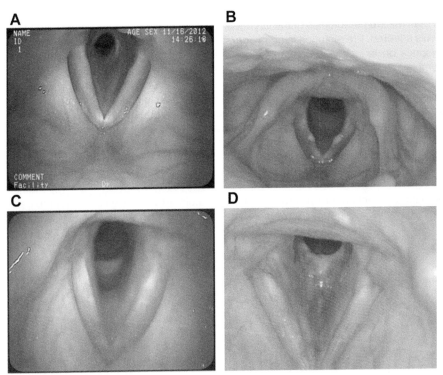

Fig. 3. (*A*) Isolated subglottic disease. This is the classically described subglottic stenosis that begins below the edges of the thyroid cartilage, involving the space occupied by the cricoid ring. Vocal folds are mobile, and symptoms are primarily shortness of breath. (*B*) Isolated glottic disease. (*C*) Infraglottic fibrosis with normal subglottis, including airway and voice symptoms secondary to fibrosis and swelling. (*D*) Involvement of the vocal folds and subglottis with fibrosis, narrowing, and reduced vocal fold motion. Symptoms include airway and voice symptoms.

are required to sustain airway patency.[41] Medical management has the potential to prevent or delay restenosis. Although prior studies suggested good outcomes with dilatation and intralesional steroids alone,[42] current treatment guidelines recommend immunosuppressive therapy for the management of actively inflamed subglottic stenosis.[43] It should be noted that subglottic stenosis can be both slow to respond and refractory to treatment; therefore, careful monitoring over a period of sustained treatment is important.

Sarcoidosis

Manifestations of sarcoidosis in the head and neck are present in approximately 9% of patients with sarcoidosis.[44] Laryngeal involvement is documented in only 1% to 5% of patients. Despite this, laryngeal sarcoidosis can sometimes be the initial (or only) site of involvement. Within the larynx, there is a predilection for the supraglottis and then subglottis (**Fig. 4**).[44] Presenting symptoms of hoarseness, dyspnea, stridor, dysphagia, and cough may be relatively mild despite extensive tissue involvement. In addition to systemic treatment, smaller lesions are amenable to intralesional steroid injection. Larger lesions leading to airway compromise can be treated surgically with laser-facilitated resection to facilitate a patent airway.

Relapsing Polychondritis

RP can lead to pathologies of the laryngeal cartilage framework with various anatomic levels affected. Presentation is often non-specific, with hoarseness, cough, wheezing, dyspnea on exertion, stridor, and tenderness of the larynx as common presenting complaints. Unlike disease processes that primarily affect the mucosa, there is a potential role for imaging through dedicated neck computed tomography.[45] Similarly, a pulmonary function test might demonstrate a non-reversible, obstructive pattern secondary to the collapse and stenosis of the airways. The primary change seen on histologic biopsy is loss of the mucopolysaccharide matrix that is followed by a reactive perichondrial mixed inflammatory matrix.[46] Surgical intervention is required only in cases where there is airway compromise.

Rheumatoid Arthritis

With its predilection for synovial tissue, rheumatoid arthritis (RA) can affect the cartilaginous joints within the larynx leading to hoarseness, dysphagia, globus sensation,

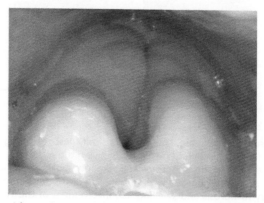

Fig. 4. Sarcoidosis, with a turban epiglottis, edema of the arytenoids—making it difficult to see the airway.

and, occasionally, stridor.[47] Estimates of laryngeal involvement range from 13% to 75% of patients with RA.[48] Inflammation can result in tenderness and erythema of the arytenoids; chronic inflammation can result in ankylosis of the cricoarytenoid joint, resulting in impairment of vocal fold movement, which can be life-threatening if bilateral. Apart from the involvement of the joint, rheumatoid nodules can develop on the vocal fold (**Fig. 5**). Surgical intervention is reserved for symptomatic nodules or treatment of a fixed cricoarytenoid joint.

Pemphigus and Pemphigoid

Although classically encountered through their dermatologic manifestations, the loosening of the epiderma–dermal junction in pemphigus can result in laryngeal presentations. Pemphigus classically presents with flaccid bullae, compared to the tenser plaques seen in pemphigoid. Isolated laryngeal involvement is rare, but nasal and laryngeal involvement can be quite widespread among patients with pemphigus (up to 49% in one review).[49] Laryngeal involvement often leads to hoarseness. The more flaccid lesions in the pemphigus will traditionally slough off when exposed to pressure (positive Nikolsky sign) of leaving a "tan, fibrous base with a halo of erythema" behind at the site of the lesion.[50] Histologic examination of a biopsy will reveal intraepithelial acantholysis that is subepithelial with involvement of the basement membrane.

Idiopathic Subglottic Stenosis

Although subglottic stenosis can result from myriad etiologies (including trauma and rheumatic disorders), approximately one in 400,000 people annually develop subglottic stenosis without an identifiable cause. There is an extensive female sex predilection, with the majority occurring in the third to fifth decades of life.[51] A rigorous history focusing on prior trauma to the airway (including intubations), as well as

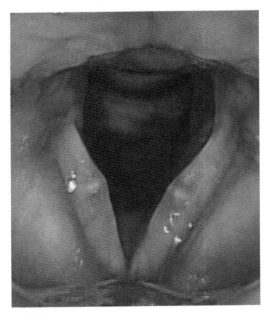

Fig. 5. Rheumatoid nodules.

evaluation of previously discussed etiologies is required. Treatment of idiopathic subglottic stenosis is primarily surgical as discussed above. Some experts suggest inhaled glucocorticoids and control of esophageal reflux[52] as adjunctive therapies.

Summary

Persistence of laryngeal or airway symptoms in a patient with a known rheumatologic condition warrants laryngeal evaluation with laryngoscopy. Computed tomography (CT) imaging is most helpful for conditions affecting the cartilage, such as RP. The most common sites of involvement differ between conditions with GPA—most commonly affecting the subglottis; sarcoid—the supraglottis; and rheumatoid arthritis—the arytenoids and vocal fold. Serologies can be helpful to confirm a suspicion but can sometimes be negative. A surgical biopsy can be useful in demonstrating laryngeal involvement. Surgical dilation with intralesional corticosteroid injections and systemic treatment of the underlying disease are the mainstays of therapy. Adjunct resection may be required to address persistent lesions, or if involvement threatens airway patency.

SUMMARY

Early recognition of otologic, sinonasal, and laryngeal manifestations of rheumatic diseases is critical to limit disease damage and improve quality of life. In addition to recognizing systemic symptoms of autoimmune disease, providers can glean clues to the underlying etiology from audiometry, endoscopic examination, and imaging of the affected areas. Because ENT manifestations can be treated with topical, systemic, and surgical approaches, collaboration between ENT and rheumatology physicians in caring for this patient population is paramount.

CLINICS CARE POINTS

- Because ENT manifestations often result in damage to the affected organ, distinguinshing between active disease and damage is critical to choosing the right treatment.
- Rheumatology involvement is important in the treatment of idiopathic inflammatory ENT disease that is responsive to immunosuppression such as Autoimmune Ear Disease, chondritis and inflammatory supraglottitis among others.

DISCLOSURE

The authors have nothing to disclose.

REFERENCES

1. Ruckenstein MJ. Autoimmune inner ear disease. Curr Opin Otolaryngol Head Neck Surg 2004;12(5):426–30.
2. Ciorba A, Corazzi V, Bianchini C, et al. Autoimmune inner ear disease (AIED): A diagnostic challenge. Int J Immunopathol Pharmacol 2018;32. https://doi.org/10.1177/2058738418808680.
3. Moscicki RA, San Martin JE, Quintero CH, et al. Serum antibody to inner ear proteins in patients with progressive hearing loss. Correlation with disease activity and response to corticosteroid treatment. JAMA 1994;272(8):611–6.

4. Broughton SS, Meyerhoff WE, Cohen SB. Immune-mediated inner ear disease: 10-year experience. Semin Arthritis Rheum 2004;34(2):544–8.

5. Harris JP, Weisman MH, Derebery JM, et al. Treatment of corticosteroid-responsive autoimmune inner ear disease with methotrexate: a randomized controlled trial. JAMA 2003;290(14):1875–83.

6. Buniel MC, Geelan-Hansen K, Weber PC, et al. Immunosuppressive therapy for autoimmune inner ear disease. Immunotherapy 2009;1(3):425–34.

7. Gluth MB, Baratz KH, Matteson EL, et al. Cogan syndrome: a retrospective review of 60 patients throughout a half century. Mayo Clin Proc 2006;81(4):483–8.

8. Vollertsen RS, McDonald TJ, Younge BR, et al. Cogan's syndrome: 18 cases and a review of the literature. Mayo Clin Proc 1986;61(5):344–61.

9. García Berrocal JR, Vargas JA, Vaquero M, et al. Cogan's syndrome: an oculo-audiovestibular disease. Postgrad Med 1999;75(883):262–4.

10. Naini AS, Ghorbani J, Montazer S, et al. Otologic Manifestations and Progression in Patients with Wegener's granulomatosis: A Survey in 55 Patients. Iranian Journal of Otorhinolaryngology 2017;29(95):327.

11. Rasmussen N. Management of the ear, nose, and throat manifestations of Wegener granulomatosis: an otorhinolaryngologist's perspective. Curr Opin Rheumatol 2001;13(1):3–11.

12. McCaffrey Tv, McDonald TJ, Facer GW, et al. Otologic manifestations of Wegener's granulomatosis. Otolaryngol Head Neck Surg 1980;88(5):586–93.

13. Hybels RL, Rice DH. Neuro-otologic manifestations of sarcoidosis. Laryngoscope 1976;86(12):1873–8.

14. Stephens SDG, Luxon L, Hinchcliffe R. Immunological disorders and auditory lesions. Audiology : Official Organ of the International Society of Audiology 1982; 21(2):128–48.

15. Kent PD, Michet CJ, Luthra HS. Relapsing polychondritis. Curr Opin Rheumatol 2004;16(1):56–61.

16. Maciaszczyk K, Durko T, Waszczykowska E, et al. Auditory function in patients with systemic lupus erythematosus. Auris Nasus Larynx 2011;38(1):26–32.

17. Roverano S, Cassano G, Paira S, et al. Asymptomatic sensorineural hearing loss in patients with systemic lupus erythematosus. J Clin Rheumatol 2006;12(5): 217–20.

18. Karatas E, Onat AM, Durucu C, et al. Audiovestibular disturbance in patients with systemic lupus erythematosus. Otolaryngology-Head Neck Surg (Tokyo) 2007; 136(1):82–6.

19. Anyah A, Mistry D, Kevern E, et al. Idiopathic Sudden Sensorineural Hearing Loss: Average Time Elapsed Before Presentation to the Otolaryngologist and Effectiveness of Oral and/or Intratympanic Steroids in Late Presentations. Cureus 2017;9(12). https://doi.org/10.7759/CUREUS.1945.

20. Wu CM, Lee KJ, Chang SL, et al. Recurrence of idiopathic sudden sensorineural hearing loss: a retrospective cohort study. Otol Neurotol 2014;35(10):1736–41.

21. Cannady SB, Batra PS, Koening C, et al. Sinonasal Wegener granulomatosis: a single-institution experience with 120 cases. Laryngoscope 2009;119(4):757–61.

22. Prokopakis E, Nikolaou V, Vardouniotis A, et al. Nasal manifestations of systemic diseases. B-ENT 2013;9(3):171–84.

23. B D, CA L, R S. Sinonasal imaging findings in granulomatosis with polyangiitis (Wegener granulomatosis): A systematic review. American Journal of Rhinology & Allergy 2017;31(1). https://doi.org/10.2500/AJRA.2017.31.4408.

24. Maguchi S, Fukuda S, Takizawa M. Histological findings in biopsies from patients with cytoplasmic-antineutrophil cytoplasmic antibody (cANCA)-positive

Wegener's granulomatosis. Auris Nasus Larynx 2001;28(Suppl). https://doi.org/10.1016/S0385-8146(01)00072-4.

25. Bacciu A, Buzio C, Giordano D, et al. Nasal polyposis in Churg-Strauss syndrome. Laryngoscope 2008;118(2):325–9.

26. Gulati S, Krossnes B, Olofsson J, et al. Sinonasal involvement in sarcoidosis: a report of seven cases and review of literature. Eur Arch Oto-Rhino-Laryngol 2012;269(3):891–6.

27. Aloulah M, Manes RP, Ng YH, et al. Sinonasal manifestations of sarcoidosis: a single institution experience with 38 cases. International Forum of Allergy & Rhinology 2013;3(7):567–72.

28. Trimarchi M, Gregorini G, Facchetti F, et al. Cocaine-induced midline destructive lesions: clinical, radiographic, histopathologic, and serologic features and their differentiation from Wegener granulomatosis. Medicine 2001;80(6):391–404.

29. Mirzaei A, Zabihiyeganeh M, Haqiqi A. Differentiation of Cocaine-Induced Midline Destructive Lesions from ANCA-Associated Vasculitis. Iranian Journal of Otorhinolaryngology 2018;30(100):309.

30. McGrath MM, Isakova T, Rennke HG, et al. Contaminated cocaine and antineutrophil cytoplasmic antibody-associated disease. Clin J Am Soc Nephrol : CJASN 2011;6(12):2799–805.

31. Zeuner M, Straub RH, Rauh G, et al. Relapsing polychondritis: clinical and immunogenetic analysis of 62 patients. J Rheumatol 1997;24(1):96–101. https://pubmed.ncbi.nlm.nih.gov/9002018/.

32. Hamano H, Kawa S, Horiuchi A, et al. High serum IgG4 concentrations in patients with sclerosing pancreatitis. N Engl J Med 2001;344(10):732–8.

33. Wilson CP, Brownlee BP, el Rassi ET, et al. Sinonasal immunoglobin G4—related disease: case report and review. Clinical Case Reports 2021;9(12):e05095.

34. Born H, Rameau A. Hoarseness. Med Clin 2021;105(5):917–38.

35. McCarty EB, Chao TN. Dysphagia and Swallowing Disorders. Med Clin 2021; 105(5):939–54.

36. Astor FC, Eidelman FJ, Hanft KL, et al. Laryngeal manifestations of vasculitic disease. South Med J 1998;91(6):588–91.

37. Stachler RJ, Francis DO, Schwartz SR, et al. Clinical Practice Guideline: Hoarseness (Dysphonia) (Update). Otolaryngology-Head Neck Surg (Tokyo) 2018; 158(1_suppl):S1–42.

38. Fijolek J, Wiatr E, Gawryluk D, et al. Intratracheal Dilation-injection Technique in the Treatment of Granulomatosis with Polyangiitis Patients with Subglottic Stenosis. J Rheumatol 2016;43(11):2042–8.

39. Mokhtari TE, Miller LE, Jayawardena ADL, et al. Eosinophilic Granulomatosis With Polyangiitis: An Unusual Case of Pediatric Subglottic Stenosis. Laryngoscope 2021;131(3):656–9.

40. Langford CA, Sneller MC, Hallahan CW, et al. Clinical features and therapeutic management of subglottic stenosis in patients with Wegener's granulomatosis. Arthritis Rheum 1996;39(10):1754–60.

41. del Pero MM, Jayne D, Chaudhry A, et al. Long-term outcome of airway stenosis in granulomatosis with polyangiitis (Wegener granulomatosis): an observational study. JAMA Otolaryngology– Head & Neck Surgery 2014;140(11):1038–44.

42. Hoffman GS, Thomas-Golbanov CK, Chan J, et al. Treatment of subglottic stenosis, due to Wegener's granulomatosis, with intralesional corticosteroids and dilation. J Rheumatol 2003;30(5):1017–21. PMID: 12734898.

43. Chung SA, Langford CA, Maz M, et al. 2021 American College of Rheumatology/ Vasculitis Foundation Guideline for the Management of Antineutrophil Cytoplasmic Antibody-Associated Vasculitis. Arthritis Care Res 2021;73(8):1088–105.
44. Ellison DE, Canalis RF. Sarcoidosis of the head and neck. Clin Dermatol 1986; 4(4):136–42.
45. Damiani JM, Levine HL. Relapsing polychondritis–report of ten cases. Laryngoscope 1979;89(6 Pt 1):929–46.
46. Reina COC, Iriarte MTG, Reyes FJB, et al. When is a biopsy justified in a case of relapsing polychondritis? J Laryngol Otol 1999;113(7):663–5.
47. Woo P, Mendelsohn J, Humphrey D. Rheumatoid nodules of the larynx. Otolaryngology-Head Neck Surg (Tokyo) 1995;113(1):147–50.
48. Beirith SC, Ikino CMY, Pereira IA. Laryngeal involvement in rheumatoid arthritis. Brazilian Journal of Otorhinolaryngology 2013;79(2):233–8.
49. Hale EK, Bystryn JC. Laryngeal and nasal involvement in pemphigus vulgaris. J Am Acad Dermatol 2001;44(4):609–11.
50. Wallner LJ, Alexander RW. PEMPHIGUS OF THE LARYNX. Laryngoscope 1964; 74(4):575–86.
51. Aravena C, Almeida FA, Mukhopadhyay S, et al. Idiopathic subglottic stenosis: a review. J Thorac Dis 2020;12(3):1100.
52. Jindal JR, Milbrath MM, Hogan WJ, et al. Gastroesophageal reflux disease as a likely cause of "idiopathic" subglottic stenosis. Ann Otol Rhinol Laryngol 1994; 103(3):186–91.

Kawasaki Disease and Multisystem Inflammatory Syndrome in Children
Common Inflammatory Pathways of Two Distinct Diseases

Magali Noval Rivas, PhD[a,b], Moshe Arditi, MD[a,b,c],*

KEYWORDS

- SARS-CoV-2 • Kawasaki disease • Superantigen • Superantigen-like motif
- Toxic shock syndrome • Multisystem inflammatory syndrome in children

KEY POINTS

- While multisystem inflammatory syndrome in children (MIS-C) and Kawasaki disease (KD) are considered 2 distinctive diseases triggered by different infectious agents, these 2 entities share inflammatory characteristics. They may belong to the same umbrella of inflammatory disorders but differ in many aspects of etiology, demography, epidemiology, clinical and laboratory findings, and pathology.
- The intensity of the inflammatory response and long-term cardiovascular sequelae diverge between KD and MIS-C. Whereas MIS-C presents as a more intense inflammatory syndrome, myocardial dysfunction, and cardiogenic shock, KD vasculitis is associated with pathologic changes in the coronary arteries and long-term cardiovascular sequelae.
- Intravenous immunoglobulin (IVIG) is efficient in treating both MIS-C and patients with KD; however, affected patients need to be followed over time to monitor the emergence or persistence of cardiovascular sequelae.

INTRODUCTION

Kawasaki disease (KD) is a febrile pediatric systemic vasculitis of unknown origin, usually affecting children younger than five years.[1] KD can result in coronary artery aneurysms (CAAs) in ≈ 25% of untreated children, and it is the leading cause of acquired

[a] Division of Infectious Diseases and Immunology, Department of Pediatrics, Guerin Children's at Cedars-Sinai Medical Center, Los Angeles, CA, USA; [b] Department of Biomedical Sciences, Infectious and Immunologic Diseases Research Center (IIDRC), Cedars-Sinai Medical Center, Los Angeles, CA, USA; [c] Smidt Heart Institute, Cedars-Sinai Medical Center, Los Angeles, CA, USA
* Corresponding author. 8700 Beverly Boulevard, Davis Building, Rooms D4024, D4025, D4027, Los Angeles, CA 90048.
E-mail address: moshe.arditi@cshs.org

Rheum Dis Clin N Am 49 (2023) 647–659
https://doi.org/10.1016/j.rdc.2023.03.002
0889-857X/23/© 2023 Elsevier Inc. All rights reserved.

heart disease in children in developed countries.[1] Multiple aspects of this pediatric illness are not completely understood, including the causative agent(s), the immune mechanisms underlying KD pathogenesis, and the potential long-term cardiovascular sequelae. Multisystem hyperinflammatory syndrome in children (MIS-C) is a novel pediatric illness that emerged during the COVID-19 pandemic.[2–8] While in most children SARS-CoV-2 infection is asymptomatic or results in mild symptoms, a subset of infected children develops MIS-C, which presents as fever, hypotension, gastrointestinal (GI) symptoms, and myocardial dysfunction.[2–8] Initially, MIS-C was called a "Kawasaki-like" disease due to mucocutaneous symptoms and the overlap of some clinical features.[3,5] Indeed, overlapping clinical features, including conjunctional injection, mucositis, and swelling of the hands and feet, hint that MIS-C and KD may belong to the same spectrum of inflammatory disorders. However, the observed epidemiological, pathological, inflammatory, and immunological differences between MIS-C and KD indicate that these 2 diseases are different entities[2,8–10] **(Fig. 1)**. Here, we review the recent advances in KD and MIS-C research.

Viral Triggers as a Shared Etiology Between Multisystem Inflammatory Syndrome in Children and Kawasaki Disease

MIS-C is a postacute hyperinflammatory syndrome that develops after either SARS-CoV-2 infection or exposure. Most patients with MIS-C have serologic evidence of previous SARS-CoV-2 infection or exposure 2 to 6 weeks before disease onset.[2–8,10] In contrast, although KD's clinical presentation and epidemiology hint toward an infectious origin, the causative agent(s) remain unidentified today.[11,12] Patients with KD do not respond to antibiotic treatment, often given pre-KD diagnosis during the acute

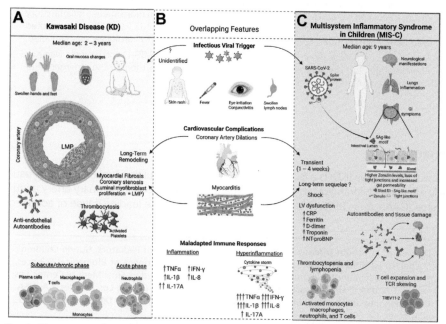

Fig. 1. Divergent and overlapping features of KD and MIS-C. (*A*) Clinical, pathological, and immunological features specific to KD. (*B*) Clinical, pathological, and immunological features that overlap between KD and MIS-C. (*C*) Clinical, pathological, and immunological features specific to MIS-C. (Created with BioRender.com.)

phase, indicating that KD triggering agent(s) might be of viral origin rather than bacterial.[12]

Multisystem clinical findings common to MIS-C and KD, such as rash, fever, GI tract abnormalities, swollen lymph nodes, headaches, and fatigue, also overlap with clinical manifestations triggered by other pediatric viral illnesses.[1,12] Associations between common respiratory viruses, including coronaviruses, and KD development have been previously reported.[13,14] However, they were not confirmed in follow-up studies.[15–17] For example, intracytoplasmic inclusion bodies detected in ciliated bronchial epithelium tissues from patients with KD, months to years after acute KD, support the hypothesis of a viral causative agent.[12,18] Serological profiling did not detect differences in antiviral antibody profiles between acute KD and control patients.[19] However, another study identified a protein epitope targeted by antibodies produced in patients with KD during the acute phase of the disease.[18] Although the source of this protein epitope remains unidentified, the authors hypothesized the possibility of a novel, uncharacterized virus.[18] The infectious agent hypothesis is further supported by the observation that KD incidence decreased in multiple areas when mitigation measures were implemented to control the spread of COVID-19.[20,21]

Epidemiological Differences Between Kawasaki Disease and Multisystem Inflammatory Syndrome in Children

Key epidemiological differences differentiate KD and MIS-C. First, KD incidence is approximately 25 per 100,000 children under five years in the US,[1] whereas a cross-sectional study of a large US cohort of patients with MIS-C estimated MIS-C incidence to be ≈ 2 per 100,000 in individuals younger than 21 years.[22] Most KD cases occur in patients younger than five years,[1] while the median age of MIS-C is 9 years.[22] Although rare, KD can also occur in adults and usually presents with fewer electrocardiographic abnormalities and CAAs than pediatric KD.[23] A rare multisystem inflammatory syndrome, called MIS-A, is also reported in adults and is highly similar to MIS-C.[24] KD prevalence is consistently greater in males (1.5 male-to-female ratio in the US).[1] In MIS-C, while the proportion of males and females is 1:1 between the ages of 0 to 4 years, it increases and reaches 2:1 for patients between 18 and 20 years.[22]

KD incidence is higher in Asian countries such as Japan, South Korea, China, and Taiwan than in the USA and Europe.[1] In contrast, reports of MIS-C in East Asia are limited,[25,26] and in the US, the incidence of MIS-C is higher in children from Hispanic or Black ethnicities and the lowest in Asian children.[22,27] The variation in the incidence of both KD and MIS-C among ethnic groups may be at least in part related to genetic predisposition. Indeed, single-nucleotide polymorphisms (SNPs) in various genes, such as ITPKC, CASP3, FCGR2A, ORAI1, BLK, and CD40 are associated with increased susceptibility to KD.[11,28] Genetic analysis from a limited number of patients with MIS-C identified rare variants in genes associated with autoimmunity pathways and regulation of inflammatory responses, which may potentially predispose to MIS-C.[29–31]

Several studies indicate that HLA class I alleles are associated with MIS-C.[32–34] The expansion of Vβ11-2+ T cells in patients with MIS-C correlates with inflammatory markers and MIS-C severity.[33–36] Severe patients with MIS-C with Vβ11-2+ T cell expansion share a combination of 3 HLA class I alleles (A02, B35, and C04).[33] The same combination was detected in patients with MIS-C from an Italian and an American cohort, however, they were not associated with disease severity.[32,34] While these observations were not reproduced in another cohort,[36] the combination of these 3 HLA classes I alleles might confer increased susceptibility to MIS-C, which may explain the rarity of MIS-C and why the disease disproportionately affects specific ethnicities.

Clinical, Biological, and Pathological Findings of Kawasaki Disease and Multisystem Inflammatory Syndrome in Children

Using data collected from retrospective cohorts of patients with KD, several studies have compared the clinical, biological, and pathological characteristics of patients with MIS-C and KD.[2,37–40] In the absence of a specific test to identify KD, the diagnosis is based on the presence of persistent fever lasting more than five days and 4 of 5 primary clinical criteria: changes in the extremities, erythematous rash, conjunctivitis, cracked lips and strawberry tongue, and cervical lymphadenopathy.[1] Only ≈30% of patients with MIS-C meet these criteria for complete KD.[39] Patients with MIS-C have higher levels of C-reactive protein (CRP), ferritin, D-dimer, troponin, and N-terminal pro-brain natriuretic peptide (NT-proBNP) than patients with KD, indicating hyperinflammation and potential cardiovascular involvement.[2,37,38] However, compared with patients with KD, children with MIS-C have lower lymphocyte and platelet counts.[2,37–40]

Patients with MIS-C commonly present with prominent cardiac involvement manifested by left ventricular (LV) systolic and diastolic dysfunction, myocardial inflammation, and coronary artery dilations.[41,42] LV dysfunction is more severe in patients with MIS-C than in patients with KD.[41] However, KD can also lead to myocarditis, which is associated with arrhythmias and may result in long-term fibrosis.[1,11,43] Coronary arteries are predominantly affected during KD and may result in dilation and aneurysms.[1,11] Children with MIS-C have fewer coronary artery abnormalities than patients with KD and they are almost always transient and resolve rapidly over time.[38,39,41,44] In patients with KD, the small and moderate CAAs can take 2 years to regress to standard lumen size.[45] The prompter resolution of cardiovascular complications after the MIS-C acute phase suggests they may result from hyperinflammation associated with capillary leakage and vasodilation rather than immune infiltrations damaging the myocardium.[46]

Immune Responses During Kawasaki Disease and Multisystem Inflammatory Syndrome in Children

Immunophenotyping studies have revealed that immune dysregulation, cytokine storm, and increased the activation of immune cells are hallmarks of MIS-C, and these correlate with disease severity.[34,36,47–49] Notably, elevated cytokines include IL-6, IL-10, TNF-α, IFN-γ, IL-1β, IL-1RA, and soluble CD25.[34–36,40,50,51] While acute KD is also associated with high levels of IL-1β, TNF-α, IFN-γ, IL-10, and IL-8,[36,52–54] concentrations of these cytokines appear higher during MIS-C.[55] IL-1β plays a crucial role in KD development. Clinical trials are currently ongoing to test the efficacy of Anakinra, an IL-1 receptor antagonist (IL-1Ra), for patients with KD refractory to IVIG treatment.[56,57] IL-17A plasma levels and the proportions of circulating Th17 T cells are increased during acute KD and may be involved in KD pathogenesis.[58] IL-17A is also elevated in MIS-C, however, to a lesser degree than in KD.[37]

Dysregulated cellular and humoral immune responses occur in MIS-C, including reductions in the proportions of plasmacytoid dendritic cells (pDCs),[49,59] monocytes,[47] and natural killer (NK) cells.[47,59] NK cells from patients with MIS-C upregulate the expression of several cytotoxic genes,[59] and monocytes from children with MIS-C upregulate alarmin-related S100A genes, indicative of an activated phenotype.[59] Similarly, monocytes from patients with KD also upregulate the S100A proteins, *IL1B*, and *TNF* transcripts.[60] The frequency of neutrophils and monocytes expressing the activation marker CD64 increases during the acute phase of the MIS-C.[47,48] Neutrophils from patients with MIS-C exhibit higher rates of spontaneous release of neutrophil extracellular traps (NETs), which may be a driver of MIS-C vascular inflammation and endothelial damage.[61] Neutrophils are similarly implicated in the early phase of CAAs formation in KD[62] and the spontaneous release of NETs by neutrophils is also enhanced in patients with KD.[63]

A hallmark of patients with MIS-C is lymphopenia, which affects both CD4[+] and CD8[+] T cells,[37,48,49,59] which is not usually observed in KD.[9] Patients with MIS-C show increased frequencies of activated and proliferating T cells[37,47–49,59]; activated CD8[+] T cells express the fractalkine receptor CX3CR1, which can interact with fractalkine-expressing vascular endothelium and may potentiate vascular endothelial damage.[49] Patients with MIS-C also exhibit elevated frequencies of plasmablast cells.[34,35,49,59] The frequency of circulating activated B cells and plasmablasts is also increased during KD.[64]

The presence of autoantibodies targeting ubiquitously expressed antigens and self-antigens has been reported in multiple cohorts of patients with MIS-C.[34,37,47,50,59] A high proportion of patients with MIS-C also express autoantibodies targeting the endogenous IL-1 receptor antagonist (IL-1Ra).[65] The expansion of B cells during KD acute may similarly lead to autoimmune responses and the production of autoantibodies.[64] Indeed, the presence of antibodies targeting type III collagen, myosin, alpha-enolase, and anti-endothelial antibodies is also observed in KD.[64] Nevertheless, further studies are still required to determine the specific role of autoantibodies in both MIS-C and KD.

The Superantigen Hypothesis and Expansion of TRBV11-2 T Cell Clonotypes in Multisystem Inflammatory Syndrome in Children

Superantigens (SAgs) are microbial proteins able to activate large fractions of T cells non-specifically by cross-linking major histocompatibility complex (MHC) class II molecules at the surface of antigen-presenting cells (APCs) with T cell Receptor (TCR) β-chains (Vβ) at their variable domain.[66] Vβ skewing with junctional diversity indicates SAg involvement.[66] Over-activation of T cells by SAg results in an uncontrolled release of chemokines and proinflammatory cytokines and underlies toxic shock syndrome (TSS). KD shares some clinical features with SAg-mediated diseases, including fever, desquamating rash, and SAgs have been considered as potential KD triggers. While a few studies reported the expansion of different Vβ T cell populations during acute KD, this has not been confirmed by follow-up studies on independent cohorts of patients with KD.[67–69] Additionally, the development of coronary artery abnormalities, a hallmark of KD, is rarely associated with SAg-mediated disease.[70] In contrast, patients with TSS present with severe GI symptoms, myocardial cardiogenic shock, and neurological manifestations.[70] These symptoms are infrequent in KD and more commonly reported during MIS-C.[2–9,71,72]

Computational studies comparing SARS-CoV-2 with bacterial toxins revealed the presence of a motif in SARS-CoV-2 Spike protein subunit S1 that harbors high sequence and structural similarities with a segment of staphylococcal enterotoxin B (SEB), a bacterial SAg.[73] This SAg-like motif is an insertion, $P_{681}RRA_{684}$ (PRRA), unique to SARS-CoV-2 and adjacent to the furin cleavage site between the S1 and S2 subunits.[71–73] In silico modeling indicates this insert has a propensity to bind to TCRs and MHC Class II.[33,50,71–74] Studies in mice and hamsters show that SARS-CoV-2 mutations resulting in the deletion of the S1-S2 furin cleavage site result in attenuated disease.[75,76] Furthermore, supporting the potential involvement of the SAg-like motif in SARS-CoV-2 pathogenesis, incubation of SARS-CoV-2 with the 6D3 anti-SEB mAb inhibited cellular viral infection in vitro.[74]

TCR repertoire sequencing performed on independent cohorts of patients with MIS-C indicate TCRVβ skewing and expansion of TRBV11-2 (Vβ21.3[+]) T cell clonotypes, suggestive of superantigenic stimulation.[33–36,59] This *TRBV11-2* enrichment affects both CD4$^+$ and CD8$^+$ T cells, is transient, and returns to baseline after MIS-C resolution.[34–36,59] Expansion of *TRBV11-2* clonotypes correlates with disease severity and cytokine storm.[33–36] Severe patients with MIS-C with TRBV11-2 T cell expansion also exhibit more robust autoantibodies responses, a solid imprint of antigenic selection in their BCR repertoires, and increased usage of autoantibody-associated IGHV genes.[50] *In silico* modeling indicates that TRBV11-2 engages in a CDR3-independent interaction with the polybasic insert "PRRA" in the SARS-CoV-2 SAg-like motif.[33,73]

Autopsy studies of fatal MIS-C cases indicate the sustained presence of SARS-CoV-2 in multiple tissues, including lung, heart, brain, and intestinal tissues.[77–80] Yonker and colleagues[81] observed the prolonged presence of SARS-CoV-2 RNA in the GI tract of patients with MIS-C weeks after initial exposure and elevated levels of Zonulin and other markers indicative of increased intestinal permeability. This suggests that the GI tract may act as a viral reservoir for SARS-CoV-2. Increased intestinal permeability might be permissive for SARS-CoV-2 antigens to breach the intestinal barrier and enter the systemic circulation.[81] Indeed, patients with MIS-C with a severe clinical phenotype and TBRV11-2 expansion have higher levels of circulating S1, which contains the SARS-CoV-2 SAg-like motif.[81] These data support the hypothesis that MIS-C is a unique disease entity driven by the SAg-like motif in SARS-CoV-2 Spike.

Long-Term Sequelae of Kawasaki Disease and Multisystem Inflammatory Syndrome in Children

Vascular inflammation stemming from acute KD can result in long-term cardiovascular sequelae and ischemic heart diseases.[11,43,82] Up to ≈7% of IVIG-treated children with KD will develop coronary artery abnormalities, which may progress to stenosis, occlusion, and/or thrombosis over time.[83] A history of KD during childhood is associated with an increased prevalence of abnormal electrocardiogram (ECG).[84] Long-term KD complications include coronary artery stenosis and calcification, myocardial infarction, fibrosis, and long-term systolic or diastolic dysfunction, and may predispose to premature atherosclerosis.[11,43,82,83,85]

While the cardiovascular manifestations of acute MIS-C improve rapidly, little is known regarding the long-term outcomes, and myocardial inflammation could lead to long-term sequelae such as fibrosis and scaring.[42] Potential long-term outcomes in patients with MIS-C are documented in a few studies.[44,46,86–89] A multicenter follow-up study of US children that developed MIS-C indicates that some symptoms, such as fatigue, weakness, activity impairment, and headache may persist beyond 2 months after hospitalization.[87] In another cohort of patients with MIS-C, six months after acute disease, markers of systemic inflammation returned to baseline, electrocardiograms were normal, GI symptoms were absent, and minimal functional neurological impairment was observed.[89] However, in this study, 18 of the 40 patients exhibited a reduced functional exercise capacity six months post-MIS-C. Whether this resulted from MIS-C or involved other factors, such as a sedentary lifestyle, remains unclear.[89] Additional and extended studies are still required to determine the long-term impacts of MIS-C on cardiovascular function, and a multicenter observational cohort study (COVID MUSIC study) is currently ongoing.[86]

Decreased Incidence of Multisystem Inflammatory Syndrome in Children with SARS-CoV-2 Variants of Concern and Vaccination

Since the beginning of the COVID-19 pandemic, several SARS-CoV-2 variants of concern (VOCs) have been characterized as the virus evolves.[90] *Omicron*, which exhibits more than 30 amino acid substitutions, quickly became the dominant circulating variant in 2022, raising potential concerns about increased MIS-C incidence. However, MIS-C severity and incidence dramatically decreased during the *Omicron* wave compared with *Alpha* and *Delta* waves.[91,92] Indeed, since June 2022, the number of MIS-C cases reported to the CDC has been dramatically reduced.[27] Multiple parameters may account for such a decrease in MIS-C frequency, including the strong association between children's vaccination (Pfizer-BioNTech) and prevention of MIS-C,[93] prior SARS-CoV-2 infections and induction of immune memory, better management, and, potentially, mutations in the *Omicron* variant itself.[91,92] Indeed, mutations in SARS-CoV-2 Spike may explain disease severity differences between variants. The highly pathogenic *Delta* harbors a Spike mutation, P681R, which becomes more polybasic in nature and is further cleaved by the acidic motif furin, releasing higher amounts of the shed S1 subunit.[94] On the other hand, the relatively less pathogenic *Omicron* harbors several mutations in Spike that result in inefficient use of TMPRSS2, suboptimal S1/S2 cleavage, and reduced levels of shed S1.[95] Since the SAg-like motif is in the S1 SARS-CoV-2 subunit, these findings may potentially support the SAg hypothesis of MIS-C and may explain the significant reduction of MIS-C incidence during the Omicron wave, in addition to vaccines-induced protection.

SUMMARY

Several clinical features overlap between MIS-C and KD. These 2 entities share inflammatory characteristics, indicating that MIS-C and KD may belong to the same broad umbrella of inflammatory disorders involving the master cytokine IL-1β,[96] but differ in many aspects of etiology, demography, epidemiology, clinical and laboratory findings, as well as pathology. The intensity of the inflammatory response and long-term cardiovascular sequelae diverge between KD and MIS-C. Whereas MIS-C presents with a more intense inflammatory syndrome, KD vasculitis is associated with pathologic changes in the coronary arteries and associated with long-term cardiovascular sequelae. The 2 to 6 weeks delay between SARS-CoV-2 exposure and MIS-C development may account for the development of the autoinflammatory response involving dysregulated B and T cell responses, plasmablast differentiation, and autoantibody production.[50,72] While the general hypothesis is that KD is triggered by a viral infectious agent(s), the causative agents remain unidentified, and whether KD can be considered a postinfectious syndrome, like MIS-C, remains unclear. In conclusion, the data available so far support the hypothesis that MIS-C and KD belong to the same broad spectrum of inflammatory disorders but with clearly distinct etiopathology, presentation, and long-term consequences.

CLINICS CARE POINTS

- MIS-C and KD are considered 2 distinctive diseases triggered by different infectious agents. However, these 2 entities share inflammatory characteristics. It is, therefore, not surprising that both diseases respond well to IVIG ± steroids. Furthermore, anti-IL-1 receptor therapies, such as Anakinra, are expected to treat these 2 conditions efficiently.

- KD is associated with the development of coronary artery aneurysms and later coronary remodeling with luminal myofibroblast proliferation that leads to coronary stenosis, ischemia, and myocardial fibrosis as long-term sequelae. Children with MIS-C should also be followed longitudinally to determine if any long-term complications will emerge.

- COVID-19 vaccinations is associated with decreased MIS-C incidence and should be encouraged among all eligible age groups.

DISCLOSURE

The authors have nothing to disclose.

FUNDING

We gratefully acknowledge support from NIH awards R01AI072726 to M. Arditi, R01HL139766 and R01HL159297 to MNR, R01AI157274 to M. Arditi and MNR.

REFERENCES

1. McCrindle BW, Rowley AH, Newburger JW, et al. Diagnosis, treatment, and long-term management of Kawasaki disease: a scientific statement for health professionals from the American Heart Association. Circulation 2017;135(17):e927–99.
2. Whittaker E, Bamford A, Kenny J, et al. Clinical characteristics of 58 children with a pediatric inflammatory multisystem syndrome temporally associated with SARS-CoV-2. JAMA 2020;324(3):259–69.
3. Verdoni L, Mazza A, Gervasoni A, et al. An outbreak of severe Kawasaki-like disease at the Italian epicentre of the SARS-CoV-2 epidemic: an observational cohort study. Lancet 2020;395(10239):1771–8.
4. Cheung EW, Zachariah P, Gorelik M, et al. Multisystem inflammatory syndrome related to COVID-19 in previously healthy children and adolescents in New York City. JAMA 2020;324(3):294–6.
5. Toubiana J, Poirault C, Corsia A, et al. Kawasaki-like multisystem inflammatory syndrome in children during the covid-19 pandemic in Paris, France: prospective observational study. BMJ 2020;369:m2094.
6. Riphagen S, Gomez X, Gonzalez-Martinez C, et al. Hyperinflammatory shock in children during COVID-19 pandemic. Lancet 2020;395(10237):1607–8.
7. Belhadjer Z, Méot M, Bajolle F, et al. Acute heart failure in multisystem inflammatory syndrome in children in the context of global SARS-CoV-2 pandemic. Circulation 2020;142(5):429–36.
8. Feldstein LR, Rose EB, Horwitz SM, et al. Multisystem inflammatory syndrome in U.S. children and adolescents. N Engl J Med 2020;383(4):334–46.
9. Rowley AH. Multisystem inflammatory syndrome in children (MIS-C) and Kawasaki disease: two different illnesses with overlapping clinical features. J Pediatrics 2020. https://doi.org/10.1016/j.jpeds.2020.06.05.
10. Godfred-Cato S, Abrams JY, Balachandran N, et al. Distinguishing multisystem inflammatory syndrome in children from COVID-19, Kawasaki Disease and toxic shock syndrome. Pediatr Infect Dis J 2022. https://doi.org/10.1097/inf.0000000000003449.
11. Soni PR, Noval Rivas M, Arditi M. A comprehensive update on Kawasaki Disease vasculitis and myocarditis. Curr Rheumatol Rep 2020;22(2):6.
12. Rowley AH. Is Kawasaki disease an infectious disorder? Int J Rheum Dis 2018; 21(1):20–5.
13. Esper F, Shapiro ED, Weibel C, et al. Association between a novel human coronavirus and Kawasaki disease. J Infect Dis 2005;191(4):499–502.
14. Chang L-Y, Lu C-Y, Shao P-L, et al. Viral infections associated with Kawasaki disease. J Formos Med Assoc 2014;113(3):148–54.
15. Ebihara T, Endo R, Ma X, et al. Lack of association between New Haven coronavirus and Kawasaki disease. J Infect Dis 2005;192(2):351–2 [author reply: 353].
16. Belay ED, Erdman DD, Anderson LJ, et al. Kawasaki disease and human coronavirus. J Infect Dis 2005;192(2):352–3 [author reply: 353].

17. Dominguez SR, Anderson MS, Glodé MP, et al. Blinded case-control study of the relationship between human coronavirus NL63 and Kawasaki syndrome. J Infect Dis 2006;194(12):1697–701.

18. Rowley AH, Baker SC, Arrollo D, et al. A protein epitope targeted by the antibody response to Kawasaki Disease. J Infect Dis 2020;222(1):158–68. https://doi.org/10.1093/infdis/jiaa066.

19. Quiat D, Kula T, Shimizu C, et al. High-throughput screening of Kawasaki Disease sera for antiviral antibodies. J Infect Dis 2020;222(11):1853–7. https://doi.org/10.1093/infdis/jiaa253.

20. Kang J-M, Kim Y-E, Huh K, et al. Reduction in Kawasaki Disease after nonpharmaceutical interventions in the COVID-19 era: a nationwide observational study in Korea. Circulation 2021;143(25):2508–10.

21. Burney JA, Roberts SC, DeHaan LL, et al. Epidemiological and clinical features of Kawasaki disease during the COVID-19 pandemic in the United States. JAMA Netw Open 2022;5(6):e2217436.

22. Belay ED, Abrams J, Oster ME, et al. Trends in geographic and temporal distribution of us children with multisystem inflammatory syndrome during the COVID-19 Pandemic. JAMA Pediatr 2021;175(8):837–45.

23. Gomard-Mennesson E, Landron C, Dauphin C, et al. Kawasaki disease in adults: report of 10 cases. Medicine 2010;89(3):149–58.

24. Morris SB, Schwartz NG, Patel P, et al. Case series of multisystem inflammatory syndrome in adults associated with SARS-CoV-2 infection - United Kingdom and United States, March-August 2020. MMWR Morb Mortal Wkly Rep 2020;69(40):1450–6.

25. Hisamura M, Asai H, Sakata N, et al. Multisystem inflammatory syndrome in children: a case report from Japan. Cureus 2022;14(3):e23682. https://doi.org/10.7759/cureus.23682.

26. Mohri Y, Shimizu M, Fujimoto T, et al. A young child with pediatric multisystem inflammatory syndrome successfully treated with high-dose immunoglobulin therapy. IDCases 2022;28:e01493.

27. CDC. Health Department-Reported Cases of Multisystem Inflammatory Syndrome in Children (MIS-C) in the United States. Available at: https://covidcdcgov/covid-data-tracker/#mis-national-surveillance. Accessed November 7, 2022.

28. Onouchi Y. The genetics of Kawasaki disease. Int J Rheum Dis 2018;21(1):26–30.

29. Lee PY, Platt CD, Weeks S, et al. Immune dysregulation and multisystem inflammatory syndrome in children (MIS-C) in individuals with haploinsufficiency of SOCS1. J Allergy Clin Immunol 2020;146(5):1194–200.e1.

30. Chou J, Platt CD, Habiballah S, et al. Mechanisms underlying genetic susceptibility to multisystem inflammatory syndrome in children (MIS-C). J Allergy Clin Immunol 2021;148(3):732–8.e1.

31. Benamar M, Chen Q, Chou J, et al. The Notch1/CD22 signaling axis disrupts Treg function in SARS-CoV-2-associated multisystem inflammatory syndrome in children. J Clin Invest. 2023 Jan 3;133(1):e163235. doi: 10.1172/JCI163235.

32. Conway SR, Lazarski CA, Field NE, et al. SARS-CoV-2-Specific T cell responses are stronger in children with multisystem inflammatory syndrome compared to children with uncomplicated SARS-CoV-2 infection. original research. Front Immunol 2022;12. https://doi.org/10.3389/fimmu.2021.793197.

33. Porritt RA, Paschold L, Rivas MN, et al. HLA class I-associated expansion of TRBV11-2 T cells in multisystem inflammatory syndrome in children. J Clin Invest 2021;131(10). https://doi.org/10.1172/jci146614.

34. Sacco K, Castagnoli R, Vakkilainen S, et al. Immunopathological signatures in multisystem inflammatory syndrome in children and pediatric COVID-19. Nat Med 2022. https://doi.org/10.1038/s41591-022-01724-3.

35. Hoste L, Roels L, Naesens L, et al. TIM3+ TRBV11-2 T cells and IFNγ signature in patrolling monocytes and CD16+ NK cells delineate MIS-C. J Exp Med 2022; 219(2). https://doi.org/10.1084/jem.20211381.

36. Moreews M, Le Gouge K, Khaldi-Plassart S, et al. Polyclonal expansion of TCR Vbeta 21.3(+) CD4(+) and CD8(+) T cells is a hallmark of Multisystem Inflammatory Syndrome in Children. Sci Immunol 2021;6(59). https://doi.org/10.1126/sciimmunol.abh1516.

37. Consiglio CR, Cotugno N, Sardh F, et al. The immunology of multisystem inflammatory syndrome in children with COVID-19. Cell 2020;183(4):968–81.e7.

38. Cattalini M, Della Paolera S, Zunica F, et al. Defining Kawasaki disease and pediatric inflammatory multisystem syndrome-temporally associated to SARS-CoV-2 infection during SARS-CoV-2 epidemic in Italy: results from a national, multicenter survey. Pediatr Rheumatol 2021;19(1):29.

39. Cherqaoui B, Koné-Paut I, Yager H, et al. Delineating phenotypes of Kawasaki disease and SARS-CoV-2-related inflammatory multisystem syndrome: a French study and literature review. Rheumatology 2021;60(10):4530–7.

40. Esteve-Sole A, Anton J, Pino-Ramirez RM, et al. Similarities and differences between the immunopathogenesis of COVID-19-related pediatric multisystem inflammatory syndrome and Kawasaki disease. J Clin Invest 2021;131(6). https://doi.org/10.1172/jci144554.

41. Matsubara D, Kauffman HL, Wang Y, et al. Echocardiographic Findings in Pediatric Multisystem Inflammatory Syndrome Associated With COVID-19 in the United States. J Am Coll Cardiol 2020;76(17):1947–61.

42. Henderson LA, Canna SW, Friedman KG, et al. American College of Rheumatology Clinical Guidance for Multisystem Inflammatory Syndrome in Children Associated With SARS-CoV-2 and Hyperinflammation in Pediatric COVID-. Arthritis Rheumatol 2022;74(4):e1–20 19: Version 3.

43. Gordon JB, Kahn AM, Burns JC. When children with Kawasaki disease grow up: myocardial and vascular complications in adulthood. J Am Coll Cardiol 2009; 54(21):1911–20.

44. Farooqi KM, Chan A, Weller RJ, et al. Longitudinal outcomes for multisystem inflammatory syndrome in children. Pediatrics 2021;148(2). https://doi.org/10.1542/peds.2021-051155.

45. Advani N, Sastroasmoro S, Ontoseno T, et al. Long-term outcome of coronary artery dilatation in Kawasaki disease. Ann Pediatr Cardiol 2018;11(2):125–9.

46. Capone CA, Misra N, Ganigara M, et al. Six month follow-up of patients with multisystem inflammatory syndrome in children. Pediatrics 2021;148(4). https://doi.org/10.1542/peds.2021-050973.

47. Gruber CN, Patel RS, Trachtman R, et al. Mapping systemic inflammation and antibody responses in multisystem inflammatory syndrome in children (MIS-C). Cell 2020;183(4):982–95.e14.

48. Carter MJ, Fish M, Jennings A, et al. Peripheral immunophenotypes in children with multisystem inflammatory syndrome associated with SARS-CoV-2 infection. Nat Med 2020;26(11):1701–7.

49. Vella LA, Giles JR, Baxter AE, et al. Deep immune profiling of MIS-C demonstrates marked but transient immune activation compared to adult and pediatric COVID-19. Sci Immunol 2021;6(57). https://doi.org/10.1126/sciimmunol.abf7570.

50. Porritt RA, Binek A, Paschold L, et al. The autoimmune signature of hyperinflammatory multisystem inflammatory syndrome in children. J Clin Invest 2021; 131(20). https://doi.org/10.1172/jci151520.

51. Lapp SA, Abrams J, Lu AT, et al. Serologic and cytokine signatures in children with multisystem inflammatory syndrome and coronavirus disease 2019. Open Forum Infect Dis 2022;9(3). https://doi.org/10.1093/ofid/ofac070.

52. Furukawa S, Matsubara T, Jujoh K, et al. Peripheral blood monocyte/macrophages and serum tumor necrosis factor in Kawasaki disease. Clin Immunol Immunopathol 1988;48(2):247–51.

53. Matsubara T, Furukawa S, Yabuta K. Serum levels of tumor necrosis factor, interleukin 2 receptor, and interferon-gamma in Kawasaki disease involved coronary-artery lesions. Clin Immunol Immunopathol 1990;56(1):29–36.

54. Lin CY, Lin CC, Hwang B, et al. The changes of interleukin-2, tumour necrotic factor and gamma-interferon production among patients with Kawasaki disease. Eur J Pediatr 1991;150(3):179–82.

55. Ghosh P, Katkar GD, Shimizu C, et al. An Artificial Intelligence-guided signature reveals the shared host immune response in MIS-C and Kawasaki disease. Nat Commun 2022;13(1):2687.

56. Tremoulet AH, Jain S, Kim S, et al. Rationale and study design for a phase I/IIa trial of anakinra in children with Kawasaki disease and early coronary artery abnormalities (the ANAKID trial). Contemp Clin Trials 2016;48:70–5.

57. Koné-Paut I, Tellier S, Belot A, et al. Phase II open label study of anakinra in intravenous immunoglobulin-resistant Kawasaki disease. Arthritis Rheumatol 2021; 73(1):151–61. https://doi.org/10.1002/art.41481.

58. Jia S, Li C, Wang G, et al. The T helper type 17/regulatory T cell imbalance in patients with acute Kawasaki disease. Clin Exp Immunol 2010;162(1):131–7.

59. Ramaswamy A, Brodsky NN, Sumida TS, et al. Immune dysregulation and autoreactivity correlate with disease severity in SARS-CoV-2-associated multisystem inflammatory syndrome in children. Immunity 2021;54(5):1083–95.e7.

60. Wang Z, Xie L, Ding G, et al. Single-cell RNA sequencing of peripheral blood mononuclear cells from acute Kawasaki disease patients. Nat Commun 2021; 12(1):5444.

61. Boribong BP, LaSalle TJ, Bartsch YC, et al. Neutrophil profiles of pediatric COVID-19 and multisystem inflammatory syndrome in children. Cell Rep Med 2022;3(12):100848.

62. Takahashi K, Oharaseki T, Naoe S, et al. Neutrophilic involvement in the damage to coronary arteries in acute stage of Kawasaki disease. Pediatr Int 2005;47(3): 305–10.

63. Yoshida Y, Takeshita S, Kawamura Y, et al. Enhanced formation of neutrophil extracellular traps in Kawasaki disease. Pediatr Res 2020. https://doi.org/10.1038/s41390-019-0710-3.

64. Hicar MD. Antibodies and immunity during Kawasaki disease. Review. Frontiers Cardiovasc Medicine 2020;7(94). https://doi.org/10.3389/fcvm.2020.00094.

65. Pfeifer J, Thurner B, Kessel C, et al. Autoantibodies against interleukin-1 receptor antagonist in multisystem inflammatory syndrome in children: a multicentre, retrospective, cohort study. Lancet Rheumatol 2022;4(5):e329–37.

66. Li H, Llera A, Emilio L, et al. The structural basis of t cell activation by superantigens. Annu Rev Immunol 1999;17(1):435–66.

67. Sakaguchi M, Kato H, Nishiyori A, et al. Characterization of CD4+ T helper cells in patients with Kawasaki disease (KD): preferential production of tumour

necrosis factor-alpha (TNF-alpha) by V beta 2- or V beta 8- CD4+ T helper cells. Clin Exp Immunol 1995;99(2):276–82.

68. Pietra BA, De Inocencio J, Giannini EH, et al. TCR V beta family repertoire and T cell activation markers in Kawasaki disease. J Immunol 1994;153(4):1881–8.

69. Mancia L, Wahlstrom J, Schiller B, et al. Characterization of the T-cell receptor V-beta repertoire in Kawasaki disease. Scand J Immunol 1998;48(4):443–9.

70. Paris AL, Herwaldt LA, Blum D, et al. Pathologic findings in twelve fatal cases of toxic shock syndrome. Ann Intern Med 1982;96(6 Pt 2):852–7.

71. Noval Rivas M, Porritt RA, Cheng MH, et al. COVID-19-associated multisystem inflammatory syndrome in children (MIS-C): A novel disease that mimics toxic shock syndrome-the superantigen hypothesis. J Allergy Clin Immunol 2021; 147(1):57–9.

72. Noval Rivas M, Porritt RA, Cheng MH, et al. Multisystem inflammatory syndrome in children and long COVID: the SARS-CoV-2 viral superantigen hypothesis. Front Immunol 2022;13:941009.

73. Cheng MH, Zhang S, Porritt RA, et al. Superantigenic character of an insert unique to SARS-CoV-2 spike supported by skewed TCR repertoire in patients with hyperinflammation. Proc Natl Acad Sci U S A 2020;117(41):25254–62.

74. Cheng MH, Porritt RA, Rivas MN, et al. A monoclonal antibody against staphylococcal enterotoxin B superantigen inhibits SARS-CoV-2 entry in vitro. Structure 2021;29(9):951–62.e3.

75. Johnson BA, Xie X, Bailey AL, et al. Loss of furin cleavage site attenuates SARS-CoV-2 pathogenesis. Nature 2021;591(7849):293–9.

76. Lau S-Y, Wang P, Mok BW-Y, et al. Attenuated SARS-CoV-2 variants with deletions at the S1/S2 junction. Emerg Microb Infect 2020;9(1):837–42.

77. Dolhnikoff M, Ferreira Ferranti J, de Almeida Monteiro RA, et al. SARS-CoV-2 in cardiac tissue of a child with COVID-19-related multisystem inflammatory syndrome. Lancet Child Adolesc Heal 2020;4(10):790–4.

78. Duarte-Neto AN, Caldini EG, Gomes-Gouvêa MS, et al. An autopsy study of the spectrum of severe COVID-19 in children: From SARS to different phenotypes of MIS-C. EClinicalMedicine 2021;35:100850.

79. Mayordomo-Colunga J, Vivanco-Allende A, López-Alonso I, et al. SARS-CoV-2 Spike protein in intestinal cells of a patient with coronavirus disease 2019 multisystem inflammatory syndrome. J Pediatr 2022;243:214–8.e5.

80. Taweevisit M, Chindamporn A, Sujjavorakul K, et al. Multisystem inflammatory syndrome in children (MIS-C) showing disseminated aspergillosis, cytomegalovirus reactivation and persistent SARS-COV-2: Case report with autopsy review. Pathol Res Pract 2022;238:154106.

81. Yonker LM, Gilboa T, Ogata AF, et al. Multisystem inflammatory syndrome in children is driven by zonulin-dependent loss of gut mucosal barrier. J Clin Invest 2021;131(14). https://doi.org/10.1172/jci149633.

82. Kato H, Sugimura T, Akagi T, et al. Long-term consequences of Kawasaki disease. A 10- to 21-year follow-up study of 594 patients. Circulation 1996;94(6): 1379–85.

83. Gordon JB, Daniels LB, Kahn AM, et al. The spectrum of cardiovascular lesions requiring intervention in adults after Kawasaki disease. JACC Cardiovasc Interv 2016;9(7):687–96.

84. Hirata S, Nakamura Y, Matsumoto K, et al. Long-term consequences of Kawasaki disease among first-year junior high school students. Arch Pediatr Adolesc Med 2002;156(1):77–80.

85. Muneuchi J, Joo K, Morihana E, et al. Detectable silent calcification in a regressed coronary artery aneurysm of a young adult with a history of Kawasaki disease. Pediatr Cardiol 2008;29(1):195–7.

86. Truong DT, Trachtenberg FL, Pearson GD, et al. The NHLBI Study on Long-terM OUtcomes after the Multisystem Inflammatory Syndrome In Children (MUSIC): Design and Objectives. Am Heart J 2022;243:43–53.

87. Maddux AB, Berbert L, Young CC, et al. Health impairments in children and adolescents after hospitalization for acute COVID-19 or MIS-C. Pediatrics 2022; 150(3). https://doi.org/10.1542/peds.2022-057798.

88. Davies P, du Pré P, Lillie J, et al. One-year outcomes of critical care patients post-COVID-19 multisystem inflammatory syndrome in children. JAMA Pediatr 2021; 175(12):1281–3.

89. Penner J, Abdel-Mannan O, Grant K, et al. 6-month multidisciplinary follow-up and outcomes of patients with paediatric inflammatory multisystem syndrome (PIMS-TS) at a UK tertiary paediatric hospital: a retrospective cohort study. Lancet Child Adolesc Health 2021;5(7):473–82.

90. Barouch DH. Covid-19 vaccines — immunity, variants, boosters. N Engl J Med 2022. https://doi.org/10.1056/NEJMra2206573.

91. Levy N, Koppel JH, Kaplan O, et al. Severity and incidence of multisystem inflammatory syndrome in children during 3 SARS-CoV-2 Pandemic Waves in Israel. JAMA 2022;327(24):2452–4.

92. Holm M, Espenhain L, Glenthøj J, et al. Risk and Phenotype of Multisystem Inflammatory Syndrome in Vaccinated and Unvaccinated Danish Children Before and During the Omicron Wave. JAMA Pediatr 2022;176(8):821–3.

93. Zambrano LD, Newhams MM, Olson SM, et al. Effectiveness of BNT162b2 (Pfizer-BioNTech) mRNA vaccination against multisystem inflammatory syndrome in children among persons aged 12-18 years - United States, July-December 2021. MMWR Morb Mortal Wkly Rep 2022;71(2):52–8.

94. Liu Y, Liu J, Johnson BA, et al. Delta spike P681R mutation enhances SARS-CoV-2 fitness over Alpha variant. Cell Rep 2022;39(7):110829.

95. Meng B, Abdullahi A, Ferreira I, et al. Altered TMPRSS2 usage by SARS-CoV-2 Omicron impacts infectivity and fusogenicity. Nature 2022;603(7902):706–14.

96. Gül A. Dynamics of inflammatory response in autoinflammatory disorders: autonomous and hyperinflammatory states. Front Immunol 2018;9:2422.

Multisystem Inflammatory Syndrome in Children and Kawasaki Disease

A Spectrum of Postinfectious Hyperinflammatory Disease

Lauren Ambler Robinson, MD[a,b], Marissa Dale, MD[c,d],
Mark Gorelik, MD[e,*]

KEYWORDS

- Kawasaki disease • MIS-C • Vasculitis • COVID-19

KEY POINTS

- Kawasaki disease (KD) and the multisystem inflammatory syndrome in children (MIS-C) share many clinical features, and many patients meet diagnostic criteria for both conditions.
- Both KD and MIS-C are monophasic hyperinflammatory conditions that occur in children following likely infectious triggers.
- Cardiac manifestations are common in both KD and MIS-C, with coronary artery aneurysms being most prevalent in KD and myocarditis with ventricular dysfunction being most prevalent in MIS-C.
- Immunomodulatory therapy is the mainstay of treatment for both KD and MIS-C, and with prompt treatment, outcomes are favorable.
- Pathophysiology of these hyperinflammatory conditions is incompletely understood.

Multisystem Inflammatory Syndrome in Children (MIS-C) and Kawasaki Disease (KD): Overlapping Entities on a Spectrum of Post-infectious Hyperinflammatory Disease.

[a] Department of Medicine, Pediatric Rheumatology, Hospital for Special Surgery, New York, NY, USA; [b] Department of Pediatric Rheumatology, 535 East 70th Street, New York, NY 10021, USA; [c] Department of Pediatrics, Columbia University Medical Center, New York, NY, USA; [d] Morgan Stanley Children's Hospital, 3959 Broadway Central 5th Floor, New York, NY 10032, USA; [e] Division of Allergy, Immunology, and Rheumatology, Department of Pediatrics, Columbia University Medical Center, College of Physicians and Surgeons Building, P&S 10-451, 630 West 168th Street, New York NY 10032, USA
* Corresponding author.
E-mail address: mg4082@cumc.columbia.edu

Rheum Dis Clin N Am 49 (2023) 661–678
https://doi.org/10.1016/j.rdc.2023.03.003
0889-857X/23/© 2023 Elsevier Inc. All rights reserved.

INTRODUCTION
Kawasaki Disease: Brief Overview

Kawasaki Disease (KD) is one of the most common vasculitides in the pediatric population and is encountered regularly by the general pediatrician. First described as an acute febrile illness in the 1950s in Japan,[1] it was not until 1970 that the link between KD and coronary artery aneurysms was clearly established.[2,3] Although the pathophysiology of KD remains incompletely understood, it is widely thought to be triggered by infection in a genetically susceptible host. The hallmark clinical features are fever, rash, conjunctivitis, lymphadenopathy, mucocutaneous changes, and hand/foot edema followed by periungual desquamation. The incidence of coronary artery aneurysms in KD, which occurs in up to 25% of untreated cases, has decreased to ~5% with the use of high-dose intravenous immunoglobulin (IVIG) as standard treatment.[4,5]

Multisystem Inflammatory Syndrome in Children: Brief Overview

The entity now known as Multisystem Inflammatory Syndrome in Children (MIS-C) was first described in March 2020, when pediatric hospitals saw an abrupt increase in cases of a systemic febrile illness often characterized by shock[6] and clinical features of KD[7,8] in temporal relationship to the SARS-CoV-2 pandemic. The most common clinical features include fever, rash, conjunctivitis, abdominal pain, and myocarditis often leading to shock and multiorgan failure if untreated. Although the pathogenesis remains incompletely understood, most cases occur between 4 and 6 weeks of SARS-CoV-2 infection, as is reflected in the case definition,[9] and thus suggest a pathogenic postinfectious immune response. Treatment with various immunosuppressive therapies has been used with success, including glucocorticoids, IVIG, interleukin-1 (IL-1) and tumor necrosis factor-α (TNF-α) blockade.[10] With prompt immunosuppressive treatment, the vast majority of children make a full recovery without currently known long-term sequelae.[11] Finally, and importantly, cases of MIS-C have fallen precipitously since arrival of the "Omicron" and subsequent "Omicron" daughter strains. In fact, in the authors' institution (NewYork–Presbyterian Hospital), it appears that there have been essentially no new cases of MIS-C since the Omicron strain replaced Delta and other pre-Delta SARS-CoV-2 strains.

A Unique Opportunity

MIS-C and KD are, in some senses, a study in contrasts. Although KD has been well described for more than 50 years and the therapeutics used to treat KD have remained relatively static since the 1980s, MIS-C is a relative infant in the family of human disease and remains without a validated set of diagnostic criteria or well-studied methods of treatment. Nevertheless, MIS-C with its overt similarity to KD has provided a unique opportunity to study and enhance the understanding of its much older sibling, in both terms of the similar features and contrasting aspects of these diseases. For instance, despite generally excellent medium- and long-term outcomes, nearly half of patients with MIS-C become critically ill during their hospitalization and require intensive care and broad immunosuppression, whereas patients with KD rarely develop shock (with the notable exception of Kawasaki Shock Syndrome). The as-yet unknown answer to why MIS-C is uniquely associated with a shock phenotype, whereas KD is rarely so, may inform upon critical concepts regarding the nature of shock and inflammation itself. As another example, MIS-C vascular aneurysms tend to resolve or remodel very quickly, whereas those of KD are long-lived. Here again, understanding how differences in molecular biology may result in these varied phenotypes could shed light on these basic mechanisms of disease.

Thus, given the clinical overlaps between KD and MIS-C, there is a unique opportunity to study these diseases in parallel with the possibility of understanding pathogenic and immunologic mechanisms that may be shared. Elucidation of the immunopathogenesis of these diseases has the potential to further scientific understanding of hyperinflammatory syndromes and could lead to discovery of targeted therapies that would further reduce morbidity and mortality.

An Important Barrier to Critical Comparisons of Kawasaki Disease and Multisystem Inflammatory Syndrome in Children

Before a critical comparison between the clinical phenotypes and pathophysiology of MIS-C and KD can be made, it is important to note that there is no universally used classification or diagnostic criteria for MIS-C. Although case definitions have been put forth by the World Health Organization and Centers for Disease Control and Prevention (CDC), many published cohorts have used alternative inclusion or diagnostic criteria, making generalizability and direct comparison challenging. One of the most apparent inconsistencies is in the proportion of patients with laboratory-confirmed exposure to SARS-CoV-2. Different cohorts contain widely variable proportions of patients without either confirmed prior infection, positive reverse transcription polymerase chain reaction, or positive SARS-CoV-2 serology.[12–15] The inclusion of patients without laboratory-confirmed evidence of prior SARS-CoV-2 infection potentially allows for inclusion of patients who do not truly have MIS-C but rather have an alternative febrile illness. Furthermore, a sizable percentage, up to 40% in some cohorts, of patients diagnosed with MIS-C fulfill either complete or incomplete American Heart Association diagnostic criteria for KD.[13,15] In these cases, it is likely not possible to definitively parse out a single diagnosis.

EPIDEMIOLOGY

The exact incidence of MIS-C compared with overall COVID-19 cases in children remains somewhat uncertain owing to a lack of central SARS-CoV-2 testing registry for children and limited access to pediatric testing early in the pandemic. Studies have demonstrated that MIS-C appears to be a relatively rare complication of COVID-19 in children. Based on CDC surveillance data from March 2020 to January 2021 for individuals less than 21 years of age, cumulative MIS-C incidence was approximately 2 per 100,000 individuals.[16]

Although initial reports of MIS-C emerged from the United Kingdom in April 2020, cases have now been reported almost worldwide.[6,17] There have been strikingly few reports of MIS-C from China and other Asian countries despite these areas being early pandemic hot spots.[18,19] KD, however, has a well-established higher incidence in children living in East Asia and children with Asian ancestry living in other areas of the world. Rates of KD vary country to country, from 25 per 100,000 children younger than 5 years of age in the United States to more than 250 per 100,000 in Japan.[20,21]

In contrast to KD, children of Asian heritage account for a small number of MIS-C cases. Rates of MIS-C are disproportionately higher in black and Hispanic populations.[15,22] This discrepancy is likely multifactorial with disparities in social determinants of health contributing to SARS-CoV-2 exposure risk. However, increased risk in patients from these backgrounds has been shown to extend beyond socioeconomic status.[23] This suggests that, similarly to KD, genetic risk factors may play a role in pathogenesis of MIS-C.

Age of patients also differs between KD and MIS-C. KD predominantly impacts infants and young children with 80% of patients younger than 5 years of age.[20,24] The mean incidence of patients with KD is around 3 years of age.[25,26] MIS-C most frequently strikes an entirely different age group with a median age of 8 to 9 years.[15,22] Although it is still unclear why KD is seen in higher rates in infants and younger children, one proposed explanation is that there is increased susceptibility at this age owing to immaturity of the immune system and incomplete exposure to common viruses.[27]

CLINICAL PRESENTATION
Common Clinical Features

The most common presenting symptoms in patients with MIS-C are fever (an obligate criteria, duration of $\geq$4 days in 90% of patients),[15] abdominal pain and/or diarrhea (53%–92% of patients),[13,15,22] and mucocutaneous features, such as erythematous rash or conjunctival injection (52%–74% of patients).[13,15,22] Shortly after initial clinical presentation, many patients with MIS-C develop hypotension secondary to vasoplegic and/or cardiogenic shock that usually resolves rapidly following treatment. Patients with KD also present with fever (an obligate criteria, usually lasting 11–13 days if untreated), with conjunctival injection being the most common (up to >90% of patients)[28] of the 5 diagnostic criteria, followed closely by polymorphous rash, mucosal changes, and distal extremity changes. Unilateral cervical lymphadenopathy, although 1 of the 5 diagnostic criteria for KD, is the least common finding occurring in about 60% of cases.[29] This is more frequent than in patients with MIS-C,[15] but in itself, this higher incidence of unilateral lymphadenopathy in KD is not sensitive enough as a discriminator. Although gastrointestinal (GI) manifestations are commonly reported to occur either at the time of or closely preceding presentation in patients with KD,[28–30] these manifestations are much less frequent and severe than those observed in patients with MIS-C. Up to 5% of patients with KD will develop a syndrome referred to as Kawasaki Disease Shock Syndrome (KDSS), characterized by hypotension or signs of poor perfusion. Still, the incidence of KDSS is low compared with the frequency of shock in MIS-C, which occurs in about half of all patients.[13,31]

Laboratory Findings

Certain laboratory findings are typical in patients with KD and are known to change from the acute phase of illness to the subacute phase, and finally, to convalescence. In the acute phase of illness, laboratory findings typically are notable for leukocytosis with neutrophilic predominance and bandemia, elevated inflammatory markers (C-reactive protein [CRP] and erythrocyte sedimentation rate [ESR]), and a predominantly normocytic normochromic anemia for age.[13,32] In the subacute phase of illness, often following treatment with IVIG, the white blood cell count drops with a relative increase in lymphocytes, and there is often a prominent thrombocytosis. ESR will typically remain elevated. After disease recovery, about 6 to 8 weeks following onset, laboratory parameters return to normal ranges.[33]

There are a few notable differences in the pattern of laboratory parameters between KD and MIS-C. The acute phase of MIS-C is characterized often by profound lymphopenia and either normal or low platelet count. Normocytic normochromic anemia is common as in KD but is on average a bit more severe in MIS-C. CRP levels are generally higher in patients with MIS-C. The most notable differences in laboratory parameters between MIS-C and KD are the notable elevations in ferritin, troponin, brain natriuretic peptide (BNP), and D-dimer seen in MIS-C. BNP elevation is also seen in patients with KD, but to a lesser degree than in MIS-C.[34] Although the more severe form of KD that presents with shock, KDSS, can have CBC findings similar to MIS-C, even in KDSS elevations in ferritin and troponin are rare.[13,35]

Ocular Findings

MIS-C and KD both appear to share the frequent finding of nongranulomatous anterior uveitis identified on slit-lamp examination. Both conditions have also been associated with variable incidence of keratitis and epitheliopathy. In KD, a variable incidence of anterior uveitis has been reported, from 29% to 83% of patients examined within a week of disease onset.[36,37] Anterior uveitis has also been described in several cases of MIS-C.[38,39] In both conditions, true incidence of uveitis is difficult to establish, as most patients do not undergo ophthalmologic examination; however, it is likely frequent. In the patients who have been followed with ophthalmologic examinations, the anterior uveitis in both MIS-C and KD appears to resolve quickly with systemic immunomodulatory therapy with or without the use of topical glucocorticoids. Uveitis is typically associated with other classical autoimmune phenomena, such as juvenile arthritis, Behcet syndrome, and others, and suggests the relationship between MIS-C, KD, and other autoimmune syndromes[40] **(Fig. 1)**.

Cardiac Involvement

The most common cardiac complication of KD is the development of coronary artery aneurysms, which occurred in up to 25% of patients before widespread use of IVIG treatment. Coronary artery aneurysms are also seen in patients with MIS-C, with rates of aneurysm development varying among cohorts, from 6% to 24% of all patients.[6,7,15,31,41,42] Coronary artery dilation in MIS-C is most often milder and shorter-lived than in patients with KD.[11] However, there have been several reported cases of giant aneurysms.[43–45] In addition, a recent case series describes delayed

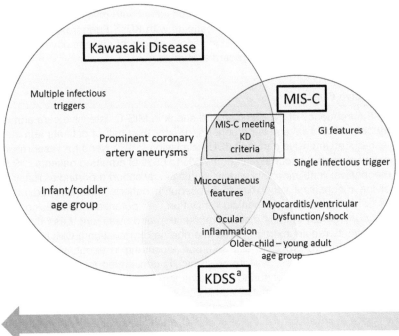

Fig. 1. Relationship of MIS-C, KDSS, and KD. [a]KDSS, Kawasaki Disease Shock Syndrome.

development of coronary aneurysms in children with MIS-C despite treatment with IVIG and corticosteroids, but responsive to infliximab.[46]

Although coronary artery dilation and aneurysm formation do occur in patients with MIS-C, the most prominent cardiac manifestations of MIS-C are myocardial inflammation and ventricular dysfunction. Biochemical evidence of myocardial inflammation or dysfunction (via elevated serum troponin or BNP) is present in 65% to 95% of cases.[31] Echocardiography in a large cohort of European patients demonstrated decreased left ventricular ejection fraction in 34% of patients with MIS-C at admission.[31] Patients with evidence of myocardial dysfunction are at highest risk for clinical shock and need for intensive care. Cardiac MRI findings in patients with MIS-C with cardiac dysfunction have demonstrated myocardial hyperemia without fibrosis.[47] Despite this high degree of myocardial inflammation and systolic dysfunction, the vast majority of patients with MIS-C have rapid recovery of systolic function, with very few reports of ongoing severe impairment of cardiac function.[31,48]

Another important feature of cardiac injury in MIS-C is electrophysiologic dysfunction.[49] A majority (two-thirds) of patients with MIS-C demonstrate electrocardiogram abnormalities and conduction abnormalities. In addition, there have been several reports of the emergence of a Brugada-like pattern on electrocardiogram at the time of diagnosis with MIS-C.[50,51]

Clinical signs of myocardial inflammation and decreased systolic function are less common in patients with KD but do occur. Many reports show that patients with KD have varying degrees of myocardial inflammation. A large cohort of patients with KD undergoing routine echocardiography as part of a treatment trial showed that 20% of patients had left ventricular dysfunction.[34] Similar to cases of ventricular dysfunction in MIS-C, the vast majority of patients have normalization of their cardiac function within days. When using more sensitive imaging techniques for myocardial inflammation, such as gallium-67 scintigraphy, findings consistent with myocardial inflammation have been identified in up to 64% of patients with KD.[52] Furthermore, autopsy specimens from patients who died of KD in various stages of disease have revealed early myocarditis followed by late myocardial fibrosis.[53]

Need for Intensive Care

Because of the frequency of hypotension and shock in MIS-C, intensive care admission is very common. In several large cohorts, greater than half of patients admitted with MIS-C required intensive care unit (ICU) admission.[13,31,54] Need for vasopressor support is very common, occurring in about 45% to 65% of admitted patients.[13,22,54] Rates of mechanical ventilation vary widely, with an early cohort reporting as many as 43% receiving mechanical ventilation.[13] Subsequent cohorts have showed much lower rates of intubation and mechanical ventilation,[15,55] potentially decreasing over time, given improvement in early disease recognition and treatment. Less than 5% of admitted patients require extracorporeal membrane oxygenation (ECMO).[15,22]

ICU admission for KD is much less common, occurring in about 3% to 7% of cases.[56–58] Nearly all of these patients are clinically considered to have KDSS and are admitted to the ICU for monitoring and management of hypotension. Vasoactive therapy is less commonly used in ICU admission for KDSS than for MIS-C. Interestingly, patients with KDSS tend to be older than patients with KD without shock, with laboratory findings similar to those found in MIS-C, such as higher CRP and neutrophil percentage as well as lower platelet count and serum albumin.[59] The use of mechanical ventilation and ECMO in the treatment of KDSS is rare but documented in case reports.[60–62]

PATHOPHYSIOLOGY
Infectious Triggers

MIS-C has a clear temporal relationship to a single infectious trigger, the SARS-CoV-2 virus. The mechanism of how SARS-CoV-2 infection leads to systemic hyperinflammation remains incompletely elucidated. There is evidence that persistence of the virus in the GI tract is associated with increased intestinal permeability and subsequent antigenemia that could trigger an immune response.[63] It has also been suggested that the spike protein of the SARS-CoV-2 virus contains a motif that functions as a superantigen, binding with high affinity to the alpha and beta chains of T-cell receptors and thus having the potential to lead to widespread T-cell activation and cytokine storm.[64] This theory is bolstered by the finding of T-cell receptor skewing suggestive of a superantigen found in adult patients with severe COVID-19 and hyperinflammation.[65]

Although no single infectious trigger has been identified for KD, there is strong evidence that infectious triggers contribute to the development of disease. Perhaps most striking is the strong seasonal variance in cases globally, suggesting exposure to infectious agents with seasonal variance.[66,67] Many infectious agents have been linked to KD, including viruses, bacteria, and fungi.[21] Recurrences are infrequent, suggesting that individuals may have a predisposition to developing this hyperinflammatory syndrome in response to only certain infectious stimuli, and that immunity may be protective. Although it has been hypothesized that KD may be driven by response to a superantigen owing to findings of T-cell receptor skewing,[68] later studies demonstrated clonal expansion of T cells and immunoglobulin A (IgA) -secreting plasma cells in the peripheral blood and tissues of patients with KD, pointing instead to a conventional antigen as an infectious trigger.[69–71] Still, there exists the possibility that certain infectious triggers could be functioning as superantigens, thus causing T-cell receptor skewing in some cohorts and not others. Study of T-cell receptor skewing specifically of patients with the KDSS phenotype, which shares more features with MIS-C and Toxic Shock Syndrome, would be of interest and could lend further evidence to the idea that these entities exist on a spectrum.

Genetic Predisposition

There is strong evidence for genetic predisposition contributing to KD pathogenesis. Siblings of patients with KD have been shown to be at significantly higher risk for the disease than the general population, and several risk alleles at different loci as well as different HLA types have been identified in different populations.[72] Certain genetic mutations have been associated with increased risk for IVIG resistance and development of coronary artery aneurysms.[73] Genetic susceptibility loci have also offered potential insights into disease pathogenesis. For instance, the ITPKC gene is a common risk locus in the Japanese population that encodes for inositol 1,4,5-triphosphate 3-kinase C.[74] Alterations in this enzyme's activity have been associated with increased activation of the NLRP3 inflammasome,[75] and this could potentially contribute to the increased IL-1 signaling found in patients with KD.[76,77] Most importantly, the wide array of risk alleles coding for proteins in various immunologic pathways in different populations points to the pathophysiologic heterogeneity of this disease.

Genetic susceptibility to MIS-C is theorized but less well established. The low incidence of MIS-C in the Asian population, despite widespread infection with SARS-CoV-2, points to the idea that risk alleles are likely to be more common in certain ethnicities and less common in others. Whole-exome sequencing on a cohort of patients with MIS-C has preliminarily revealed mutations in immunologically relevant pathways in up to 17%,[78] although these data are yet to be replicated. Furthermore, associations between HLA types and MIS-C have been described and are of particular interest because it has also been shown that certain HLA types are associated with severe acute COVID-19 with hyperinflammation in adults.[79] This is an important active area of research.

Cytokine Profiles and Proteomics

Both KD and MIS-C are characterized by "cytokine storming" with significant alteration in levels of various proinflammatory cytokines. Although the cytokine profiles are not identical, they have been shown to have very significant overlap.[14,35] Particularly, KD and MIS-C have both been shown to have elevated levels of interferon-γ (IFN-γ), TNF-α, IL-6, IL-8, IL-10, and IL-1β, although with less IL-8 dysregulation in KD.[14] In addition, proteomic analysis of patients with KD and MIS-C compared with healthy controls and patients with acute COVID-19 showed many similarities in the proteomes of MIS-C and KD.[14] It is important to note, however, that there are differences in the cytokine profiles of KD and MIS-C despite their many overlaps. For instance, IL-17A has been shown to be more elevated in KD than MIS-C, although subsequent groups demonstrated significant IL-17 elevation in patients with MIS-C.[28,65] Interestingly, several studies have found that patients with MIS-C segregate into 2 distinct groups with different cytokine profiles and disease severity/characteristics.[14,80] It is suggested that the milder KD-like phenotype of MIS-C has immunologic overlap with KD, whereas the more severe MIS-C phenotype with increased GI and neurologic involvement has a distinct immunologic pattern characterized by IFN-γ signaling and higher levels of classical complement activation.[14,80] Studies from the authors' group and others show marked upregulation of IL-27 in MIS-C, which is also known to be associated with mortality in patients with septic shock.[81,82] The idea that MIS-C may represent a spectrum of disease with varying degrees/varieties of immunologic dysregulation is further supported by the findings that cohorts of patients with MIS-C have been segregated into various categories based on clinical presentation. Proposed subcategories of MIS-C based on clinical presentation are severe MIS-C, acute COVID-19 with hyperinflammation, and a milder KD-like phenotype.[83] Study of these subcategories of MIS-C has the potential to reveal different degrees and patterns of immune dysregulation.

Immunophenotyping and Autoantibodies

Both the innate and adaptive immune systems have been implicated in the pathogenesis of KD and MIS-C. In both conditions there is increased activation of monocytes and neutrophils in the acute phase, despite no increase in overall number of monocytes and neutrophils in MIS-C.[12,84] In KD, there is expansion of CD8$^+$ T cells as well as increased numbers of antibody secreting cells, often with oligoclonal expansion suggesting response to a particular antigen.[85,86] It is suggested in KD via the presence of elevated IL-17 levels, that there is enhanced Th17 cell response compared with Th1/Th2 responses. Although MIS-C is characterized by lymphopenia, immunophenotyping has demonstrated increased activation of CD8$^+$ nonnaïve T cells, CD4$^+$ effector T cells, and central memory T cells.[12,35,87] Several groups have also identified increased IL-17 signaling in MIS-C, suggesting involvement of the Th17 pathway.[12,88]

The mechanism of vasculitis in KD and MIS-C, particularly of the coronary arteries, is not well understood. In KD, autopsy specimens of the coronaries have demonstrated presence of IgA-secreting plasma cells, and it is suggested that IgA is important in vascular damage.[64,70] Interestingly, although patients with selective IgA deficiency can manifest with KD, a case series of such patients demonstrated a relative lack of coronary artery aneurysm formation, further suggesting the importance of IgA in the development of the coronary vasculitis.[89] CD8+ T cells have also been suggested to play an important role in coronary artery inflammation, as evidence by the presence of activated CD8+ T cells in the intima of coronary lesions in KD.[90] A lack of coronary tissue sampling in MIS-C leaves the nature of coronary artery inflammation and aneurysm formation in this condition poorly understood.

In both KD and MIS-C, an endothelial protein, endoglin, has been shown to be elevated in plasma, and anti-endoglin antibodies have been also identified.[35] These antibodies are thought to represent a result of endothelial injury rather than a cause. No consistent autoantibody profile has been recognized in either KD or MIS-C. In MIS-C, most patients have serologic evidence of prior SARS-CoV-2 infection with antibodies detectable to the spike protein.[13,15,22] However, there is no evidence to date that these antibodies or circulating immune complexes are pathogenic in the disease.[80] Finally, a recent study demonstrated that in patients treated with IVIG, spurious "autoantibodies" may be detected, which in fact are derived from IVIG.[91] This suggests caution with data suggesting autoantibodies when derived from samples obtained from post-IVIG–treated patients.

TREATMENT
Immunomodulation

Initial therapeutic goals for treatment of KD are to reduce inflammation, decrease vascular damage, and prevent potential cardiac sequelae. Standard-of-care primary treatment for KD in the acute phase is IVIG as a single infusion and aspirin.[24,92] As soon as diagnosis is established, IVIG infusion should be initiated. IVIG treatment has been shown to decrease incidence of new coronary abnormalities.[93] The exact mechanism of action for IVIG in the treatment of KD is still unknown but appears to have an overall anti-inflammatory effect with many KD patients experiencing dramatic improvement in symptoms within hours of IVIG initiation.[94]

Around 10% to 20% of patients with KD will develop fever again at least 36 hours after the end of IVIG infusion and are characterized as IVIG resistant.[95] The most frequently administered second-line treatment options include a second infusion of IVIG, high-dose pulse steroids, or infliximab. The optimal choice of a second-line agent in a refractory patient with KD remains an area of research. Importantly, repeated doses of IVIG can result in hemolysis, and thus, in many cases, use of infliximab or corticosteroids may be reasonable.[92] In the case of highly refractory patients, there should be consideration of agents such as cyclosporine, anakinra or, in extreme circumstances, cyclophosphamide.

Patients with KD who are at high risk of IVIG resistance or development of coronary artery aneurysms may benefit from a stronger initial treatment regimen, such as the addition of steroids or an immunomodulatory agent.[92] Several scoring systems to predict IVIG resistance exist. However, these scoring systems have been developed in Japanese patients and have not performed as well when applied to North American populations.[95] There is growing evidence that patients with coronary artery aneurysms at time of diagnosis would benefit from primary treatment intensification to decrease aneurysm progression and expedite return to normal vessel lumen diameter.[96]

Similar to KD treatment, MIS-C treatment approaches aim to reduce exaggerated inflammatory responses. Most MIS-C treatments to date have been derived from KD and other hyperinflammatory syndromes. Initial management of patients with MIS-C depends on the constellation of presenting clinical symptoms. The most severe subset of patients with MIS-C can present in shock and with cardiovascular manifestations and should be treated with broad-spectrum antibiotics, fluid resuscitation, and if needed, inotropic support. In contrast to KD whereby approximately 5% of patients present with cardiovascular shock, large case series of MIS-C have shown that more than half of patients necessitate ICU care and may require vasopressors or inotropes.[15,22,97]

Expert consensus first-tier immunomodulatory therapy for hospitalized patients with MIS-C is IVIG in combination with low- to moderate-dose glucocorticoids.[98,99] Although the benefit of universal IVIG and glucocorticoid is not established in KD, retrospective MIS-C data have shown that this combination therapy results in more favorable outcomes than IVIG alone with decreased need for hemodynamic support and use of second-line immunomodulatory agents.[10,100,101]

Clinical improvements for patients that respond to initial treatment are typically seen within the first day of treatment. Refractory disease in MIS-C is usually described as ongoing fever, continued organ dysfunction, and uptrending inflammatory markers. For patients with refractory disease after initial treatment, second-tier options include high-dose glucocorticoids, anakinra, and infliximab. Because patients with refractory disease can decline and deteriorate quickly, intensification therapy should be initiated promptly. Second doses of IVIG, a commonly used second-line treatment in KD, are not recommended in MISC because of risk of fluid overload in the setting of cardiac dysfunction. Although not recommended in the American College of Rheumatology or National Institutes of Health current guidelines, tocilizumab has also been used in refractory MIS-C.[97] However, because of case reports suggesting lack of efficacy and in fact worsening of aneurysms associated with the use of tocilizumab in patients with KD, tocilizumab use in MIS-C should be with caution.[102]

Anticoagulation

Although there is no clear evidence that aspirin reduces coronary abnormalities in KD, it has remained as first-line treatment owing to its anti-inflammatory and antiplatelet properties. Traditionally, the initial dose of aspirin varied depending on local practice patterns from either a moderate dose of 30 to 50 mg/kg per day or a high dose of 80 to 100 mg/kg per day. Following the cessation of the acute phase, patients were then switched to low dosing (3–5 mg/kg per day) for strictly anticoagulative properties. However, recent literature has suggested that there is no benefit in terms of prevention of coronary aneurysms of high-/moderate-dose versus low-dose aspirin for patients in the acute phase of KD.[103,104] In fact, the use of high-dose aspirin preceded the use of IVIG, and at the time, was used in an attempt to suppress the inflammatory state.[105] The continued use of high-dose aspirin is a hold-over from this period, but is likely of no added benefit. Thus, new guidelines now advocate use of either high- or low-dose aspirin from the beginning of the acute phase, without a dose preference.[92]

Although there is a lack of randomized clinical trials evaluating antithrombotic regimens for prophylaxis of coronary thrombosis, standard of care is to use antiplatelet agents for small- to moderate-sized aneurysms. Patients with large or giant aneurysms are at much higher risk for thrombosis. Therefore, this subset of patients is usually treated with a combination of antiplatelet and anticoagulant therapy.

As seen in KD, patients with MIS-C are at risk for thrombotic complications, such as apical left ventricular thrombus, myocardial infarction, and venous thromboembolism. There are few data to guide prophylactic management, and thus, most commonly followed management strategies have been extrapolated from KD. For instance, low-dose aspirin is also recommended for use in patients with MIS-C until normalization of platelet count, and follow-up echocardiogram shows normal coronary arteries. Initiation of prophylactic systemic anticoagulation for hospitalized patients should be decided on an individual basis with consideration of the balance between thrombotic risk factors versus bleeding risk. Patients with MIS-C with large coronary artery aneurysm, moderate to severe left ventricular dysfunction, or documented thrombosis should receive therapeutic anticoagulation unless there are contraindications.[106]

PROGNOSIS

Full recovery in the vast majority of patients with KD and MIS-C is expected with appropriate management. Overall long-term clinical outcomes of MIS-C are not clear yet, but follow-up data over the past 2 years appear to be positive. In-hospital mortality for KD is 0.17% in the United States and less than 0.1% in Japan.[24] Mortalities for MIS-C, from large case series and CDC data, are estimated at around 1% of affected children.[97,107,108]

Degree of cardiac involvement plays a significant role in short-term morbidity and mortality for patients with both KD and MIS-C. Long-term outcomes for patients with KD with cardiac sequelae are driven by ongoing dynamic remodeling of heart tissues and vessels. Because inflammation during the acute phase of KD can affect any tissue of the heart, fibrotic changes occur in the valves and the myocardium as well, which can lead to arrhythmias, valvular dysfunction, and heart failure later in life.[109] Complete resolution of coronary aneurysms in the first 2 years after disease onset is seen in over half of vessels. Chance of aneurysm resolution depends on initial size, with a worse prognosis associated with giant aneurysms owing to increased thrombosis incidence.[110]

Even if coronary aneurysms do regress, patients are still at increased risk for development of early-onset coronary artery disease in adulthood. In fact, there are several cases of fatal and nonfatal myocardial infarctions in young adults that can be attributed to missed or undiagnosed KD cases. Coronary angiography of a subset of adults under 40 years old with suspected myocardial ischemia demonstrated that 5% of this population was found to have lesions of late KD sequelae despite no prior known history of the disease.[111]

Data on long-term cardiac outcomes for patients with MIS-C are limited, but follow-up studies over the past 2 years overall look positive. With higher rates of myocardial dysfunction in MIS-C compared with classic KD, myocardial functional defects have been the most significant cause of short-term morbidity and mortality in patients with MIS-C.[19,112] As seen in patients with KDSS who experience decreased systolic function, patients with MIS-C with systolic dysfunction typically have normalized systolic function during follow-up but may still have persistence of other echocardiogram abnormalities, such as left ventricular strain and diastolic dysfunction.[31] Persistence of these abnormalities is still of uncertain clinical significance.

Initial follow-up studies on MIS-C coronary artery abnormalities have been promising as well with case series showing either (1) complete and rapid resolution of coronary abnormalities or (2) only a minority of patients with persistent abnormalities 6 months to 1 year later.[112,113] At this time, it is unclear whether this regression in coronary abnormalities is treatment-related or merely part of the natural history of the disease. Future studies on risk of cardiovascular events will be needed as patients with MIS-C enter adulthood.

SUMMARY

The emergence of MIS-C has led to new interest and focus on postinfectious autoimmune/hyperinflammatory disease and especially KD. Many features of these 2 conditions are similar, such as presence of rash, oral mucosal changes, and palmar erythema, but the clinical similarities are not merely skin deep. As mentioned, patients with MIS-C and KD often develop uveitis and coronary aneurysms, and although rarer in KD, shock syndrome is seen in both conditions. The existence of KDSS with laboratory findings highly similar to MIS-C is perhaps the strongest suggestion that MIS-C and KD exist on a spectrum. Although there is some question as to whether a superantigen promotes a toxic shock–like phenomenon in MIS-C,[114] the presence of autoimmune features, such as uveitis and the delayed onset after infection, suggests that there is a complex interaction between superantigen and the phenotypic presentation that is more layered than classical toxic shock. The occurrence of KD in epidemic spikes is strongly suggestive of an infectious trigger,[115] much as MIS-C, which is clearly a postinfectious phenomenon. Conversely, the clarity of the postinfectious nature of MIS-C adds confidence to the postinfectious suspicions surrounding KD. Ultimately, whether MIS-C is indeed a sibling disorder of KD from a molecular and pathophysiologic state is unclear, and may never be solved, as the incidence of MIS-C is now rapidly diminished and possibly extinct following the replacement of "Delta" and previous strains with new strains of SARS-CoV-2. In turn, this decrease in MIS-C incidence with newer strains of SARS-CoV-2 may be the silver lining of this pandemic for our children.

CLINICS CARE POINTS

- Patients may meet criteria for both Kawasaki disease and multisystem inflammatory syndrome in children, and in such cases, prompt treatment with steroids and intravenous immunoglobulin (with attention to avoid volume overload in cases of ventricular dysfunction) is appropriate.
- Close monitoring of patients with multisystem inflammatory syndrome in children is warranted, as shock is common, and greater than 50% of patients will require intensive care.
- Echocardiography is needed in the evaluation of all patients with Kawasaki disease and multisystem inflammatory syndrome in children to assess for coronary artery aneurysm formation and ventricular dysfunction.
- Incidence of multisystem inflammatory syndrome in children has decreased dramatically with the emergence of post-Delta SARS-CoV-2 variants, and maintenance of a broad differential diagnosis when evaluating children with febrile illnesses is critical.

DISCLOSURE

The authors have nothing to disclose.

FUNDING

MG is supported by National Heart Lung and Blood Institute 5K08HL155033.

REFERENCES

1. Kawasaki T. [Acute febrile mucocutaneous syndrome with lymphoid involvement with specific desquamation of the fingers and toes in children]. Arerugi Allergy 1967;16(3):178–222.
2. Burns JC, Kushner HI, Bastian JF, et al. Kawasaki disease: a brief history. Pediatrics 2000;106(2):E27.
3. Kawasaki T, Kosaki F, Okawa S, et al. A new infantile acute febrile mucocutaneous lymph node syndrome (MLNS) prevailing in Japan. Pediatrics 1974;54(3):271–6.

4. Newburger JW, Takahashi M, Beiser AS, et al. A single intravenous infusion of gamma globulin as compared with four infusions in the treatment of acute Kawasaki syndrome. N Engl J Med 1991;324(23):1633–9.

5. Furusho K, Nakano H, Shinomiya K, et al. High-dose intravenous gammaglobulin for Kawasaki disease. Lancet 1984;324(8411):1055–8.

6. Riphagen S, Gomez X, Gonzalez-Martinez C, et al. Hyperinflammatory shock in children during COVID-19 pandemic. Lancet 2020;395(10237):1607–8.

7. Verdoni L, Mazza A, Gervasoni A, et al. An outbreak of severe Kawasaki-like disease at the Italian epicentre of the SARS-CoV-2 epidemic: an observational cohort study. Lancet 2020;395(10239):1771–8.

8. Viner RM, Whittaker E. Kawasaki-like disease: emerging complication during the COVID-19 pandemic. Lancet 2020;395(10239):1741–3.

9. HAN Archive - 00432 | Health Alert Network (HAN). Published September 21, 2021. Available at: https://emergency.cdc.gov/han/2020/han00432.asp. Accessed June 12, 2022.

10. McArdle AJ, Vito O, Patel H, et al. Treatment of multisystem inflammatory syndrome in children. N Engl J Med 2021;385(1):11–22.

11. Farooqi KM, Chan A, Weller RJ, et al. Longitudinal outcomes for multisystem inflammatory syndrome in children. Pediatrics 2021;148(2). e2021051155.

12. Carter MJ, Fish M, Jennings A, et al. Peripheral immunophenotypes in children with multisystem inflammatory syndrome associated with SARS-CoV-2 infection. Nat Med 2020;26(11):1701–7.

13. Whittaker E, Bamford A, Kenny J, et al. Clinical characteristics of 58 children with a pediatric inflammatory multisystem syndrome temporally associated with SARS-CoV-2. JAMA 2020;324(3):259–69.

14. Porritt RA, Binek A, Paschold L, et al. The autoimmune signature of hyperinflammatory multisystem inflammatory syndrome in children. J Clin Invest 2021; 131(20):e151520.

15. Feldstein LR, Rose EB, Horwitz SM, et al. Multisystem inflammatory syndrome in U.S. children and adolescents. N Engl J Med 2020;383(4):334–46.

16. Belay ED, Abrams J, Oster ME, et al. Trends in geographic and temporal distribution of US children with multisystem inflammatory syndrome during the COVID-19 pandemic. JAMA Pediatr 2021;175(8):837–45.

17. Jones VG, Mills M, Suarez D, et al. COVID-19 and Kawasaki disease: novel virus and novel case. Hosp Pediatr 2020;10(6):537–40.

18. Dionne A, Son MBF, Randolph AG. An update on multisystem inflammatory syndrome in children related to SARS-CoV-2. Pediatr Infect Dis J 2022;41(1):e6–9.

19. Sancho-Shimizu V, Brodin P, Cobat A, et al. SARS-CoV-2-related MIS-C: a key to the viral and genetic causes of Kawasaki disease? J Exp Med 2021;218(6): e20210446.

20. Lin MT, Wu MH. The global epidemiology of Kawasaki disease: Review and future perspectives. Glob Cardiol Sci Pract 2017;2017(3):e201720.

21. Nakamura A, Ikeda K, Hamaoka K. Aetiological significance of infectious stimuli in Kawasaki disease. Front Pediatr 2019;7:244.

22. Dufort EM, Koumans EH, Chow EJ, et al. Multisystem inflammatory syndrome in children in New York state. N Engl J Med 2020;383(4):347–58.

23. Javalkar K, Robson VK, Gaffney L, et al. Socioeconomic and racial and/or ethnic disparities in multisystem inflammatory syndrome. Pediatrics 2021;147(5). e2020039933.

24. McCrindle BW, Rowley AH, Newburger JW, et al. Diagnosis, treatment, and long-term management of Kawasaki disease: a scientific statement for health

professionals from the American Heart Association. Circulation 2017;135(17): e927–99.

25. Holman RC, Belay ED, Christensen KY, et al. Hospitalizations for Kawasaki syndrome among children in the United States, 1997-2007. Pediatr Infect Dis J 2010;29(6):483–8.

26. Uehara R, Belay ED. Epidemiology of Kawasaki disease in Asia, Europe, and the United States. J Epidemiol 2012;22(2):79–85.

27. Newburger JW, Takahashi M, Burns JC. Kawasaki disease. J Am Coll Cardiol 2016;67(14):1738–49.

28. Son MBF, Newburger JW. Kawasaki disease. Pediatr Rev 2018;39(2):78–90.

29. Sadeghi P, Izadi A, Mojtahedi SY, et al. A 10-year cross-sectional retrospective study on Kawasaki disease in Iranian children: incidence, clinical manifestations, complications, and treatment patterns. BMC Infect Dis 2021;21:368.

30. Baker AL, Lu M, Minich LL, et al. Associated symptoms in the ten days prior to diagnosis of Kawasaki disease. J Pediatr 2009;154(4):592–5.e2. https://doi.org/10.1016/j.jpeds.2008.10.006.

31. Valverde I, Singh Y, Sanchez-de-Toledo J, et al. Acute cardiovascular manifestations in 286 children with multisystem inflammatory syndrome associated with COVID-19 infection in Europe. Circulation 2021;143(1):21–32.

32. Tremoulet AH, Jain S, Chandrasekar D, et al. Evolution of laboratory values in patients with Kawasaki disease. Pediatr Infect Dis J 2011;30(12):1022–6.

33. Rowley AH, Shulman ST. Kawasaki syndrome. Clin Microbiol Rev 1998;11(3): 405–14.

34. Printz BF, Sleeper LA, Newburger JW, et al. Noncoronary cardiac abnormalities are associated with coronary artery dilation and with laboratory inflammatory markers in acute Kawasaki disease. J Am Coll Cardiol 2011;57(1):86–92.

35. Consiglio CR, Cotugno N, Sardh F, et al. The immunology of multisystem inflammatory syndrome in children with COVID-19. Cell 2020;183(4):968–81.e7.

36. Choi HS, Lee SB, Kwon JH, et al. Uveitis as an important ocular sign to help early diagnosis in Kawasaki disease. Korean J Pediatr 2015;58(10):374–9.

37. Burns JC, Joffe L, Sargent RA, et al. Anterior uveitis associated with Kawasaki syndrome. Pediatr Infect Dis 1985;4(3):258–61.

38. Öztürk C, Yüce Sezen A, Savaş Şen Z, et al. Bilateral acute anterior uveitis and corneal punctate epitheliopathy in children diagnosed with multisystem inflammatory syndrome secondary to COVID-19. Ocul Immunol Inflamm 2021;29(4): 700–4.

39. Wong Chung JERE, Engin Ö, Wolfs TFW, et al. Anterior uveitis in paediatric inflammatory multisystem syndrome temporally associated with SARS-CoV-2. Lancet Lond Engl 2021;397(10281):e10.

40. Barisani-Asenbauer T, Maca SM, Mejdoubi L, et al. Uveitis- a rare disease often associated with systemic diseases and infections- a systematic review of 2619 patients. Orphanet J Rare Dis 2012;7:57.

41. Feldstein LR, Tenforde MW, Friedman KG, et al. Characteristics and outcomes of US children and adolescents with multisystem inflammatory syndrome in children (MIS-C) compared with severe acute COVID-19. JAMA 2021;325(11): 1074–87.

42. Cheung EW, Zachariah P, Gorelik M, et al. Multisystem inflammatory syndrome related to COVID-19 in previously healthy children and adolescents in New York City. JAMA 2020;324(3):294–6.

43. Villacis-Nunez DS, Hashemi S, Nelson MC, et al. Giant coronary aneurysms in multisystem inflammatory syndrome in children associated with SARS-CoV-2 infection. JACC Case Rep 2021;3(13):1499–508.

44. Richardson KL, Jain A, Evans J, et al. Giant coronary artery aneurysm as a feature of coronavirus-related inflammatory syndrome. BMJ Case Rep 2021; 14(7):e238740.

45. Navaeifar MR, Shahbaznejad L, Sadeghi Lotfabadi A, et al. COVID-19-associated multisystem inflammatory syndrome complicated with giant coronary artery aneurysm. Case Rep Pediatr 2021;2021:8836403.

46. Nelson MC, Mrosak J, Hashemi S, et al. Delayed coronary dilation with multisystem inflammatory syndrome in children. CASE 2022;6(1):31–5.

47. Blondiaux E, Parisot P, Redheuil A, et al. Cardiac MRI of children with multisystem inflammatory syndrome (MIS-C) associated with COVID-19: case series. Radiology 2020;202288. https://doi.org/10.1148/radiol.2020202288.

48. Belhadjer Z, Méot M, Bajolle F, et al. Acute heart failure in multisystem inflammatory syndrome in children in the context of global SARS-CoV-2 pandemic. Circulation 2020;142(5):429–36.

49. Dionne A, Newburger JW. The electrocardiogram in multisystem inflammatory syndrome in children: mind your Ps and Qs. J Pediatr 2021;234:10–1.

50. Piazza I, Ali H, Ferrero P. Brugada-like pattern and myocarditis in a child with multisystem inflammatory syndrome: overlap or differential diagnosis? Eur Heart J - Case Rep. 2021;5(7):ytab289.

51. De Nigris A, Pepe A, Di Nardo G, et al. Brugada pattern in a child with severe SARS-CoV-2 related multisystem inflammatory syndrome. Pediatr Rep 2021; 13(3):504–10.

52. Matsuura H, Ishikita T, Yamamoto S, et al. Gallium-67 myocardial imaging for the detection of myocarditis in the acute phase of Kawasaki disease (mucocutaneous lymph node syndrome): the usefulness of single photon emission computed tomography. Br Heart J 1987;58(4):385–92.

53. Fujiwara H, Hamashima Y. Pathology of the heart in Kawasaki disease. Pediatrics 1978;61(1):100–7.

54. Alsaied T, Tremoulet AH, Burns JC, et al. Review of cardiac involvement in multisystem inflammatory syndrome in children. Circulation 2021;143(1):78–88.

55. Savas Sen Z, Tanir G, Gumuser Cinni R, et al. Multisystem inflammatory syndrome in children during severe acute respiratory syndrome coronavirus-2 pandemic in Turkey: a single-centre experience. J Paediatr Child Health 2022; 58(1):129–35.

56. Dominguez SR, Friedman K, Seewald R, et al. Kawasaki disease in a pediatric intensive care unit: a case-control study. Pediatrics 2008;122(4):e786–90.

57. Kanegaye JT, Wilder MS, Molkara D, et al. Recognition of a Kawasaki disease shock syndrome. Pediatrics 2009;123(5):e783–9.

58. Maddox RA, Person MK, Kennedy JL, et al. Kawasaki disease and Kawasaki disease shock syndrome hospitalization rates in the United States, 2006–2018. Pediatr Infect Dis J 2021;40(4):284–8.

59. Zheng Z, Huang Y, Wang Z, et al. Clinical features in children with Kawasaki disease shock syndrome: a systematic review and meta-analysis. Front Cardiovasc Med 2021;8:736352.

60. Zhang H, Xie L, Xiao T. Extracorporeal membrane oxygenation support for cardiac dysfunction due to Kawasaki disease shock syndrome. Front Pediatr 2019; 7:221.

61. Best D, Millar J, Kornilov I, et al. Extracorporeal membrane oxygenation for Kawasaki disease: two case reports and the Extracorporeal Life Support Organization experience 1999–2015. Perfusion 2017;32(7):609–12.

62. Liu J, Yang C, Zhang Z, et al. Kawasaki disease shock syndrome with acute respiratory distress syndrome in a child: a case report and literature review. BMC Pulm Med 2022;22(1):220.

63. Yonker LM, Gilboa T, Ogata AF, et al. Multisystem inflammatory syndrome in children is driven by zonulin-dependent loss of gut mucosal barrier. J Clin Invest 2021;131(14):149633.

64. Noval Rivas M, Wakita D, Franklin MK, et al. Intestinal permeability and IgA provoke immune vasculitis linked to cardiovascular inflammation. Immunity 2019; 51(3):508–21.e6.

65. Cheng MH, Zhang S, Porritt RA, et al. Superantigenic character of an insert unique to SARS-CoV-2 spike supported by skewed TCR repertoire in patients with hyperinflammation. Proc Natl Acad Sci U S A 2020;117(41):25254–62.

66. Burns JC, Herzog L, Fabri O, et al. Seasonality of Kawasaki disease: a global perspective. PLoS One 2013;8(9):e74529.

67. Chang RKR. Hospitalizations for Kawasaki disease among children in the United States, 1988-1997. Pediatrics 2002;109(6):e87.

68. Abe J, Kotzin BL, Jujo K, et al. Selective expansion of T cells expressing T-cell receptor variable regions V beta 2 and V beta 8 in Kawasaki disease. Proc Natl Acad Sci U S A 1992;89(9):4066–70.

69. Rowley AH, Baker SC, Arrollo D, et al. A protein epitope targeted by the antibody response to Kawasaki disease. J Infect Dis 2020;222(1):158–68.

70. Rowley AH, Eckerley CA, Jäck HM, et al. IgA plasma cells in vascular tissue of patients with Kawasaki syndrome. J Immunol Baltim Md 1950 1997;159(12): 5946–55.

71. Shulman ST, Rowley AH. Kawasaki disease: insights into pathogenesis and approaches to treatment. Nat Rev Rheumatol 2015;11(8):475–82.

72. Onouchi Y. The genetics of Kawasaki disease. Int J Rheum Dis 2018;21(1): 26–30.

73. Onouchi Y, Suzuki Y, Suzuki H, et al. ITPKC and CASP3 polymorphisms and risks for IVIG unresponsiveness and coronary artery lesion formation in Kawasaki disease. Pharmacogenomics J 2013;13(1):52–9.

74. Onouchi Y, Gunji T, Burns JC, et al. ITPKC functional polymorphism associated with Kawasaki disease susceptibility and formation of coronary artery aneurysms. Nat Genet 2008;40(1):35–42.

75. Alphonse MP, Duong TT, Shumitzu C, et al. Inositol-triphosphate 3-kinase c mediates inflammasome activation and treatment response in Kawasaki disease. J Immunol 2016;197(9):3481–9.

76. Leung DYM, Kurt-Jones E, JaneW N, et al. Endothelial cell activation and high interleukin-1 secretion in the pathogenesis of acute Kawasaki disease. Lancet 1989;334(8675):1298–302.

77. Maury CP, Salo E, Pelkonen P. Circulating interleukin-1 beta in patients with Kawasaki disease. N Engl J Med 1988;319(25):1670–1.

78. Chou J, Platt CD, Habiballah S, et al. Mechanisms underlying genetic susceptibility to multisystem inflammatory syndrome in children (MIS-C). J Allergy Clin Immunol 2021;148(3):732–8.e1.

79. Shkurnikov M, Nersisyan S, Jankevic T, et al. Association of HLA class I genotypes with severity of coronavirus disease-19. Front Immunol 2021;12. Available

at: https://www.frontiersin.org/article/10.3389/fimmu.2021.641900. Accessed June 30, 2022.

80. Esteve-Sole A, Anton J, Pino-Ramirez RM, et al. Similarities and differences between the immunopathogenesis of COVID-19-related pediatric multisystem inflammatory syndrome and Kawasaki disease. J Clin Invest 2021;131(6):144554.

81. Huang JJ, Gaines SB, Amezcua ML, et al. Upregulation of type 1 conventional dendritic cells implicates antigen cross-presentation in multisystem inflammatory syndrome. J Allergy Clin Immunol 2022;149(3):912–22.

82. Hanna WJ, Berrens Z, Langner T, et al. Interleukin-27: a novel biomarker in predicting bacterial infection among the critically ill. Crit Care Lond Engl 2015;19:378.

83. Godfred-Cato S, Bryant B, Leung J, et al. COVID-19–associated multisystem inflammatory syndrome in children — United States, March–July 2020. Morb Mortal Wkly Rep 2020;69(32):1074–80.

84. Hokibara S, Kobayashi N, Kobayashi K, et al. Markedly elevated CD64 expression on neutrophils and monocytes as a biomarker for diagnosis and therapy assessment in Kawasaki disease. Inflamm Res 2016;65(7):579–85.

85. Lindquist ME, Hicar MD. B Cells and Antibodies in Kawasaki Disease. Int J Mol Sci 2019;20(8):1834.

86. Xu M, Jiang Y, Wang J, et al. Distinct variations of antibody secreting cells and memory B cells during the course of Kawasaki disease. BMC Immunol 2019; 20(1):16.

87. Vella LA, Giles JR, Baxter AE, et al. Deep immune profiling of MIS-C demonstrates marked but transient immune activation compared to adult and pediatric COVID-19. Sci Immunol 2021;6(57):eabf7570.

88. Gruber CN, Patel RS, Trachtman R, et al. Mapping Systemic Inflammation and Antibody Responses in Multisystem Inflammatory Syndrome in Children (MIS-C). Cell 2020;183(4):982–95.e14.

89. Nishikawa T, Nomura Y, Kono Y, et al. Selective IgA deficiency complicated by Kawasaki syndrome. Pediatr Int Off J Jpn Pediatr Soc 2008;50(6):816–8.

90. Shimizu C, Toshiaki O, Takahashi K, et al. The role of TGF-β and myofibroblasts in the arteritis of Kawasaki disease. Hum Pathol 2013;44(2):189–98.

91. Burbelo PD, Castagnoli R, Shimizu C, et al. Autoantibodies against proteins previously associated with autoimmunity in adult and pediatric patients with COVID-19 and children with MIS-C. Front Immunol 2022;13:841126.

92. Gorelik M, Chung SA, Ardalan K, et al. 2021 American College of Rheumatology/Vasculitis Foundation guideline for the management of Kawasaki disease. Arthritis Care Res 2022;74(4):538–48.

93. Mori M, Miyamae T, Imagawa T, et al. Meta-analysis of the results of intravenous gamma globulin treatment of coronary artery lesions in Kawasaki disease. Mod Rheumatol 2004;14(5):361–6.

94. Burns JC, Franco A. The immunomodulatory effects of intravenous immunoglobulin therapy in Kawasaki disease. Expert Rev Clin Immunol 2015;11(7):819–25.

95. Sleeper LA, Minich LL, McCrindle BM, et al. Evaluation of Kawasaki disease risk-scoring systems for intravenous immunoglobulin resistance. J Pediatr 2011;158(5):831–5.e3.

96. Dionne A, Burns JC, Dahdah N, et al. Treatment intensification in patients with Kawasaki disease and coronary aneurysm at diagnosis. Pediatrics 2019; 143(6):e20183341.

97. Kaushik A, Gupta S, Sood M, et al. A systematic review of multisystem inflammatory syndrome in children associated with SARS-CoV-2 infection. Pediatr Infect Dis J 2020;39(11):e340–6.

98. American college of rheumatology clinical guidance for Multisystem inflammatory syndrome in children associated with SARS–CoV-2 and hyperinflammation in pediatric COVID-19: version 3 - Henderson - 2022 - arthritis & Rheumatology - Wiley Online Library Available at: https://onlinelibrary.wiley.com/doi/10.1002/art.42062. Accessed July 1, 2022.

99. Information on COVID-19 Treatment, Prevention and Research. COVID-19 Treatment Guidelines. Available at: https://www.covid19treatmentguidelines.nih.gov/. Accessed July 1, 2022.

100. Ouldali N, Toubiana J, Antona D, et al. Association of intravenous immunoglobulins plus methylprednisolone vs immunoglobulins alone with course of fever in multisystem inflammatory syndrome in children. JAMA 2021;325(9):855–64.

101. Son MBF, Murray N, Friedman K, et al. Multisystem inflammatory syndrome in children - initial therapy and outcomes. N Engl J Med 2021;385(1):23–34.

102. Nozawa T, Imagawa T, Ito S. Coronary-artery aneurysm in tocilizumab-treated children with Kawasaki's disease. N Engl J Med 2017;377(19):1894–6.

103. Chiang MH, Liu HE, Wang JL. Low-dose or no aspirin administration in acute-phase Kawasaki disease: a meta-analysis and systematic review. Arch Dis Child 2021;106(7):662–8.

104. Ito Y, Matsui T, Abe K, et al. Aspirin dose and treatment outcomes in Kawasaki disease: a historical control study in Japan. Front Pediatr 2020;8:249.

105. Ishii M, Ebato T, Kato H. History and future of treatment for acute stage Kawasaki disease. Korean Circ J 2019;50(2):112–9.

106. Whitworth H, Sartain SE, Kumar R, et al. Rate of thrombosis in children and adolescents hospitalized with COVID-19 or MIS-C. Blood 2021;138(2):190–8.

107. Bowen A, Miller AD, Zambrano LD, et al. Demographic and clinical factors associated with death among persons <21 years old with multisystem inflammatory syndrome in children-United States, February 2020-March 2021. Open Forum Infect Dis 2021;8(8):ofab388.

108. CDC. COVID Data tracker. Centers for disease control and prevention. Published March 28, 2020. Available at: https://covid.cdc.gov/covid-data-tracker. Accessed July 1, 2022.

109. Brogan P, Burns JC, Cornish J, et al. Lifetime cardiovascular management of patients with previous Kawasaki disease. Heart Br Card Soc 2020;106(6):411–20.

110. Suda K, Iemura M, Nishiono H, et al. Long-term prognosis of patients with Kawasaki disease complicated by giant coronary aneurysms: a single-institution experience. Circulation 2011;123(17):1836–42.

111. Daniels LB, Tjajadi MS, Walford HH, et al. Prevalence of Kawasaki disease in young adults with suspected myocardial ischemia. Circulation 2012;125(20):2447–53.

112. Fremed MA, Farooqi KM. Longitudinal outcomes and monitoring of patients with multisystem inflammatory syndrome in children. Front Pediatr 2022;10:820229.

113. Capone CA, Misra N, Ganigara M, et al. Six Month Follow-up of Patients With Multi-System Inflammatory Syndrome in Children. Pediatrics 2021;148(4). e2021050973.

114. Noval Rivas M, Porritt RA, Cheng MH, et al. COVID-19-associated multisystem inflammatory syndrome in children (MIS-C): A novel disease that mimics toxic shock syndrome-the superantigen hypothesis. J Allergy Clin Immunol 2021;147(1):57–9.

115. Rowley AH, Shulman ST. The Epidemiology and Pathogenesis of Kawasaki Disease. Front Pediatr 2018;6. Available at: https://www.frontiersin.org/articles/10.3389/fped.2018.00374. Accessed July 25, 2022.

Vasculitis and Pregnancy
Disease State and Management

Catherine A. Sims, MD[a],*, Bonnie L. Bermas, MD[b],
Megan E.B. Clowse, MD, MPH[c]

KEYWORDS

• Vasculitis • Women's health • Pregnancy • Birth control • Preconception counseling

KEY POINTS

• A highly effective birth control plan is recommended for all fertile women not planning to conceive in the next year.
• Personal goals and desires for pregnancy should be considered when deciding on treatment for vasculitis.
• Pregnancy complications experienced by women with vasculitis depend on the category of vasculitis (small, medium, large, and variable).
• Women with vasculitis can minimize pregnancy complications by planning pregnancy during times of quiescent disease.

INTRODUCTION

Vasculitides are a group of autoimmune diseases that cause inflammation of blood vessels leading to diverse clinical manifestations and complications. These diseases are classified according to the size of vessels affected by inflammation, ranging from small, medium, large, to variable. Although Takayasu's arteritis (TA) and Behcet's disease (BD) are the most common vasculitides diagnosed in reproductive-aged women, antineutrophil cytoplasmic antibody-associated vasculitis (AAV) and other forms of vasculitis can also occur. Each type of vasculitis has unique disease characteristics making their impacts on pregnancy and potential complications different. Vasculitis manifestations and the treatments used to control disease can impact fertility, pregnancy outcomes, fetal development, and maternal health. The prior reliance on cyclophosphamide (CYC) limited fertility in women with vasculitis, but by replacing it with non-ovarian toxic therapies, this has opened new opportunities.

[a] Division of Rheumatology, Duke University, 1021 Red Hat Lane, Durham, NC 27713, USA;
[b] University of Texas Southwestern, 2001 Inwood Road, Dallas, TX 75235, USA; [c] Division of Rheumatology & Immunology, Duke University, 40 Duke Medicine Circle Clinic 1J, Durham, NC 27713, USA
* Corresponding author.
E-mail address: catherine.sims@duke.edu

Rheum Dis Clin N Am 49 (2023) 679–694
https://doi.org/10.1016/j.rdc.2023.03.009
0889-857X/23/© 2023 Elsevier Inc. All rights reserved.

rheumatic.theclinics.com

Rheumatologists have the opportunity to incorporate family planning goals in discussions with patients to ensure therapy plans are safe and effective while taking into consideration the patient's personal preferences. This article explores the importance of planned pregnancy during quiescent disease, contraception, complications of vasculitis and pregnancy, pregnancy and lactation compatible medications, and the management of unplanned pregnancies.

Pregnancy Complications in a Patient with Vasculitis

Patients diagnosed with vasculitis during pregnancy or who conceive during active disease have poorer pregnancy outcomes including miscarriage and maternal death.[1] Assessing for disease activity depends on the type of vasculitis and prior manifestations but includes a combination of laboratory testing and imaging. **Table 1** summarizes the diagnostic modalities used to determine disease activity before conception and each disease-specific section below identifies important considerations when stratifying pregnancy risk. For example, in small vessel vasculitides, glomerulonephritis (GN) serves as a risk factor for the development of hypertension (HTN) and preeclampsia, whereas in TA, inflammation of the renal artery can lead to poor renal blood flow and subsequent HTN. Preeclampsia is defined as new onset HTN and proteinuria or new onset HTN and significant end-organ dysfunction with or without proteinuria in the last half of pregnancy or postpartum. The most important aspects of pregnancy management in women with vasculitis are planned pregnancies during well-controlled disease on pregnancy and lactation compatible medications (**Table 2**). This section discusses each major classification of vasculitis as defined by the 2012 Chapel Hill Consensus Consortium and associated pregnancy complications reported in the literature.[2]

Antineutrophil Cytoplasmic Antibody-Associated Vasculitis

Antineutrophil cytoplasmic antibody (ANCA)-associated vasculitides are small vessel vasculitides organized into three distinct diseases: granulomatosis with polyangiitis (GPA), microscopic polyangiitis (MPA), and eosinophilic GPA (EGPA). GPA can present with sinus inflammation (bloody nasal discharge, nasal crusting), hearing loss, pulmonary nodules, masses, or cavitations, pauci-immune GN, and cartilaginous involvement.[3] Disease manifestations of MPA include pauci-immune GN, lung fibrosis or interstitial lung disease, and sinonasal signs or symptoms.[4] Diagnostic criteria for EGPA include eosinophilia, obstructive airway disease, nasal polyps, extravascular eosinophilic predominant inflammation, and mononeuritis multiplex or motor neuropathy not due to radiculopathy.[5] Women with active AAV are more likely to experience poor pregnancy outcomes including preterm delivery, need for cesarean delivery, and preeclampsia.[1,6,7] Preterm delivery is defined as birth before 37 weeks gestation.

Renal Manifestations: Patients with a history of GN should be assessed with a urinalysis evaluating for proteinuria and/or hematuria and serum creatinine before conception. During pregnancy, a patient's glomerular filtration rate can increase by up to 40% to 50% with a decrease in serum creatinine around 20%.[8] Proteinuria can be quantified with a urine protein-to-creatinine ratio to establish a trend. The presence of active urinary sediment indicates renal inflammation that may require increased immunosuppression. Providers should ask female patients if they are menstruating as this will contaminate the urine sample and appear as hematuria. If GN is suspected during pregnancy, a renal biopsy can be done to confirm diagnosis. Women with GN during pregnancy should be treated with glucocorticoids, increased pregnancy compatible immunosuppression, and closely monitored for worsening renal function and HTN with frequent urinalyses, serum creatinine, and home blood pressure monitoring.

Table 1
Vasculitis and pregnancy complications organized by disease type and treatment recommendations

Types of Vasculitis	Potential Maternal and Fetal Complications[a]	Assessment of Disease Activity	Signs of Active Vasculitis	Therapies[b]
ANCA-associated vasculitis	Preeclampsia Need for cesarean delivery Preterm delivery	Urinalysis, UPC, serum creatinine, chest imaging, PFT, C-reactive protein (CRP)	Crusting rhinitis Arthralgias Diffuse alveolar hemorrhage Glomerulonephritis Subglottic stenosis Paresthesias Rash Asthma	Azathioprine Glucocorticoids Rituximab[c] CYC[c] Mepolizumab[d] Blood pressure control, daily low-dose aspirin to decrease chances of preeclampsia
Polyarteritis nodosa	Renal failure Arterial hypertension	Vascular imaging to assess for active inflammation, aneurysms, and stenoses, serum creatinine, CRP	Limb claudication/ischemia Uncontrolled HTN Rash	Azathioprine Glucocorticoids TNFi Rituximab[c] CYC[c] Blood pressure control, daily low dose aspirin to decrease chances of preeclampsia
Takayasu's arteritis	New or worsening HTN New or worsening heart disease Preeclampsia Inability to measure BP	Vascular imaging to assess for active inflammation, aneurysms, and stenoses, TTE, serum creatinine, CRP, assess BP in multiple limbs	Uncontrolled HTN New/worsening heart failure Renal insufficiency Cerebral hemorrhage CVA	Azathioprine Glucocorticoids TNFi Rituximab[c] CYC[c] Blood pressure control, daily low-dose aspirin to decrease chances of preeclampsia Anticoagulation in cases of embolic/thrombotic events

(continued on next page)

Table 1
(continued)

Types of Vasculitis	Potential Maternal and Fetal Complications[a]	Assessment of Disease Activity	Signs of Active Vasculitis	Therapies[b]
Behcet's disease	Oral/vaginal ulcerations Ocular inflammation Thrombotic risk	Determine history of thromboembolic disease Ophthalmologic examination Rule out HSV as cause of vaginal ulcerations	Oral/vaginal ulcerations Ocular inflammation Venous/arterial clots	Azathioprine Glucocorticoids (topical and systemic) TNFi Anticoagulation in cases of embolic/thrombotic events

Abbreviations: CVA, cerebrovascular accident; CYC, cyclophosphamide; HTN, hypertension; PFT, pulmonary function test; TNFi, tumor necrosis factor inhibitor; TTE, transthoracic echocardiogram; UPC, urine protein:creatinine ratio.

[a] Women with well controlled and quiescent disease at conception have lower rate of pregnancy complications.

[b] See **Table 2** for an expanded discussion on medication options and pregnancy/lactation safety data

[c] In life- or organ-threatening disease.

[d] Unknown safety profile in pregnancy/lactation.

Table 2
Medication recommendations for pregnant women with vasculitis

Recommendation	Medication	Monitoring
Strongly Recommended	Azathioprine (Imuran)	Check TPMT levels in mothers prior to initiation Consider CBC in infants as cases of mild, asymptomatic neutropenia have been reported during breastfeeding[36]
	Colchicine (Colcrys, Mitigare)	Avoid breastfeeding within 4 h of dose to minimize infant exposure
	Glucocorticoids	May continue low-dose ($\leq$10 mg/d) prednisone during pregnancy if clinically indicated and tapering higher doses to < 20 mg daily by adding pregnancy-compatible glucocorticoid sparing agents if needed Prednisone excretion into the breastmilk is low and there have been no adverse effects reported
	Certolizumab (Cimzia)	Can be continued throughout entire pregnancy and breastfeeding; does not cross placenta Small amount excreted into breastmilk that is not clinically significant
Conditionally Recommended	Tumor necrosis factor inhibitors (TNFi) Etanercept Adalimumab Golimumab Infliximab	Continue in first and second trimesters; consider holding in third trimester if disease controlled to decrease transplacental transfer Large protein molecules and immunoglobulin G (IgG) antibodies do not cross into breastmilk in high concentrations
	Calcineurin Inhibitors Tacrolimus Cyclosporine	Recommend monitoring of blood pressure. Increased risk of preterm birth and growth restriction Consider monitoring infant drug levels during breastfeeding if potential side effects
	Non-steroidal anti-inflammatory drugs (NSAIDs) Ibuprofen Naproxen Meloxicam	FDA Black Box warning against NSAID use after 20 wk due to oligohydramnios and closure of ductus arteriosus Ibuprofen is preferred over

(continued on next page)

Table 2
(continued)

Recommendation	Medication	Monitoring
	Diclofenac *Celecoxib* *Indomethacin*	aspirin and naproxen due to its extremely low levels in breastmilk, short half-life, and safe use in infants in doses much higher than those excreted in breastmilk
	Rituximab	Discontinue when pregnancy is confirmed but can continue if organ- or life-threatening disease during pregnancy Large protein molecules and IgG antibodies do not cross into breastmilk in high concentrations
Insufficient Information	Mepolizumab	Owing to its large size, the amount secreted into breastmilk is likely to be very low Emerging data that it may be safe in breastfeeding[37]
	Abatacept (Orencia)	Small amount excreted into breastmilk. One case report found no adverse effects in breastfeeding infant[38]
	Tocilizumab (Actemra)	Limited data suggests small amounts excreted into breastmilk. No adverse effects reported in infants.
Pregnancy Incompatible	Cyclophosphamide	Discontinue CYC 3 mo before conception due to high-risk for birth defects with first trimester exposure. Can be considered for life- and organ-threatening disease during the second and third trimesters. Enters breastmilk in potentially toxic amounts and has highly toxic active metabolites that add risk to the infant. Most sources consider breastfeeding to be contraindicated during CYC treatment.
	Methotrexate (Rasuvo, Otrexup)	Discontinue 1–3 mo before conception Small studies found breastmilk contains <1% of the maternal weight adjusted MTX dose which decreases within 24 h of weekly dosing.[39,40] This level of transfer is unlikely to harm an infant and monitoring the infant's complete blood

(continued on next page)

Table 2 (continued)		
Recommendation	Medication	Monitoring
		count and differential can be considered.
	Mycophenolate Mofetil (MMF, Cellcept)	Associated with cleft lip and palate, micrognathia, microtia, and auditory canal abnormalities.[41,42] Expert opinion suggests pregnancy should be delayed at least 6 wk after discontinuing mycophenolate.[43]

Pulmonary Manifestations: A certain amount of dyspnea is expected during pregnancy. However, a significant shortness of breath warrants evaluation. Respiratory manifestations of AAV include tracheal and subglottic stenosis, pulmonary cavitations, interstitial lung disease, and alveolar hemorrhage. In addition, patients with AAV are at higher risk for blood clots, and pregnancy is a prothrombotic state making pulmonary embolism a possibility.[9] Women with new or worsening shortness of breath should be evaluated for vasculitis manifestations and/or pulmonary embolism. If tracheal or subglottic stenosis is suspected, this should be evaluated before delivery as these patients require specific intubation protocols. Cardiac manifestations are more common in EGPA and can present as dyspnea.[1]

Polyarteritis Nodosa

Polyarteritis nodosa is a necrotizing arteritis of medium or small arteritis not associated with ANCA.[2] It has historically been associated with hepatitis B (HBV) and C viral (HCV) infections. With implementation of hepatitis screenings, vaccination, and education the incidence of HBV- and HCV-associated polyarteritis nodosa (PAN) has decreased. Affected medium sized blood vessels become thickened through intimal hyperplasia leading to poor blood flow and risk for thrombosis. Aneurysms can also develop leading to infarction and ischemia. The kidney is the most commonly involved organ although skin, heart, nerve, and gastrointestinal involvement can occur.[10]

Renal Artery Involvement: Pregnant women with PAN can experience renal failure and uncontrolled HTN requiring premature delivery as a life-saving measure.[11–14] During pregnancy, when suspicion arises of PAN-induced renal failure, imaging can reveal stenoses and aneurysms in addition to active inflammation. Assessing renal function with serum creatinine is also important given the physiologic changes in blood volume and renal perfusion during pregnancy.

Management of Hypertension: HTN during pregnancy increases the risk for poor placental development which can lead to pregnancy loss, preterm birth, preeclampsia, and fetal growth restriction.[15] The 2020 American College of Obstetrics and Gynecology clinical management guidelines recommend labetalol, hydralazine, and nifedipine for blood pressure control during pregnancy.[16] Angiotensin-converting enzymes (ACE) inhibitors and angiotensin II receptor blockers (ARB) should be avoided in pregnancy due to reported fetal cardiovascular malformations, miscarriage, and stillbirth.[17]

Takayasu's Arteritis

TA is an often granulomatous arteritis impacting the aorta and its major branches typically in patients less than 50 years.[2] Pregnant women with TA can experience complications including new or worsening HTN, new or worsening heart disease, and preeclampsia.[18–20] Before pregnancy, the patient's vasculature should be assessed with imaging to identify structural changes, specifically abnormalities of the renal artery or ascending aorta, which could pose complications during pregnancy. If subclavian involvement is identified, blood pressure measurements will not be reliable on that appendage creating reliance on BP measurements from the legs or contralateral arm.

Hypertension: New onset or worsening HTN is observed more frequently in women with prepregnancy renal artery involvement. Prepregnancy HTN, prepregnancy renal artery involvement, and active TA during pregnancy are associated with adverse pregnancy outcomes.[20] Vascular imaging evaluates for active inflammation, stenoses, and aneurysms. Considering the changes in blood volume and fluid shifts during pregnancy, vascular health should be evaluated before conception, if possible, to anticipate significant complications. Importantly, the authors recommend optimizing blood pressure control with pregnancy compatible medications such as labetalol, hydralazine, and nifedipine. ACE inhibitors and ARB should be avoided due to reported fetal malformations and loss of pregnancy with exposure.[17]

Cardiac Manifestations: Women with prior cardiac manifestations or structural changes of the ascending aorta and/or aortic arch that could impact cardiac function should be evaluated with a transthoracic echocardiogram (TTE) to assess heart structure and function before pregnancy. The involvement of specialists including cardiologists and cardiac anesthesia is important to provide comprehensive care.

Behcet's Disease

BD is characterized by recurrent oral and/or genital aphthous ulcerations along with ocular, cutaneous, articular, gastrointestinal, and nervous system inflammation.[2] It can also affect arteries and veins. Worsening oral ulcerations and ocular inflammation can occur during pregnancy, which may require increased topical and systemic therapy in some cases. BD that results in major internal organ involvement, structural vascular changes, and/or blood clots may increase risk. There is an increased risk for thrombotic disease in BD outside of pregnancy, but given the prothrombotic state induced by pregnancy, this risk increases. If the patient has a history of thromboembolic disease, anticoagulation should be discussed before conception. Low molecular weight heparin (LMWH) and heparin can be used safely in pregnancy. Women can inject anticoagulants into their lower abdomen throughout pregnancy. Indication, dosing, and frequency should be discussed with the patient's maternal fetal medicine (MFM) physician.

Preconception Counseling and Contraception

Rheumatologists have the opportunity to discuss family planning at each clinic visit to ensure treatment recommendations incorporate a patient's personal goals (**Fig. 1**). Using the One Key Question (https://powertodecide.org/one-key-question), "do you want to become pregnant in the next year?" is a simple and effective way to start this conversation. The Vasculitis Foundation (VF) provides handouts to discuss pregnancy and birth control options for men and women with vasculitis (https://www.vasculitisfoundation.org/vpreg/).

If the patient is interested in pregnancy, disease activity should be assessed (see **Table 1**) to ensure conception during quiescent disease and medications should be reviewed for pregnancy and lactation compatibility (see **Table 2**). Patients should be counseled on potential vasculitis and pregnancy complications and the importance of close follow-up with their rheumatologist, MFM physician, and other specialists involved. All women with a history of thromboembolic disease or those deemed

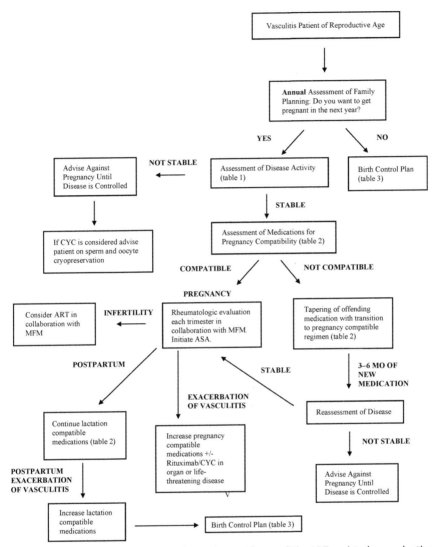

Fig. 1. Reproductive management in the patient with vasculitis. ART, assisted reproductive technology; CYC, cyclophosphamide; MFM, maternal fetal medicine.

high risk for blood clots should be anticoagulated before conception. Daily aspirin is recommended for all pregnant women with systemic lupus erythematosus (SLE) and antiphospholipid syndrome (APS) starting in the first trimester to decrease the risk of preeclampsia.[21] Although there is minimal data assessing the utility of aspirin in pregnant women with vasculitis, this recommendation should be extended to this population to mitigate the risk of preeclampsia.

If the patient is not interested in pregnancy, a birth control plan should be discussed (**Table 3**). Ideally, a patient's plan will include one of the most effective birth control options (intrauterine devices [IUD], subdermal implants, tubal ligation) to minimize unintended pregnancies and potential complications. It is important for providers to explain the different levels of effectiveness for each form of birth control. When

Table 3
Birth control options for people with vasculitis

Types of Birth Control	Effectiveness	Length of Effectiveness	Safe in Vasculitis?	Considerations
Tubal ligation	<1% pregnancies annually	Permanent	Yes	Intended for women who have no future pregnancy plans
Intrauterine device (IUD)	<1% pregnancies annually	3–10 y. Able to remove at any time	Yes	Safe to use all IUD types (copper and hormonal) in women with vasculitis
Subdermal implant	<1% pregnancies annually	3 y. Able to remove at any time	Yes	Progesterone-only. Does not increase clotting risk.
Depo-Provera *Medroxyprogesterone acetate*	6%–9% pregnancies annually	Until discontinuation; can be discontinued at any time	Maybe	Avoid in women with high risk[a] for or history of blood clots, avoid in women with osteoporosis
Pill with estrogen	6%–9% pregnancies annually	Until discontinuation; can be discontinued at any time	Maybe	Avoid in women with high risk[a] for or history of blood clots
Vaginal ring	6%–9% pregnancies annually	Until discontinuation; can be discontinued at any time	Maybe	Avoid in women with high risk[a] for or history of blood clots
Patch	6%–9% pregnancies annually	Until discontinuation; can be discontinued at any time	Maybe	Avoid in women with high risk[a] for or history of blood clots
Mini pill	6%–9% pregnancies annually	Until discontinuation; can be discontinued at any time	Yes	OK for women with clotting risk. Lower effectiveness than other hormonal options.
Condoms, spermicide, cervical caps, fertility awareness	10%–25% pregnancies annually	During intercourse	Yes	Recommend these forms of birth control be combined with more effective forms. Condoms prevent STI
Emergency contraception *Plan B*	Can reduce risk of pregnancy by 87%	Can be used up to 72 h after unprotected sex	Yes	Can be ordered online without a prescription

Abbreviation: STI, sexually transmitted infections.

[a] High risk for blood clots includes positive anticardiolipin antibody, anti-beta 2 glycoprotein antibody, and/or lupus anticoagulant.

recommending birth control to women with vasculitis, specific considerations including history of blood clots and/or presence of antiphospholipid antibodies should be taken into consideration. Emergency contraception is safe to use in all women with vasculitis up to 72 hours after unprotected sex. Obstetricians can offer emergency contraception up to 5 days after unprotected sex.

Ovarian Protection During the Use of Cyclophosphamide

CYC, once the cornerstone of vasculitis treatment, can cause ovarian insufficiency leading to infertility and/or premature menopause. To mitigate these outcomes, EULAR recommends and ACR conditionally recommends monthly gonadotropin-releasing hormone agonist therapy in women receiving monthly CYC infusions.[21] Leuprolide is traditionally dosed 3.75 mg monthly or 11.25 mg every 3 months with the first dose at least 10 days before a CYC infusion to avoid exposure during the initial surge of estrogen caused by the leuprolide. The data for this recommendation are based on studies in the oncologic population whose ovarian function remained stable with this approach.[22] The risk for ovarian failure is greater in patients over 30 years of age and those with prolonged courses of CYC. Prior data have demonstrated a direct correlation between cumulative dose of CYC and ovarian failure with a threshold above 10 g increasing the risk.[23] Although high-dose oral or intravenous (IV) CYC poses an increased risk for ovarian damage women who receive lower doses, such as the EURO-lupus protocol (500 mg IV CYC every 2 weeks for 6 doses) have little ovarian damage.[24]

Pregnancy and Vasculitis Management

The timing of pregnancy during quiescent disease while taking pregnancy compatible medications is the most important part of pregnancy planning. Rheumatologists should assess the patient at least once per trimester to evaluate for disease activity (see **Table 1**), complications, and medication adherence. Patients should also be followed by an MFM specialist and disease-specific subspecialists (cardiology, nephrology, dermatology, and so forth).

The ACR recommends keeping non-fluorinated glucocorticoids (methylprednisolone, prednisone, prednisolone, and hydrocortisone) below an equivalent of 20 mg prednisone per day, during pregnancy.[21] Long-term glucocorticoid use during pregnancy increases the risk for preterm birth, gestational HTN, gestational diabetes, prelabor rupture of membranes, and preeclampsia.[25,26] If a vasculitis flare during pregnancy warrants higher doses, they should be used for as short a time as possible and immunosuppression with steroid sparing agents should be introduced (see **Table 2**).

For example, if a woman with AAV on maintenance therapy with azathioprine develops active disease, such as pulmonary or renal manifestations, initially the dose of glucocorticoids can be increased to 1 mg/kg or the patient can be pulsed with 0.5–1g solumedrol a day. Flares that occur early in pregnancy can potentially be treated with rituximab as little of this drug gets transferred across the placenta until week 15. The addition of rituximab or CYC later in the pregnancy has been used in life- or organ-threatening situations.[27,28] There are many effective medications for vasculitis without pregnancy data. In cases of life- or organ-threatening disease, discussions with the patient and multidisciplinary team about risks and benefits of these medications may be warranted.

Active vasculitic disease during pregnancy poses a significant threat to the mother and pregnancy (see **Table 1**) denoting the importance of therapy escalation when indicated.

Family Planning in Male Patients with Vasculitis

CYC can cause infertility in men as well as mutated sperm. The cumulative dose of CYC is the main determinate for the recovery of normospermic level. Literature within the oncology population has shown the majority of men will achieve this recovery if the cumulative CYC dose was less than 7.5 g/m^2.[29,30] If a male patient plans to undergo therapy with CYC then sperm cryopreservation should be discussed and performed before initiation of therapy to preserve options for future pregnancies. Men treated with CYC should not attempt conception with a partner for 3 months following treatment due to concerns for spermatotoxicity resulting in mutated sperm.[31,32] It is safe for men to conceive with their partner on all other forms of immunosuppression including methotrexate (MTX) and mycophenolate mofetil (MMF).[33]

In men not interested in conceiving children in the future, vasectomy is the most effective form of birth control. Condoms are less effective and should be used in combination with partner contraception to decrease the risk of unplanned pregnancies. Condoms are the only form of birth control that prevent contraction of sexually transmitted infections.

Assisted Reproductive Technology

The ACR reproductive guidelines do not specifically address assisted reproductive technology (ART) in women with vasculitis, but their recommendations for women with SLE and APS can be extrapolated to women with vasculitis. It is important for providers to assess level of disease activity and risk of thrombosis before initiation of ART. If the patient is high risk for thrombosis including prior history of blood clots and/or presence of APS antibodies, anticoagulation should be discussed with MFM before initiation of ART.[21] In women with a history of blood clots, the ACR reproductive health guidelines (RHG) recommend anticoagulation with heparin or LMWH. Past vasculitis manifestations must be considered, such as diffuse alveolar hemorrhage, and the risks and benefits of anticoagulation discussed with the patient.

If a woman is planning on pregnancy during the cycle, she should be on a pregnancy compatible regimen and disease activity assessed at least every 3 months. In women undergoing egg retrieval and/or embryo freezing, all immunosuppression, except for CYC, can be continued including MMF and MTX. Embryo transfer involves an embryo transferred into the patient's own uterus. Similar to traditional conception, the woman's vasculitis should be well controlled on pregnancy compatible medications before this procedure. In surrogacy, a woman with vasculitis choses to have a different woman carry the pregnancy. This allows the woman with vasculitis to continue any immunosuppression needed to keep her vasculitis well controlled.

Managing Unplanned Pregnancies

Teratogenic exposures can result in devastating fetal anomalies that threaten the viability and health of the pregnancy. If a patient experiences an unplanned pregnancy, all teratogenic medications including MMF, MTX, CYC (see **Table 2**) should be discontinued immediately. Discussion with MFM should be initiated for diagnostic evaluation of pregnancy complications. If the patient conceived while taking MTX, folic acid 5 mg daily should be started immediately and continued throughout pregnancy. If the patient conceived while taking leflunomide, a cholestyramine washout (8g three times daily) should be started immediately and continued for 11 days. Providers should discuss the timing of conception using the patient's last menstrual period to calculate the amount of teratogenic exposure. Patients and providers can contact MotherToBaby (https://mothertobaby.org/), which is a nonprofit organization that provides evidence-based information regarding medication exposures during pregnancy and breastfeeding.

Women who conceive during active vasculitis or those diagnosed with vasculitis during pregnancy have higher risk of morbidity and mortality.[1,34,35] In these settings, pregnancy termination can act as a life- and/or organ-saving medical procedure; however, this intervention is no longer available in all states. As a result, some women with vasculitis will be required to continue pregnancies with high risk of complications including maternal death.

Women who conceive while taking medications with insufficient data (see **Table 2**) should talk to their rheumatologist about next steps in management. Biologic medications, such as tumor necrosis factor inhibitors, do not cross the placenta early in pregnancy and can be continued into the third trimester. These medications can be discontinued several weeks before delivery to the decrease risk of placental transfer. However, small molecules have the ability to cross the placenta early in pregnancy and with no data of exposure during pregnancy; the continuation of this class of medications will need to be a discussion of risks and benefits with the patient.

Resources for Patients and Health Care Providers

The VF has created a printable handout addressing birth control and pregnancy management that can be used by both patients and providers. The handout is accompanied by videos that walk through the highlights of the handout. These resources can be found at the following link: https://www.vasculitisfoundation.org/vpreg/. MotherToBaby (https://mothertobaby.org/) provides guidance to patients and providers regarding teratogenic exposures during pregnancy and/or breastfeeding. The 2020 ACR RHG and reproductive health initiative resources are available at https://www.rheumatology.org/Practice-Quality/Reproductive-Health-Initiative.

CLINICS CARE POINTS

- Disease activity, sequelae of prior disease, and organ involvement should be considered before pregnancy to determine risks, monitoring, and management.

- If a woman with vasculitis is not planning to conceive in the next year or is prescribed a teratogenic medication, a birth control plan should be discussed and implemented to decrease the risk of unplanned pregnancies and poor outcomes (see **Table 3**)

- Pregnancy outcomes are optimized in women with planned pregnancies during quiescent vasculitic disease.

- Frequently observed complications of pregnancy in women with vasculitis include intrauterine growth restriction, premature delivery, low birth weight, and need for cesarean delivery (see **Table 1**).

DISCLOSURES

Educational grant from UCB (C.A. Sims, M.E.B. Clowse), grant funding and consulting with UCB,Belgium and GSK, UpToDate author (B.L. Bermas).

REFERENCES

1. Pagnoux C, Le Guern V, Goffinet F, et al. Pregnancies in systemic necrotizing vasculitides: report on 12 women and their 20 pregnancies. Rheumatology 2011;50:953–61.

2. Jennette J, Falk R, Bacon P, et al. 2012 Revised international Chapel Hill consensus conference nomenclature of vasculitides. Arthritis Rheum 2013; 65:1–11.
3. Robson J, Grayson P, Ponte C, et al. 2022 American College of Rheumatology/ European Alliance of Associations for Rheumatology classification criteria for granulomatosis with polyangiitis. Ann Rheum Dis 2022;81:315–20.
4. Suppiah R, Robson C, Grayson C, et al. 2022 American College of Rheumatology/European Alliance of Associations for Rheumatology classification criteria for microscopic polyangiitis. Arthritis Rheumatol 2022;74:400–6.
5. Grayson P, Ponte C, Suppiah R, et al. 2022 American College of Rheumatology/ European Alliance of Associations for Rheumatology classification criteria for eosinophilic granulomatosis with polyangiitis. Ann Rheum Dis 2022;8:309–14.
6. Koukoura O, Mantas N, Linardakis H, et al. Successful term pregnancy in a patient with Wegner's Granulomatosis: case report and literature review. Fertil Steril 2008;89:457e1–5.
7. Daher A, Sauvetre G, Girszyn N, et al. Granulomatosis with polyangiitis and pregnancy: A case report and review of the literature. Obstet Med 2020;13:76–82.
8. Lopes van Balen V, van Gansewinkel T, de Haas S, et al. Maternal kidney function during pregnancy: systematic review and meta-analysis. Ultrasound Obstet Gynecol 2019;54:297–307.
9. Merkel P, Lo G, Holbrook J, et al. Brief communication: high incidence of venous thrombotic events among patients with Wegener Granulomatosis: the Wegener's clinical occurrence of thrombosis (WeCLOT) Study. Ann Intern Med 2005;142: 620–6.
10. Stanton M, Tiwari V. Polyarteritis nodosa. StatPearls [Internet]. Treasure Island (FL): StatPearls Publishing; 2022.
11. Owen J, Hauth JC. Polyarteritis nodosa in pregnancy: a case report and brief literature review. Am J Obstet Gynecol 1989;160:606–7.
12. Pitkin RM. Polyarteritis nodosa. Clin Obstet Gynecol 1983;26:579–86.
13. Janin-Mercier A, Beyvin A, Pablo M, et al. Cutaneous periarteritis nodosa occurring during pregnancy. Acta Derm Venereol 1982;62:256–8.
14. Fredi M, Lazzaroni M, Tani C, et al. Polyarteritis Nodosa in Pregnancy. Ochsner J 2018;18:94–7.
15. Agrawal A, Wenger N. Hypertension During Pregnancy. Curr Hypertens Rep 2020;27:64.
16. Gestational Hypertension and Preeclampsia: ACOG Practice Bulletin, Number 222. Obstet Gynecol 2020;135:e237–60.
17. Buawangpong N, Teekachunhatean S, Koonrungsesomboon N. Adverse pregnancy outcomes associated with first-trimester exposure to angiotensin-converting enzyme inhibitors or angiotensin II receptor blockers: A systematic review and meta-analysis. Pharmacol Res Perspect 2020;8:e00644.
18. Matsumura A, Moriwaki R, Numano F. Pregnancy in Takayasu arteritis from the view of internal medicine. Heart Vessels Suppl 1992;7:125–32.
19. Gatto M, Iaccarino L, Canova M, et al. Pregnancy and vasculitis: a systematic review of the literature. Autoimmun Rev 2012;11:A447–59.
20. He S, Li Z, Zhang G, et al. Pregnancy outcomes in Takayasu arteritis patients. Semin Arthritis Rheum 2022;55:152016.
21. Sammaritano L, Bermas B, Chakravarty E, et al. 2020 American College of Rheumatology (ACR) guideline for the management of reproductive health in rheumatic and musculoskeletal diseases. Arthritis Rheum 2020;72:529–56.

22. Moore H, Unger J, Phillips A, et al. Goserelin for Ovarian Protection During Breast-Cancer Adjuvant Chemotherapy. N Engl J Med 2015;372:923–32.

23. Mok C, Lau C, Wong R. Risk factors for ovarian failure in patients with systemic lupus erythematosus receiving cyclophosphamide therapy. Arthritis Rheum 1998;41:831–7.

24. Tamirou F, Husson S, Gruson D, et al. Brief Report: The Euro-lupus low-dose intravenous cyclophosphamide regimen does not impact the ovarian reserve, as measured by serum levels of anti-müllerian hormone. Arthritis Rheumatol 2017; 69:1267–71.

25. Committee on Obstetric Practice and Society for Maternal Fetal Medicine. Immune modulating therapies in pregnancy and lactation. Obstet Gynecol 2019; 133:287–95.

26. Palmsten K, Bandoli G, Watkins J, et al. Oral corticosteroids and risk of preterm birth in the California medicaid program. J Allergy Clin Immunol Pract 2021;9: 375–84.e5.

27. Pefanis A, Williams D, Skrzypek H, et al. A case of ANCA-associated vasculitis presenting de novo in pregnancy, successfully treated with rituximab. Obstet Med 2020;13:41–4.

28. Harris C, Marin J, Beaulieu M. Rituximab induction therapy for de novo ANCA associated vasculitis in pregnancy: a case report. BMC Nephrol 2018;19:152.

29. Smart E, Lopes F, Rice S, et al. Chemotherapy drugs cyclophosphamide, cisplatin and doxorubicin induce germ cell loss in an in vitro model of the prepubertal testis. Sci Rep 2018;8:1773.

30. Meistrich M, Wilson G, Brown B, et al. Impact of cyclophosphamide on long-term reduction in sperm count in men treated with combination chemotherapy for Ewing and soft tissue sarcomas. Cancer 1992;70:2703–12.

31. Wyrobek A, Schmid T, Marchetti F. Relative susceptibilities of male germ cells to genetic defects induced by cancer chemotherapies. J Natl Cancer Inst Monogr 2005;34:31–5.

32. Stahl P, Stember D, Hsiao W, et al. Indications and strategies for fertility preservation in men. Clin Obstet Gynecol 2010;53:815–27.

33. Mouyis M, Flint J, Giles I. Safety of anti-rheumatic drugs in men trying to conceive: A systematic review and analysis of published evidence. Semin Arthritis Rheum 2019;48:911–20.

34. Cetinkaya R, Odabas A, Gursan N, et al. Microscopic polyangiitis in a pregnant woman. South Med J 2002;95:1441–3.

35. Clowse M, Richeson R, Pieper C, et al. Vasculitis Clinical Research Consortium. Pregnancy outcomes among patients with vasculitis. Arthritis Care Res 2013;65: 1370–4.

36. Drugs and Lactation Database. (LactMed) 2022 [Internet]Available at: https://www.ncbi.nlm.nih.gov/books/NBK501922/.

37. Middleton P, Gade E, Aguilera C, et al. ERS/TSANZ Task Force Statement on the management of reproduction and pregnancy in women with airways diseases. Eur Respir J 2020;55:1901208.

38. Saito J, Yakuwa N, Takai C, et al. Abatacept concentrations in maternal serum and breast milk during breastfeeding and an infant safety assessment: A case study. Rheumatology 2019;58:1692–4.

39. Delaney S, Colantonio D, Ito S. Methotrexate in breast milk. Birth Defects Res 2017;109:711.

40. Baker T, Datta P, Rewers-Felkins K, et al. High-dose methotrexate treatment in a breastfeeding mother with placenta accreta: a case report. Breastfeed Med 2018;13:450–2.
41. Sifontis N, Coscia L, Constantinescu S, et al. Pregnancy outcomes in solid organ transplant recipients with exposure to mycophenolate mofetil or sirolimus. Transplantation 2006;82:1698–702.
42. Perez-Aytes A, Ledo A, Boso V, et al. In utero exposure to mycophenolate mofetil: a characteristic phenotype? Am J Med Genet 2008;146A:1–7.
43. Coscia L, Armenti D, King R, et al. Update on the teratogenicity of maternal mycophenolate mofetil. J Pediatr Genet 2015;4:42–55.

Managing Immunosuppression in Vasculitis Patients in Times of Coronavirus Disease 2019

Sebastian E. Sattui, MD, MS[a], Zachary S. Wallace, MD, MSc[b,c,d,*]

KEYWORDS

• Vasculitis • COVID-19 • Immunosuppression • Risk mitigation

KEY POINTS

- Patients with vasculitis are among those at greatest risk for COVID-19 and severe outcomes, though outcomes have improved following the introduction of effective vaccinations and anti-viral treatments.
- Certain patients with vasculitis who are treated with B cell depletion and cyclophosphamide, are at especially high risk for blunted responses to vaccination and breakthrough infection, including severe disease.
- Identification of a form of pre-exposure prophylaxis effective against currently circulating variants is important for providing additional protection for patients who use B cell depletion and other strong immunosuppressants.

INTRODUCTION

The coronavirus disease 2019 (COVID-19) pandemic, caused by the severe acute respiratory syndrome coronavirus 2 (SARS-CoV-2), has represented a major challenge to health care systems worldwide. Since the beginning of the pandemic, patients living with rheumatic diseases have been appropriately considered high risk due to their immunocompromised status associated with the use of antirheumatic drugs, a higher burden of comorbidities as well as the hyper-inflammatory and -coagulable states associated with rheumatic disease and COVID-19.[1] Among those with rheumatic disease, patients with vasculitis have been of particular concern given their burden of comorbidities (eg, lung disease, renal disease), typical demographics (eg, older age), and frequent use of highly immunosuppressive treatments (ie, high dose glucocorticoids, B-cell depleting therapies), all of which predispose to severe COVID-19.

[a] Division of Rheumatology and Clinical Immunology, University of Pittsburgh, BST S723, 3500 Terrace Street, Pittsburgh, PA 15261, USA; [b] Harvard Medical School, Boston, MA, USA; [c] Clinical Epidemiology Program, Mongan Institute, Massachusetts General Hospital, 100 Cambridge Street, 16th Floor, Boston, MA 02114, USA; [d] Division of Rheumatology, Allergy, and Immunology, Department of Medicine, Massachusetts General Hospital, Boston, MA USA
* Corresponding author.
E-mail address: zswallace@mgh.harvard.edu

Rheum Dis Clin N Am 49 (2023) 695–711
https://doi.org/10.1016/j.rdc.2023.03.007
0889-857X/23/© 2023 Elsevier Inc. All rights reserved.

Since the beginning of the pandemic, large collaborative efforts including clinical trial platforms and large registries have led to significant improvement in the outcomes of COVID-19 with the establishment of management protocols, repurposing of existing drugs, and discovery of new therapeutics.[2,3] The rapid development of highly effective vaccines against SARS-CoV-2 also reduced the risk of COVID-19 and severe disease (eg, hospitalization, death) in the general population. Similar benefits have also been observed in individuals with rheumatic diseases.[4] However, the blunted response to SARS-CoV-2 vaccines in patients receiving antirheumatic drugs has left certain patients (eg, patients on B-cell depleting therapies) at high risk for severe disease, even with the recommended booster regimen.[5] Therefore, the ongoing spread and evolution of new SARS-CoV-2 variants continue to impact treatment decisions, including the role of mitigating strategies (eg, pre-exposure prophylaxis), the risks and benefits of different antirheumatic drugs, and recommendations regarding shielding practices (eg, social distancing, masking) for patients with vasculitis.

The aim of this review is to summarize the existing evidence on risks and outcomes of COVID-19 infection in patients with systemic vasculitis, highlighting some of the current challenges involved in the management of these conditions during the ongoing pandemic. We will also review the efficacy of COVID-19 vaccination and other mitigation strategies and discuss their implementation in the management of patients with vasculitis.

OUTCOMES OF CORONAVIRUS DISEASE 2019 IN PATIENTS WITH VASCULITIS

Although with some variability, large population-based and health care system studies, as well as meta-analyses incorporating these studies, have observed an increased risk of both COVID-19 infection and severe COVID-19 (eg, hospitalization, intensive care admission, death) in patients with systemic rheumatic diseases when compared to the general population.[6,7] Importantly though, general risk factors for severe COVID-19 among patients with rheumatic disease are similar to those in general population (eg, age, comorbidities). In a large population-based study investigating the risk of COVID-19 hospitalization risk in patients with specific systemic rheumatic diseases, patients with vasculitis were found to have the highest risk for hospitalization compared to controls (odds ratio [OR] 2.07, 95% confidence interval [CI] 1.06, 4.06).[8] This increased risk was mostly driven by comorbidities and demographics given the observed attenuation in these associations after adjustment for these factors.

Though susceptible to selection bias, some registry-based studies have examined COVID-19 outcomes in patients with vasculitis.[9,10] In the COVID-19 Global Rheumatology Alliance (GRA) registry analysis of 1020 patients with vasculitis and polymyalgia rheumatica, increased risk of poor outcomes (ie, hospitalization, mechanical ventilation, or death) was associated with older age, male sex, higher burden of comorbidities, prednisone-equivalent doses over 10 mg/d, and moderate or high-severe disease activity at baseline.[10] Reassuringly, rates of poor outcomes improved during the study period following June 15, 2020.

Among patients with vasculitis, similar risk factors (eg, age, male sex, and comorbidities) as in the general population seem to identify those at particularly high risk of poor outcomes of COVID-19. However, the risk of severe outcomes and associated risk factors may vary between different forms of vasculitis (**Table 1**). For instance, those with ANCA-associated vasculitis (AAV), may be at higher risk for worse outcomes compared with patients without vasculitis given higher reported point estimates for severe disease and mortality.[10] Among patients with ANCA-associated vasculitis, risk factors for more severe disease include older age, chronic kidney disease, moderate or high-severe

Table 1
Risk factors for severe COVID-19 infection in patients with vasculitis

Risk Factors	
Non-Modifiable	Older age
	Race/ethnicity
	Male sex
	Comorbidities (chronic kidney disease in AAV)
	Obesity (GCA)
Modifiable	High disease activity
	Use of rituximab or cyclophosphamide
	High dose glucocorticoids

Abbreviations: AAV, ANCA-associated vasculitis; GCA, giant cell arteritis.

disease activity at baseline, and treatment with higher glucocorticoid doses, cyclophosphamide, and/or rituximab. The increased risk for poor outcomes with rituximab and other B-cell depleting therapies has been reported in multiple conditions and poses an important risk to patients with AAV given the pivotal role of rituximab both in remission induction and maintenance of remission.[7,11,12] Higher rates of severe outcomes have also been observed in patients with giant cell arteritis (GCA).[10] The demographics (eg, older age) and frequent use of high dose glucocorticoids likely contribute to the higher rates of poor outcomes in this patient population.[13]

Unlike GCA and AAV, registry and cohort studies studying outcomes of COVID-19 infection in patients with Behcet's syndrome have overall shown a lower rate of complications with COVID-19 infection and somewhat lower mortality.[10,14,15] As seen with other systemic rheumatic diseases including case reports of other forms of vasculitis, one study did report flares of Behcet's during COVID-19 infection in up to 43% of patients, however, there was no signal for increased thrombotic events.[14,16–18] Outside of few case reports, little is known about outcomes of COVID-19 infection in patients with other forms of vasculitis. In the COVID-19 GRA analysis, the majority of patients with other forms of vasculitis did not require hospitalization, though 21 (14.2%) were reported to have died from COVID-19.[10] Interpreting absolute mortality rates from registry-based studies is challenging because the denominator (eg, all with infection) is unknown.

Reassuringly, outcomes of COVID-19 infection have continued to improve in those with rheumatic disease, including vasculitis, during the pandemic, and the risk of severe infection in patients with COVID-19 is largely observed in those who remain unvaccinated.[4] However, breakthrough infections (eg, COVID-19 infection after SARS-CoV-2 vaccination) have been found to occur at higher rates in immunocompromised patients, especially those using anti-rheumatic drugs such as B-cell depleting therapies and anti-metabolites, which are known to blunt the immune response and leave many with no detectable antibody response.[19,20] Although large population-based studies have shown similar severity in breakthrough infections between patients with systemic rheumatic disease when compared to the general population, severe infection and death do occur and remain a significant concern in vasculitis patients on these treatments.[19,21,22]

IMPACT OF CORONAVIRUS DISEASE 2019 PANDEMIC ON PATIENTS WITH VASCULITIS

The COVID-19 pandemic significantly affected patients with vasculitis who endorsed specific concerns and changed behaviors regarding accessing health care and use of vasculitis treatments. A survey of the Vasculitis Patients Powered Research Network (VPPRN), an online cohort of vasculitis patients, done during the earlier months of the pandemic (April-May 2020) reported a high level of concern in patients, which was associated with the use of immunosuppression, older age, female sex, and comorbid pulmonary disease.[23] Interruption of medication, without consultation with a clinician, reported by 10.5% of patients and up to 29% of patients on rituximab avoided their infusions. Both demographic and regional differences were noted with regards to the uptake of telemedicine visits among patients with vasculitis. A survey of GCA and polymyalgia rheumatica patients from the UK and the Netherlands also reported a high frequency of anxiety, isolation, depression, and concerns regarding the use of immunosuppressive treatments.[24]

A subsequent study of a larger internet-based cohort of patients with rheumatic diseases, which included VPPRN patients, explored anti-rheumatic drug interruptions in patients from March 2020 to May 2021.[25] An association between self-reported anxiety and medication interruptions was reported, and although the rate of antirheumatic drug interruption decreased throughout the study period, an increase was observed during follow-up in periods characterized by COVID-19 surges. Interruptions in treatments were associated with an increased risk of flares. These findings highlight the ongoing impact of the pandemic on patients with vasculitis and other rheumatic diseases, even as outcomes improve. Patient education regarding disease management and COVID-19 mitigation strategies as well as interventions focused on securing early access to care and treatments should remain a priority for clinicians and health care systems.

CORONAVIRUS DISEASE 2019 VACCINATION IN PATIENTS WITH VASCULITIS

The rapid development of effective COVID-19 vaccines has been one of the pivotal events of the pandemic. Widespread use of different forms of COVID-19 vaccines has been employed including mRNA vaccines (eg, BNT162b2 [Pfizer-BioNtech], mRNA-1273 [Moderna]), viral-vector vaccines (eg, ChAdOx1 [Astra-Zeneca], Ad26.COV2.S [Johnson & Johnson]), inactivated virus vaccines (eg, Sinovac and Sinopharm), and protein-subunit vaccines (eg, NVX-CoV2373 [Novavax]). Unfortunately, patients with systemic rheumatic diseases were generally excluded from the initial trials, even though this population was among those most in need of effective vaccines given their risk for severe disease. While our understanding of the effectiveness of vaccination in patients with vasculitis and other rheumatic diseases treated with immunosuppression has improved since they were introduced to the general population, there remain concerns and knowledge gaps regarding the impact of immunosuppression on the immune response (eg, cellular, antibody, antibody function).[5]

In contrast to immunocompetent hosts in whom seroconversion following SARS-CoV-2 vaccination is nearly universally observed, studies have reported lower rates of seroconversion, lower antibody titers, and reduced neutralization in many users of antirheumatic drugs.[26–29] Seropositivity rates between 85 and 94% after initial series have been reported in patients with systemic rheumatic diseases.[29–32] Few studies have reported specific findings in patients with vasculitis. Seropositivity rates of 82.6% (38/46) and 55% (87/159) after initial regimen (1 dose of Ad26.COV2.S or 2 doses of mRNA vaccine, or 2 doses of BNT162b2 or ChAdOx1, respectively) have been reported in 2 separate studies of AAV patients, and rituximab was associated with lack of response in both studies.[33,34] In a study of patients with GCA, seroconversion after initial regimen with BNT162b2 was reported in 93.8% of patients; all patients with impaired serological response were on methotrexate.[35]

Lack of seroconversion has been strongly associated with the use of specific medications such as B-cell depleting therapies as well as antimetabolites such as cyclophosphamide, mycophenolate mofetil, azathioprine, and methotrexate (**Table 2**).[29,36–38] Other antirheumatic drugs including Janus Kinase (JAK) inhibitors and tumor necrosis-α (TNF-α) inhibitors may also impact antibody responses.[29,39] With regards to glucocorticoids, their effect on seroconversion is still unclear since they are typically combined with other antirheumatic drugs. However, some studies have shown decreases in seroconversion associated with glucocorticoids, including one large cohort study that showed lower antibody titers, compared to immunocompetent controls, in patients receiving low doses of prednisone (<7.5 mg/d).[29]

Seroconversion is thought to correlate with neutralizing antibody titers and cellular response. However, one large US study found lower neutralization titers against the delta variant in patients receiving TNF-α monotherapy, despite adequate seroconversion.[29] With regards to cellular response, studies in patients on B-cell depleting agents have shown spike-specific CD4 T-cell response in patients even in the absence of seroconversion. However, it seems that these spike-specific CD4 T-cells might have an impaired function, which might explain the observations of increased breakthrough infections, including severe COVID-19, in vaccinated patients on B-cell depleted therapies.[40,41] One single-center study of patients with GCA showed a lack of neutralization activity in 16% and decreased cellular response in 30% of patients, despite robust seroconversion.[42] The clinical significance of these findings requires further investigation to facilitate better approaches to stratifying risk and advising mitigation strategies.[43]

Enhancing Vaccine Response

SARS-CoV-2 vaccine boosters, both third and fourth boosters, have been shown to improve antibody response in patients with systemic rheumatic diseases.[44,45] Decreased risk of infection in systemic rheumatic disease patients with a third booster dose has been observed in one large population study.[46] Improvement in seroconversion has also been reported in patients with AAV after a third booster dose, including B-cell depleted patients at the time of the initial series.[47,48] However, this might not be the case for all patients on B-cell depleting therapies since lack of response, including the formation of neutralizing antibodies, has been reported even

Table 2
Anti-rheumatic drugs used for the treatment of vasculitis and their association with antibody response to SARS-CoV-2 vaccination

Significantly Reduce Antibody Response	Probably Reduce Antibody Response	May Not Affect Antibody Response
Rituximab	TNF-α inhibitors	IL-6 inhibitors
Cyclophosphamide	Janus kinase inhibitors	Apremilast
Methotrexate	Abatacept	Colchicine
Azathioprine		
Mycophenolate		
Leflunomide		
Glucocorticoids		

Abbreviations: IL, interleukin; TNF, tumor necrosis factor.

after COVID-19 vaccine booster. In part, some of these differences may have to do with the timing of vaccination relative to B cell depletion therapy. Therefore, although COVID-19 vaccine boosters can certainly enhance response, certain patients with systemic rheumatic diseases remain at high risk for COVID-19.

Given the known effect of some antirheumatic drugs on COVID-19 vaccine response, temporarily holding antirheumatic drugs (eg, as in the case of daily medications) or delaying retreatment (eg, as in the case of rituximab and other medications administered by infusion or subcutaneous injection) has been recommended by some. While this was empirically recommended based on previous experience with other vaccinations, two recent studies, one including patients using methotrexate and the other including mycophenolate mofetil users, found that temporarily holding medication was associated with an improved antibody response after vaccination.[49,50] Flares were reported in the mycophenolate mofetil study, highlighting the importance of individualized assessment to guide these strategies. With regards to rituximab, studies have shown that longer periods from the last rituximab dosing as well as B-cell reconstitution are strong predictors of seroconversion after COVID-19 vaccination.[37,38,51] In light of this evidence, the American College of Rheumatology has continued to recommend strategies to optimize vaccine response in patients on antirheumatic drugs.[52]

Flares and Coronavirus Disease 2019 Vaccination

A large physician-reported registry of 5121 patients with systemic rheumatic disease reported flares in 4.4% of patients, with only 1.5% of cases requiring changes in medications.[53] In the COVID-19 GRA Vaccine survey which included 2860 participants, flares that required medication changes were reported by 4.6% of patients.[54] A subsequent survey, which included 5619 participants, reported a similar rate of flares requiring medication changes (4.9%).[55] Risk of flares was higher in patients with specific rheumatic diseases such as systemic lupus erythematosus and polymyalgia rheumatica, when compared to rheumatoid arthritis, and in patients with a history of a previous serious reaction to other vaccines, as well as female sex. Overall, the risk of severe flare after COVID-19 vaccination seems to be relatively low. Although emerging case reports have reported either flares of pre-existing vasculitis or even new cases of vasculitis,[56,57] the benefits of vaccination in patients with vasculitis and other systemic rheumatic diseases clearly exceeds the risks, and vaccination should be encouraged in all patients.

ONGOING CHALLENGES IN THE MANAGEMENT OF PATIENTS WITH VASCULITIS
Rituximab

The greatest challenge to the use of rituximab during the COVID-19 pandemic has been the increasing recognition of its impact on the immune response to infection[7,10,11,58,59] as well as on the immunogenicity of COVID-19 vaccines.[22,29,37,60] Because of the associated higher risks for severe COVID-19 and reduced vaccine efficacy, a number of patients and clinicians have had to weigh these risks against the important benefits of rituximab for patients with vasculitis. Indeed, prior to the pandemic, a number of clinical trials had established the superior efficacy of routine retreatment with B cell depletion for reducing the risk of relapse in AAV.[61–63] The COVID-19 pandemic and the risks associated with B cell depletion during this time have forced many to reconsider the prioritization of continuous B cell depletion for maintaining remission in AAV. Decisions regarding the use of rituximab to treat vasculitis during the COVID-19 pandemic require shared decision making by the patient and clinician. Factors to consider when making these choices include the patient's history of AAV (eg, treatment history, organ involvement, and damage), prior COVID-19 immunity (eg, vaccination prior to rituximab, prior infection), the use of pre-exposure prophylaxis (see later in discussion), and the patient's values.

Cyclophosphamide

Like rituximab, cyclophosphamide leads to B cell depletion and has an impact on T cell function as well. This combination leaves patients vulnerable to both severe infection as well as a blunted immune response to vaccination. Given the less frequent use of cyclophosphamide in contemporary practice, there is scant data on COVID-19 outcomes in patients receiving cyclophosphamide.[10,64] In contrast to B cell depleting therapies, however, the use of cyclophosphamide is often limited to short durations to minimize toxicities and the half-life of oral or intravenous formulations is much shorter. To minimize COVID-19 risk, the dose and duration of cyclophosphamide should be minimized as much as possible and, when used, risk mitigating strategies discussed later in this discussion should be implemented. It may be ideal to delay vaccination until cyclophosphamide is discontinued.

Prolonged Viral Shedding and Within Host Viral Evolution

A growing number of reports describe prolonged viral shedding and within-host viral evolution among patients with COVID-19 who had prior exposure to rituximab and cytotoxic therapies.[65–70] Given the frequent use of rituximab, cyclophosphamide, and other potent immunosuppression for vasculitis, it is important to consider this population at risk for prolonged viral shedding and within-host viral evolution because of the associated implications for individual patient management and public health. Patients treated with rituximab, cyclophosphamide, or other strong immunosuppressants may be recommended to extend their quarantine during an acute infection and consider themselves contagious beyond the recommended 5-10 day window. Prolonged viral shedding in patients with vasculitis may predispose them to within-host viral evolution during which mutations may develop against monoclonal antibodies or antivirals, as has been previously described.[65] Additional studies are needed to understand the frequency of these events as well as ways to prevent them.

These observations highlight the substantial impact of the impaired immune response in vasculitis patients treated with rituximab and other immunosuppressants. Without an appropriate immune response, viral control may be difficult to attain and this likely contributes to the more frequent severe acute outcomes observed in these patients, such as hospitalization, mechanical ventilation, and death, as described above. Indeed, previous studies have found that some patients with COVID-19 who had prior exposure to rituximab mounted no detectable antibody response to SARS-CoV-2 which is known to be important for controlling viral replication.[59] This highlights the important role that monoclonal antibodies against SARS-CoV-2 may have for patients with vasculitis who are strongly immunosuppressed and unlikely to mount an antibody response. Earlier in the pandemic effective monoclonal antibodies were an important treatment for this patient population. Unfortunately, there are currently no effective monoclonal antibodies against the Omicron variant.

Equity

The COVID-19 pandemic has illuminated many of the ongoing racial and ethnic disparities in health and access to healthcare that exist in the United States and around the world. Racial and ethnic minorities in the United States, including patients who identify as Black or African American or Hispanic, have been found to have a higher risk for

COVID-19 as well as severe outcomes.[71] This has also been observed in patients with rheumatic diseases, including patients with vasculitis.[72] Clinicians should be aware of these disparities and identify opportunities to help their patients with vasculitis get better access to testing, pre-exposure prophylaxis, antiviral treatments, and risk mitigating strategies (eg, masking, social distancing).

Post-Acute Sequelae of Coronavirus Disease 2019 or Long Coronavirus Disease 2019

Postacute sequelae of COVID-19 (PASC) or "Long COVID" is now a well-recognized complication of COVID-19, defined as symptoms of COVID-19 that persist or develop at least 28 days after the onset of acute infection.[73–77] Common symptoms of PASC include fatigue, myalgia and arthralgia, loss of sense of smell or taste, dyspnea, headaches, and brain fog. Other manifestations of PASC include complications such as new-onset diabetes, chronic kidney disease, and other manifestations of end-organ damage. The etiology of PASC is poorly understood but hypotheses include alterations in inflammatory cytokine profiles,[78] cellular immune responses,[79] reactivation of chronic viral infections,[80] and autoantibody formation.[81,82] Given the heterogeneity of PASC, it is plausible that distinct etiologies may be associated with different hosts recovering from acute illness. Given the association of vasculitis and its treatments with poor acute COVID-19 outcomes, it is possible that this population is more vulnerable to PASC but there is scarce data on this topic. Previous studies have suggested that while anyone recovering from COVID-19, even asymptomatic patients, can develop PASC, those with more severe acute infections tend to be at higher risk. Patients and clinicians should be aware that persistent or new symptoms developing in vasculitis patients after acute infection resolution may reflect PASC and will need to be distinguished from those attributable to the underlying vasculitis. There are no known effective treatments for PASC as of spring 2023.

MITIGATION STRATEGIES

As discussed, many of the immunosuppressives used to treat vasculitis blunt the immune response to COVID-19 vaccination, leaving this population quite vulnerable to COVID-19, including severe disease. Masking, social distancing, and other measures were widely adopted early in the pandemic to reduce the risk of COVID-19. However, it is increasingly impractical for many to continue these measures indefinitely. These strategies may have negative effects on mental health,[83] including in patients with rheumatic disease,[84] and can make it difficult for patients to carry on their necessary activities of daily living, such as working, attending medical appointments, or caring for themselves and their families. Moreover, many governments have dropped requirements for masking, vaccination, or social distancing which further increase the risk for patients with vasculitis when they are in public. Alternative approaches are therefore needed to keep patients with vasculitis safe during the ongoing pandemic (**Fig. 1**).

Preexposure Prophylaxis

The pharmacologic options for preexposure prophylaxis (PrEP) against COVID-19 remain limited. As of early 2023, no longer authorized for the only US Food and Drug Administration-authorized treatment to prevent COVID-19 in patients who are immunosuppressed. This treatment is a combination of 2 Fc-modified human monoclonal antibodies that have preserved efficacy against SARS-CoV-2 variants, including Omicron and its subvariants. The Fc-modifications are meant to extend

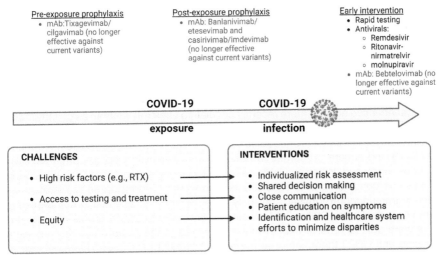

Fig. 1. Ongoing challenges and mitigation strategies in the management of vasculitis patients during the COVID-19 pandemic. COVID-19, coronavirus disease 2019; mAb, monoclonal antibody; RTX, rituximab. (Created with BioRender.com.)

the half-life, in contrast to other monoclonal antibodies that have been used during the pandemic to treat acute infection and have a shorter half-life. Tixagevimab/cilgavimab was originally studied as PrEP in a randomized clinical trial that enrolled unvaccinated patients who were at increased risk of an inadequate response to vaccination, including immunosuppressed patients (PROVENT trial)[85]; however, only 3.3% of patients enrolled in this trial received immunosuppressive treatment prior to enrollment. Other patients were included in the trial because of other factors that contribute to the risk of poor vaccine response (eg, obesity, cardiovascular disease). In PROVENT, the use of tixagevimab/cilgavimab vs placebo was associated with a 82.8% (95% CI 65.8%-91.4%) reduction in the relative risk of COVID-19 over 6 months.[85] Ongoing clinical trials investigating an updated monoclonal antibody for pre-exposure prophylaxis are enrolling more immunosuppressed patients who remain the most vulnerable populations.

The published data from PROVENT reported outcomes through August 29, 2021, a period characterized by the dominance of pre-Omicron SARS-CoV-2 variants. To further assess the effectiveness of tixagevimab/cilgavimab against early Omicron variants and among immunocompromised patients, an observational retrospective cohort study from Israel compared the risk of COVID-19 among patients who received tixagevimab/cilgavimab vs those who did not.[86] All patients included in the study had been invited to receive tixagevimab/cilgavimab as part of a nationwide campaign for patients at high risk but not all participated. Among those invited to participate in the program (n = 5,124), 825 received tixagevimab/cilgavimab and 43.9% of them qualified for tixagevimab/cilgavimab because they had received anti-CD20 treatment in the previous 6 months. Of note, a large portion of patients in this study was receiving anti-CD20 treatment as part of therapy for lymphoma; it is unclear how many had vasculitis or other immune-mediated inflammatory diseases being treated with anti-CD20 monoclonals. In contrast to PROVENT, the majority of patients in this observational study had previously received at least one COVID-19 vaccine. In a multivariable adjusted analysis, those who received tixagevimab/cilgavimab had a 49% lower odds of COVID-19 infection compared with not receiving tixagevimab/cilgavimab (OR 0.51, 95% CI 0.30–0.84). Additionally, there was a strong benefit associated with tixagevimab/cilgavimab vs not receiving tixagevimab/cilgavimab when assessing severe COVID-19 (OR 0.08, 95% CI 0.01–0.54). While there are important limitations to this study related to its design and the way it handled potential confounding, the findings did support the effectiveness and importance of tixagevimab/cilgavimab for reducing the risk of COVID-19 during the early Omicron period. Unfortunately, this treatment is no longer effective against more recently circulating Omicron variants as of early 2023.

Collectively, the available data suggests that there is likely to be an important and ongoing role for monoclonal antibodies such as tixagevimab/cilgavimab for preventing COVID-19 and severe outcomes in patients with vasculitis who are often severely immunosuppressed. When available, recommendations suggest that tixagevimab/cilgavimab be considered in many patients who would be considered moderately-to-severely immunocompromised, not only those who have received B cell depleting therapies in the United States.[87] Many centers ran have started programs whereby patients were able to receive tixagevimab/cilgavimab at the same time that they were receiving anti-CD20 therapies or at the time of another clinical encounter. Tixagevimab/cilgavimab was well-tolerated but there was a risk of an injection site reaction and/or hypersensitivity reaction.[88] Additionally, based on some observations during its development program, there was an associated warning regarding a potentially higher risk of cardiovascular events associated with tixagevimab/cilgavimab. In our practice, have considered the potential benefits of tixagevimab/cilgavimab to outweigh these potential risks, except in patients with high risk of cardiovascular disease. The implementation of pre-exposure prophylaxis will need to be reassessed when it is available again.

Postexposure Prophylaxis

Postexposure prophylaxis (PEP) has also been used to prevent COVID-19 in immunosuppressed patients exposed to COVID-19. Similar to PrEP, options available for PEP have been limited to monoclonal antibodies.[89,90] The experience using monoclonal antibodies as PEP, however, has illuminated the challenges associated with this approach in the face of SARS-CoV-2 evolution towards variants with resistance to treatments, including monoclonal antibodies. As of the spring 2023, there are no longer monoclonal antibody treatments authorized for use as postexposure prophylaxis because current SARS-CoV-2 variants in circulation have resistance to previously authorized treatments.[87,89,90] Previously, bamlanivimab/etesevimab and casirivimab/imdevimab had been authorized for use as PEP in patients at high risk for severe COVID-19.

Access to Testing and Treatment

It is critical that patients with vasculitis be counseled to reach out to their providers if they are exposed to COVID-19 or test positive for COVID-19. We counsel our patients to keep a supply of rapid antigen tests at home, if they have access to these tests, and to contact us immediately if they test positive. Indeed, the early initiation of antiviral therapy with remdesevir,[91] ritonavir-boosted nirmatrelvir,[92,93] or molnupiravir,[94] is critical for reducing the risk of severe disease in patients with vasculitis who are often on treatments or have comorbidities associated with a higher risk of severe disease.[87] However, the evidence supporting the efficacy of bebtelovimab is limited.

According to most recent US National Institutes of Health guidance,[87] ritonavir-boosted nirmatrelvir or remdesevir are preferred over molnupiravir bebtelovimab because of the stronger efficacy data supporting their use. Of note, it is important to review the drug-drug interactions associated with ritonavir-boosted nirmatrelvir. For patients with vasculitis, it is important to know that there are potential interactions of ritonavir-boosted nirmatrelvir with glucocorticoids, colchicine, avacopan, and cyclophosphamide. In these instances, ritonavir-boosted nirmatrelvir may increase exposure to the metabolites of glucocorticoids and cyclophosphamide, leading to higher risk of toxicities.

One must also consider the dose reduction needed for patients with an estimated glomerular filtration rate (eGFR) of 30-60 mL/min; ritonavir-boosted nirmatrelvir is contraindicated in patients with an eGFR < 30 mL/min, due to the renal excretion of nirmatrelvir,[95] which has relevance for many patients living with vasculitis. Similarly, the safety of remdesivir for patients with an eGFR < 30 mL/min is controversial and large safety studies are lacking. Both the drug itself and its carrier (sulfobutylether-β-cyclodextrin) may contribute to kidney injury.[5] Therefore, the use of remdesivir in patients with an eGFR < 30 mL/min or who are receiving dialysis should be done so in collaboration with infectious disease and nephrology experts.

SUMMARY

The COVID-19 pandemic has substantially impacted the lives of patients living with vasculitis and has imposed a number of challenges for the management of vasculitis. Many patients with vasculitis remain at higher risk for COVID-19 and severe outcomes, despite advances such as vaccines, antivirals, and other management strategies. In part, this increased risk is because many of the medications that are highly effective for vasculitis, such as rituximab, also interfere with the immune response to vaccination and infection. When available, the use of pre and postexposure treatment, as well as access to early diagnosis and treatment for those infected are essential for reducing the risk of severe COVID-19 in patients with vasculitis. Patients and clinicians can use the expanding data on outcomes of COVID-19 in patients with vasculitis in the context of evolving COVID-19 and vasculitis management strategies to make decisions together regarding their vasculitis care in this uncertain time. Moving forward, clinical trials of therapeutics that enroll patients with vasculitis and others who use immunosuppression are needed to inform management strategies.

CLINICS CARE POINTS

- Patients with vasculitis, especially those with comorbidities or using rituximab or cyclophosphamide, are at increased risk for severe COVID-19 and poor outcomes.
- Early diagnosis and initiation of treatment are important for improving outcomes in this vulnerable population.
- Vaccination may not be as effective in patients with vasculitis, especially those using rituximab, cyclophosphamide, and other immunosuppressives.

SOURCE(S) OF SUPPORT IN THE FORMS OF GRANTS OR INDUSTRIAL SUPPORT

Dr S.E. Sattui is supported by the Rheumatology Research Foundation RISE Pilot Award and the Bristol-Myers Squibb Foundation, United States Winn Career Development Award outside of the submitted work. Dr Z.S. Wallace is funded by NIH, United States/NIAMS, United States [K23AR073334, R01 AR080659-01 and R03AR078938] and the Rheumatology Research Foundation, United States [K Supplement].

CONFLICTS OF INTEREST

Dr S.E. Sattui reports research support from AstraZeneca, United States. Dr Z.S. Wallace reports research support from Bristol-Myers Squibb, United States and Principia/Sanofi and consulting fees from Zenas Biopharma, Horizon, Sanofi, Shionogi, Viela Bio, and MedPace.

REFERENCES

1. Grainger R, Kim AHJ, Conway R, et al. COVID-19 in people with rheumatic diseases: risks, outcomes, treatment considerations. Nat Rev Rheumatol 2022; 18(4):191–204.
2. Normand ST. The recovery platform. N Engl J Med 2021;384(8):757–8.
3. Robinson PC, Yazdany J, Machado PM. Global research collaboration in a pandemic-challenges and opportunities: the COVID-19 Global Rheumatology Alliance. Curr Opin Rheumatol 2021;33(2):111–6.
4. Kawano Y, Patel NJ, Wang X, et al. Temporal trends in COVID-19 outcomes among patients with systemic autoimmune rheumatic diseases: from the first wave through the initial Omicron wave. Ann Rheum Dis 2022;81(12):1742–9.
5. Friedman MA, Curtis JR, Winthrop KL. Impact of disease-modifying antirheumatic drugs on vaccine immunogenicity in patients with inflammatory rheumatic and musculoskeletal diseases. Ann Rheum Dis 2021;80(10):1255–65.
6. Conway R, Grimshaw AA, Konig MF, et al. SARS-CoV-2 infection and COVID-19 outcomes in rheumatic diseases: a systematic literature review and meta-analysis. Arthritis Rheumatol 2022;74(5):766–75.
7. MacKenna B, Kennedy NA, Mehrkar A, et al. Risk of severe COVID-19 outcomes associated with immune-mediated inflammatory diseases and immune-modifying therapies: a nationwide cohort study in the OpenSAFELY platform. The Lancet Rheumatology 2022;4(7):e490–506.
8. Eder L, Croxford R, Drucker AM, et al. COVID-19 hospitalizations, intensive care unit stays, ventilation, and death among patients with immune-mediated inflammatory diseases compared to controls. J Rheumatol 2022;49(5):523–30.
9. Rutherford MA, Scott J, Karabayas M, et al. Risk factors for severe outcomes in patients with systemic vasculitis and COVID-19: A Binational, Registry-Based Cohort Study. Arthritis Rheumatol 2021;73(9):1713–9.
10. Sattui SE, Conway R, Putman MS, et al. Outcomes of COVID-19 in patients with primary systemic vasculitis or polymyalgia rheumatica from the COVID-19 Global Rheumatology Alliance physician registry: a retrospective cohort study. The Lancet Rheumatology 2021;3(12):e855–64.
11. Patel NJ, D'Silva KM, Hsu TY, et al. Coronavirus disease 2019 outcomes among recipients of Anti-CD20 monoclonal antibodies for immune-mediated diseases: a comparative cohort study. ACR Open Rheumatol 2022;4(3):238–46.
12. Andersen KM, Bates BA, Rashidi ES, et al. Long-term use of immunosuppressive medicines and in-hospital COVID-19 outcomes: a retrospective cohort study using data from the National COVID Cohort Collaborative. The Lancet Rheumatology 2022;4(1):e33–41.
13. Vieira M, Comarmond C, Labreuche J, et al. COVID-19 outcomes in giant cell arteritis and polymyalgia rheumatica versus rheumatoid arthritis: a national, multi-center, cohort study. J Autoimmun 2022;132:102868.
14. Ozcifci G, Aydin T, Atli Z, et al. The incidence, clinical characteristics, and outcome of COVID-19 in a prospectively followed cohort of patients with Behçet's syndrome. Rheumatol Int 2022;42(1):101–13.

15. Polat B, Erden A, Güven SC, et al. COVID-19 in patients with Behçet's disease: outcomes and rate of Behçet's exacerbations in a retrospective cohort. Mod Rheumatol 2022;32(2):455–9.
16. Di Iorio M, Cook CE, Vanni KMM, et al. DMARD disruption, rheumatic disease flare, and prolonged COVID-19 symptom duration after acute COVID-19 among patients with rheumatic disease: a prospective study. Semin Arthritis Rheum 2022;55:152025.
17. Ozcan S, Sonmez O, Karaca C, et al. ANCA-associated vasculitis flare might be provoked by COVID-19 infection: a case report and a review of the literature. Clinical Kidney Journal 2022;15(11):1987–95.
18. Valero C, Baldivieso-Achá JP, Uriarte M, et al. Vasculitis flare after COVID-19: report of two cases in patients with preexistent controlled IgA vasculitis and review of the literature. Rheumatol Int 2022;42(9):1643–52.
19. Boekel L, Stalman EW, Wieske L, et al. Breakthrough SARS-CoV-2 infections with the delta (B.1.617.2) variant in vaccinated patients with immune-mediated inflammatory diseases using immunosuppressants: a substudy of two prospective cohort studies. The Lancet Rheumatology 2022;4(6):e417–29.
20. Sun J, Zheng Q, Madhira V, et al. Association between immune dysfunction and COVID-19 breakthrough infection after SARS-CoV-2 vaccination in the US. JAMA Intern Med 2022;182(2):153–62.
21. Liew J, Gianfrancesco M, Harrison C, et al. SARS-CoV-2 breakthrough infections among vaccinated individuals with rheumatic disease: results from the COVID-19 Global Rheumatology Alliance provider registry. RMD Open 2022;8(1):1–11.
22. Calabrese CM, Kirchner E, Husni EM, et al. Breakthrough SARS-CoV-2 infections in immune mediated disease patients undergoing B cell depleting therapy: A retrospective cohort analysis. Arthritis Rheumatol 2022;74(12):1906–15.
23. Banerjee S, George M, Young K, et al. Effects of the COVID-19 pandemic on patients living with vasculitis. ACR Open Rheumatol 2021;3(1):17–24.
24. Mackie SL, Brouwer E, Conway R, et al. Clinical pathways for patients with giant cell arteritis during the COVID-19 pandemic: an international perspective. The Lancet Rheumatology 2021;3(1):e71–82.
25. Dharia T, Venkatachalam S, Baker JF, et al. Medication interruptions and subsequent disease flares during the COVID-19 pandemic: a longitudinal online study of patients with rheumatic disease. Arthritis Care Res 2022;74(5):733–40.
26. Anderson EJ, Rouphael NG, Widge AT, et al. Safety and immunogenicity of SARS-CoV-2 mRNA-1273 vaccine in older adults. N Engl J Med 2020;383(25):2427–38.
27. Sadoff J, Le Gars M, Shukarev G, et al. Interim results of a phase 1-2a trial of Ad26.COV2.S Covid-19 vaccine. N Engl J Med 2021;384(19):1824–35.
28. Walsh EE, Frenck RW Jr, Falsey AR, et al. Safety and immunogenicity of two RNA-based Covid-19 vaccine candidates. N Engl J Med 2020;383(25):2439–50.
29. Deepak P, Kim W, Paley MA, et al. Effect of immunosuppression on the immunogenicity of mRNA vaccines to SARS-CoV-2 : a prospective cohort study. Ann Intern Med 2021;174(11):1572–85.
30. Boekel L, Steenhuis M, Hooijberg F, et al. Antibody development after COVID-19 vaccination in patients with autoimmune diseases in the Netherlands: a substudy of data from two prospective cohort studies. The Lancet Rheumatology 2021;3(11):e778–88.
31. Furer V, Eviatar T, Zisman D, et al. Immunogenicity and safety of the BNT162b2 mRNA COVID-19 vaccine in adult patients with autoimmune inflammatory

rheumatic diseases and in the general population: a multicentre study. Ann Rheum Dis 2021;80(10):1330–8.

32. Simon D, Tascilar K, Fagni F, et al. SARS-CoV-2 vaccination responses in untreated, conventionally treated and anticytokine-treated patients with immune-mediated inflammatory diseases. Ann Rheum Dis 2021;80(10):1312–6.

33. Carruthers JE, Wells J, Gupta A, et al. Response to vaccination against SARS-CoV-2 in patients with antineutrophil cytoplasmic antibody-associated vasculitis with renal involvement. Front Med 2021;8:817845.

34. Floyd L, Elsayed ME, Seibt T, et al. SARS-CoV-2 vaccine response in patients with antineutrophil cytoplasmic autoantibody-associated vasculitis. Kidney International Reports 2022;7(3):629–32.

35. Delvino P, Bartoletti A, Cassaniti I, et al. Impact of immunosuppressive treatment on the immunogenicity of mRNA COVID-19 vaccine in vulnerable patients with giant cell arteritis. Rheumatology 2022;61(2):870–2.

36. Haberman RH, Herati R, Simon D, et al. Methotrexate hampers immunogenicity to BNT162b2 mRNA COVID-19 vaccine in immune-mediated inflammatory disease. Ann Rheum Dis 2021;80(10):1339–44.

37. Jinich S, Schultz K, Jannat-Khah D, et al. B cell reconstitution is strongly associated With COVID-19 vaccine responsiveness in rheumatic disease patients who received treatment with rituximab. Arthritis Rheumatol 2022;74(5):776–82.

38. Schumacher F, Mrdenovic N, Scheicht D, et al. Humoral immunogenicity of COVID-19 vaccines in patients with inflammatory rheumatic diseases under treatment with Rituximab: a case-control study (COVID-19VacRTX). Rheumatology 2022;61(10):3912–8.

39. Haberman RH, Um S, Axelrad JE, et al. Methotrexate and TNF inhibitors affect long-term immunogenicity to COVID-19 vaccination in patients with immune-mediated inflammatory disease. The Lancet Rheumatology 2022;4(6):e384–7.

40. Moor MB, Suter-Riniker F, Horn MP, et al. Humoral and cellular responses to mRNA vaccines against SARS-CoV-2 in patients with a history of CD20 B-cell-depleting therapy (RituxiVac): an investigator-initiated, single-centre, open-label study. Lancet Rheumatology 2021;3(11):e789–97.

41. Prendecki M, Clarke C, Edwards H, et al. Humoral and T-cell responses to SARS-CoV-2 vaccination in patients receiving immunosuppression. Ann Rheum Dis 2021;80(10):1322–9.

42. Monti S, Fornara C, Delvino P, et al. Immunosuppressive treatments selectively affect the humoral and cellular response to SARS-CoV-2 in vaccinated patients with vasculitis. Rheumatology 2022;62(2):726–34.

43. Ferri C, Ursini F, Gragnani L, et al. Impaired immunogenicity to COVID-19 vaccines in autoimmune systemic diseases. High prevalence of non-response in different patients' subgroups. J Autoimmun 2021;125:102744.

44. Connolly CM, Teles M, Frey S, et al. Booster-dose SARS-CoV-2 vaccination in patients with autoimmune disease: a case series. Ann Rheum Dis 2022;81(2):291–3.

45. Teles M, Connolly CM, Frey S, et al. Attenuated response to fourth dose SARS-CoV-2 vaccination in patients with autoimmune disease: a case series. Ann Rheum Dis 2022;81(5):738–40.

46. Bieber A, Sagy I, Novack L, et al. BNT162b2 mRNA COVID-19 vaccine and booster in patients with autoimmune rheumatic diseases: a national cohort study. Ann Rheum Dis 2022;81(7):1028–35.

47. Kant S, Azar A, Geetha D. Antibody response to COVID-19 booster vaccine in rituximab-treated patients with anti-neutrophil cytoplasmic antibody-associated vasculitis. Kidney Int 2022;101(2):414–5.

48. Speer C, Töllner M, Benning L, et al. Third COVID-19 vaccine dose with BNT162b2 in patients with ANCA-associated vasculitis. Ann Rheum Dis 2022; 81(4):593–5.
49. Arumahandi de Silva AN, Frommert LM, Albach FN, et al. Pausing methotrexate improves immunogenicity of COVID-19 vaccination in elderly patients with rheumatic diseases. Ann Rheum Dis 2022;81(6):881–8.
50. Connolly CM, Chiang TP, Boyarsky BJ, et al. Temporary hold of mycophenolate augments humoral response to SARS-CoV-2 vaccination in patients with rheumatic and musculoskeletal diseases: a case series. Ann Rheum Dis 2022; 81(2):293–5.
51. Stefanski AL, Rincon-Arevalo H, Schrezenmeier E, et al. B Cell Numbers Predict Humoral and Cellular Response Upon SARS-CoV-2 Vaccination Among Patients Treated With Rituximab. Arthritis Rheumatol 2022;74(6):934–47.
52. Curtis JR, Johnson SR, Anthony DD, et al. American College of Rheumatology Guidance for COVID-19 Vaccination in Patients With Rheumatic and Musculoskeletal Diseases: Version 4. Arthritis Rheumatol 2022;74(5):e21–36.
53. Machado PM, Lawson-Tovey S, Strangfeld A, et al. Safety of vaccination against SARS-CoV-2 in people with rheumatic and musculoskeletal diseases: results from the EULAR Coronavirus Vaccine (COVAX) physician-reported registry. Ann Rheum Dis 2022;81(5):695–709.
54. Sattui SE, Liew JW, Kennedy K, et al. Early experience of COVID-19 vaccination in adults with systemic rheumatic diseases: results from the COVID-19 global rheumatology alliance vaccine survey. RMD Open 2021;7(3):1–10.
55. Rider LG, Parks CG, Wilkerson J, et al. Baseline factors associated with self-reported disease flares following COVID-19 vaccination among adults with systemic rheumatic disease: results from the COVID-19 global rheumatology alliance vaccine survey. Rheumatology 2022;61(Si2):Si143–50.
56. Shakoei S, Kalantari Y, Nasimi M, et al. Cutaneous manifestations following COVID-19 vaccination: A report of 25 cases. Dermatol Ther 2022;35(8):e15651.
57. Visentini M, Gragnani L, Santini SA, et al. Flares of mixed cryoglobulinaemia vasculitis after vaccination against SARS-CoV-2. Ann Rheum Dis 2022;81(3): 441–3.
58. Cook C, Patel NJ, D'Silva KM, et al. Clinical characteristics and outcomes of COVID-19 breakthrough infections among vaccinated patients with systemic autoimmune rheumatic diseases. Ann Rheum Dis 2022;81(2):289–91.
59. D'Silva KM, Serling-Boyd N, Hsu TY, et al. SARS-CoV-2 antibody response after COVID-19 in patients with rheumatic disease. Ann Rheum Dis 2021;80(6):817–9.
60. Mrak D, Simader E, Sieghart D, et al. Immunogenicity and safety of a fourth COVID-19 vaccination in rituximab-treated patients: an open-label extension study. Ann Rheum Dis 2022;81(12):1750–6.
61. Guillevin L, Pagnoux C, Karras A, et al. Rituximab versus azathioprine for maintenance in ANCA-associated vasculitis. N Engl J Med 2014;371(19):1771–80.
62. Charles P, Terrier B, Perrodeau E, et al. Comparison of individually tailored versus fixed-schedule rituximab regimen to maintain ANCA-associated vasculitis remission: results of a multicentre, randomised controlled, phase III trial (MAINRIT-SAN2). Ann Rheum Dis 2018;77(8):1143–9.
63. Charles P, Perrodeau É, Samson M, et al. Long-term rituximab use to maintain remission of antineutrophil cytoplasmic antibody-associated vasculitis: a randomized trial. Ann Intern Med 2020;173(3):179–87.
64. Ugarte-Gil MF, Alarcón GS, Izadi Z, et al. Characteristics associated with poor COVID-19 outcomes in individuals with systemic lupus erythematosus: data

from the COVID-19 Global Rheumatology Alliance. Ann Rheum Dis 2022;81(7): 970–8.

65. Choudhary MC, Crain CR, Qiu X, et al. Severe acute respiratory syndrome coronavirus 2 (SARS-CoV-2) sequence characteristics of coronavirus disease 2019 (COVID-19) persistence and reinfection. Clin Infect Dis 2022;74(2):237–45.

66. Choi B, Choudhary MC, Regan J, et al. Persistence and evolution of SARS-CoV-2 in an immunocompromised host. N Engl J Med 2020;383(23):2291–3.

67. Avanzato VA, Matson MJ, Seifert SN, et al. Case study: prolonged infectious SARS-CoV-2 shedding from an asymptomatic immunocompromised individual with cancer. Cell 2020;183(7):1901–12.e1909.

68. Meiring S, Tempia S, Bhiman JN, et al. Prolonged shedding of severe acute respiratory syndrome coronavirus 2 (SARS-CoV-2) at high viral loads among hospitalized immunocompromised persons living with human immunodeficiency virus (hiv), south africa. Clin Infect Dis 2022;75(1):e144–56.

69. Xu K, Chen Y, Yuan J, et al. Factors associated with prolonged viral RNA shedding in patients with coronavirus disease 2019 (COVID-19). Clin Infect Dis 2020;71(15):799–806.

70. Aydillo T, Gonzalez-Reiche AS, Aslam S, et al. Shedding of viable SARS-CoV-2 after immunosuppressive therapy for cancer. N Engl J Med 2020;383(26):2586–8.

71. Tai DBG, Shah A, Doubeni CA, et al. The Disproportionate Impact of COVID-19 on Racial and Ethnic Minorities in the United States. Clin Infect Dis 2021;72(4): 703–6.

72. Gianfrancesco MA, Leykina LA, Izadi Z, et al. Association of race and ethnicity with COVID-19 outcomes in rheumatic disease: data from the COVID-19 global rheumatology alliance physician registry. Arthritis Rheumatol 2021;73(3):374–80.

73. Morin L, Savale L, Pham T, et al. Four-month clinical status of a cohort of patients after hospitalization for COVID-19. JAMA 2021;325(15):1525–34.

74. Daugherty SE, Guo Y, Heath K, et al. Risk of clinical sequelae after the acute phase of SARS-CoV-2 infection: retrospective cohort study. BMJ (Clinical Research ed). 2021;373:n1098.

75. Al-Aly Z, Xie Y, Bowe B. High-dimensional characterization of post-acute sequelae of COVID-19. Nature 2021;594(7862):259–64.

76. Lerner AM, Robinson DA, Yang L, et al. Toward Understanding COVID-19 Recovery: National Institutes of Health Workshop on Postacute COVID-19. Ann Intern Med 2021;174(7):999–1003.

77. Nalbandian A, Sehgal K, Gupta A, et al. Post-acute COVID-19 syndrome. Nature MEDICINE 2021;27(4):601–15.

78. Peluso MJ, Lu S, Tang AF, et al. Markers of Immune Activation and Inflammation in Individuals With Postacute Sequelae of Severe Acute Respiratory Syndrome Coronavirus 2 Infection. J Infect Dis 2021;224(11):1839–48.

79. Visvabharathy L, Hanson B, Orban Z, et al. Neuro-COVID long-haulers exhibit broad dysfunction in T cell memory generation and responses to vaccination. medRxiv 2021.

80. Gold JE, Okyay RA, Licht WE, et al. Investigation of Long COVID Prevalence and Its Relationship to Epstein-Barr Virus Reactivation. Pathogens 2021;10(6):763.

81. Knight JS, Caricchio R, Casanova JL, et al. The intersection of COVID-19 and autoimmunity. J Clin Invest 2021;131(24).

82. Woodruff MC, Walker TA, Truong AD, et al. Evidence of persisting autoreactivity in post-acute sequelae of SARS-CoV-2 infection. medRxiv 2021. 2021.2009.2021. 21263845.

83. Aknin LB, Andretti B, Goldszmidt R, et al. Policy stringency and mental health during the COVID-19 pandemic: a longitudinal analysis of data from 15 countries. Lancet Public Health 2022;7(5):e417–26.
84. Cook C, Cox H, Fu X, et al. Perceived risk and associated shielding behaviors in patients with rheumatoid arthritis during the Coronavirus 2019 Pandemic. ACR Open Rheumatol 2021;3(12):834–41.
85. Levin MJ, Ustianowski A, De Wit S, et al. Intramuscular AZD7442 (Tixagevimab-Cilgavimab) for Prevention of Covid-19. N Engl J Med 2022;386(23):2188–200.
86. Kertes J, David SSB, Engel-Zohar N, et al. Association between AZD7442 (tixa-gevimab-cilgavimab) administration and SARS-CoV-2 infection, hospitalization and mortality. Clin Infect Dis 2022;76(3):e126-e132.
87. Health NIo. COVID-19 Treatment Guidelines Panel. Coronavirus Disease 2019 (COVID-19) Treatment Guidelines. Available at: https://www.covid19treatment guidelines.nih.gov/. Accessed August 29, 2022, 2022.
88. FDA. Fact Sheet for Patients, Parents And Caregivers Emergency Use Authoriza-tion (EUA) of EVUSHELD™ (tixagevimab co-packaged with cilgavimab) for Coro-navirus Disease 2019 (COVID-19) 2022; Available at: https://www.fda.gov/media/154702/download. Accessed August 29, 2022, 2022.
89. O'Brien MP, Forleo-Neto E, Musser BJ, et al. Subcutaneous REGEN-COV anti-body combination to prevent Covid-19. N Engl J Med 2021;385(13):1184–95.
90. Kuritzkes DR. Bamlanivimab for prevention of COVID-19. JAMA 2021;326(1):31–2.
91. Gottlieb RL, Vaca CE, Paredes R, et al. Early remdesivir to prevent progression to severe Covid-19 in outpatients. N Engl J Med 2022;386(4):305–15.
92. Arbel R, Wolff Sagy Y, Hoshen M, et al. Nirmatrelvir use and severe Covid-19 out-comes during the omicron surge. N Engl J Med 2022;387(9):790–8.
93. Hammond J, Leister-Tebbe H, Gardner A, et al. Oral nirmatrelvir for high-risk, nonhospitalized adults with Covid-19. N Engl J Med 2022;386(15):1397–408.
94. Jayk Bernal A, Gomes da Silva MM, Musungaie DB, et al. Molnupiravir for oral treatment of Covid-19 in nonhospitalized patients. N Engl J Med 2022;386(6):509–20.
95. Hiremath S, McGuinty M, Argyropoulos C, et al. Prescribing nirmatrelvir/ritonavir for COVID-19 in advanced CKD. Clin J Am Soc Nephrol 2022;17(8):1247–50.

The Future of Vasculitis
A Manifesto

Paul A. Monach, MD, PhD

KEYWORDS

- Vasculitis • Giant cell arteritis • ANCA-associated vasculitis • Takayasu arteritis
- Clinical trials • Biomarkers

KEY POINTS

- Advances in quality of care for patients with vasculitis will continue to rely on a combination of clinical trials, registries, analysis of large collections of electronic health records, laboratory investigation, and consensus documents produced through international communication and collaboration.
- "Long-shot" prospects for paradigm shifts in care include autoantigen-specific immune-cell targeting, manipulation of the microbiome, and expansion of regulatory T cells.
- Patient involvement in advancing care is expanding through development and use of patient-reported outcomes in trials and through contributions to consensus guidelines and trial design.
- Simplified and innovative approaches to trial design will be essential to allow greater access of patients to expert vasculitis centers both for trial participation and clinical care.

INTRODUCTION

Writing on "the future of vasculitis" carries the near-certainty of being proved wrong in the future. However, the high risk of failure is mitigated by the impossibility of being wrong *right now*. Hence, this topic is appealing to someone who is fond of making predictions and unable to conceive of any adverse personal consequence of making bad ones. My goal is not to predict what results of research will be but to predict the directions in which research might go, which really means advocating where research *should* go, in the hope that the better ideas I propose will garner further support than they already have.

Unfortunately, two of the predictions I can make with greatest confidence are that progress in diagnosis and treatment of vasculitis will require research and that research will require funding. For the foreseeable future, governments will spend progressively more on health care, defense, the consequences of climate change, and interest on debt. Given the current state of politics and public opinion in the United States, there is reason for concern.

Rheumatology Section, VA Boston Healthcare System, 150 South Huntington Avenue, Boston, MA 01230, USA
E-mail address: Paul.Monach@va.gov

Rheum Dis Clin N Am 49 (2023) 713–729
https://doi.org/10.1016/j.rdc.2023.03.014
0889-857X/23/Published by Elsevier Inc.

Proceeding from there requires postulating that research in rare diseases will obtain sufficient interest to receive ongoing funding, but not so much interest that the details are determined by elected officials or political appointees. I can postulate with confidence that patients with vasculitis will continue to value, seek out, and praise the expertise of their physicians.

I will start with a few predictions of things that will *not* happen, without defending them.

1. People will not be told, from their genotypes, microbiome analysis, or any other information, whether they will or will not get vasculitis.
2. Our patients will not be able to get artificial or laboratory-grown kidneys or retinas to replace the ones lost to vasculitis—or not anytime soon.
3. Medicine will not become so "personalized" that the safest and most effective treatment plan can be determined and provided up-front by any practitioner from the objective data.
4. More generally, we will not be replaced by Artificial Intelligence algorithms—ever.

The consequence, of course, is simply that people who specialize in vasculitis will continue to add value, as determined by the patients and the colleagues who refer them.

BASIC AND TRANSLATIONAL RESEARCH
Animal Models of Vasculitis

The bigger and more fundamental the advance, the harder it is to predict, especially in basic science. What can be said with some confidence is that incremental advance in understanding of different forms of vasculitis will be made using animal models of anti-neutrophil cytoplasmic antibody (ANCA)-associated vasculitis (AAV), small-vessel immune-complex vasculitis (reverse passive Arthus reaction), and large-vessel vasculitis induced using *Candida* or *Lactobacillus* extracts or using transplant and explant models of giant cell arteritis (GCA).[1] These models have already led to one major (and to me, unexpected) advance in treatment of human AAV, namely the use of avacopan to block the receptor for the complement fragment C5a (C5aR).[2] Additional promising drug targets will undoubtedly be identified for GCA and be extrapolated for study in Takayasu's arteritis (TAK).

Target Autoantigens

The identification of pathogens or autoantigens underlying different vasculitides remains a plausible goal and would be clinically relevant. However, it is sobering that no such advance has been made since discoveries of ANCA and hepatitis C virus as the antigen in most cases of mixed cryoglobulinemia, despite tremendous improvements in screening technologies. Antibodies are easier to identify than T cells and are likely the causes of disease in all forms of small-vessel vasculitis associated with immune complexes. Diseases found to be associated with HLA class II alleles are promising for the likely existence of target antigens shared among patients with the allele. Recently, IgA vasculitis was associated with HLA alleles, specifically HLA-DRB1*01 seen in multiple European and East Asian populations.[3–5]

It is not yet known whether polyarteritis nodosa (PAN) has any HLA association, and even if it does, that association might give more credence to a search for autoantigens recognized by T cells rather than antibodies—a much more technically difficult process. It must also be acknowledged that the robust association of GCA with HLA-DRB1*04[6] has not led to the identification of target antigens, but improved technology to screen for T-cell-recognized antigens would make such a search more feasible. Parenthetically, diseases associated with HLA class I alleles might indicate a poorly understood dysregulation of innate immunity rather than (or in addition to) association with antigens presented to CD8+ T cells. Ankylosing spondylitis and Behcet's syndrome exhibit features of excessive inflammation without an obvious need to invoke an adaptive immune response.

Microbiome

In very general terms, the microbiomes of different organ systems will continue to be studied in vasculitis and many other diseases,[7-11] and results will lead to more sophisticated interpretations as more patients with more diseases are studied and compared with better methods. The big step, one of the best candidates for a "holy grail" of research in autoimmune and inflammatory diseases, would be manipulation of the microbiome as a treatment of existing disease. Any advance made in a more common disease, such as rheumatoid arthritis or psoriasis, should be immediately considered for pilot studies in vasculitis in which dysbiosis is evident. Although the adverse effects of antibiotics on dysbiosis are well-known, greater understanding of the effects of specific antibiotics could lead to targeted investigation about whether the use of certain antibiotics contributes to poor disease control and need for ongoing immunosuppressive therapy.

Hemato-Inflammatory Diseases

My other general prediction is that additional "hemato-inflammatory" diseases will be discovered, following the seminal discovery of VEXAS (vacuoles, E1 enzyme, X-linked, autoinflammatory, somatic) syndrome.[12] Before that an association of myelodysplastic syndrome (MDS) with Behcet's and gastrointestinal involvement,[13] especially MDS with trisomy 8, had been described sufficiently often that it is a semantic question whether to say that MDS can "mimic" or "cause" Behcet's. It is not far-fetched to propose that within 10 years, patients with PAN, relapsing polychondritis, late-onset Behcet's, or unusual inflammatory syndromes will undergo a panel of genetic screening tests including UBA1, ADA2, other specific genes not yet discovered, and cytogenetics.

Biomarkers

Although much of my own research in vasculitis has focused on biomarkers of active vasculitis, those studies have led me conclude that research on biomarkers should not be directed toward determining low-level disease activity, but rather toward predicting the future events of relapse and remission and contributing to definitions of subsets of named diseases.

Biomarkers are not needed to distinguish highly active vasculitis from remission, which is where most of the findings have been made and is a sensible place to start.[14] Trying to distinguish mildly active disease from remission is much more challenging, as the gold standard of "clinician's assessment" is acknowledged up-front to be faulty, otherwise the research would not be needed. Biomarkers are expected to be less abnormal in milder disease, and direct effects of age, sex, other medical conditions, and especially medications can rise to the level of making results unimpressive or uninterpretable.[15,16]

Identifying which organs are currently being damaged is clinically important and plausible. Progress has been made in improving on urinalysis for interpretation of activity in the kidney,[17-19] and I anticipate a combination of urinary biomarkers being added to routine clinical assessment within 10 years. The assessment of ongoing damage in other organs for which symptoms, physical examination, and laboratory or other testing is often insufficient to distinguish active disease from previous damage—such as the peripheral and central nervous systems—is plausible.[20] A note of caution comes from the finding that muscle involvement in small-vessel vasculitis usually produces no elevation of creatine kinase.[21]

Distinguishing active vasculitis from infection would seem to be feasible and is obviously of great clinical importance. However, to the extent that there have been comparisons, the main result has been to provide caution in interpreting mildly elevated procalcitonin—a test now in wide use in the United States—as evidence of infection in patients with Kawasaki disease or AAV.[22–24] Personally, I doubt that combinations of cytokines and chemokine signatures will prove to have adequate ability to discriminate between infection and vasculitis. The approach most likely to bear fruit would be to await new biomarkers proposed to be specific for infection, such as procalcitonin, and then test them in patients with active vasculitis.

Biomarker and imaging studies in which the outcome being assessed is objective and determined well after the measurement of the biomarker are more promising. Circulating proteins or gene-expression patterns have been associated with response to treatment[25] and especially with relapse risk, such as myeloperoxidase (MPO)-ANCA versus proteinase-3 (PR3)-ANCA in AAV,[26] IL-6 in GCA,[27] and gene-expression signatures in AAV.[28] Large-vessel imaging in large-vessel vasculitis seems likely to be refined for more routine and standardized clinical use.[29,30] However, so far these results only shift probabilities modestly. The most promising future role of biomarkers may be in the definition of subsets of vasculitides,[31] as results could easily be combined with clinical and imaging assessments and could lead to the choice of treatment based on subset, or, if medical research can afford another term arisen like a phoenix from the ashes of ancient Greek, "Pharmacophenomics."

CLINICAL OBSERVATIONAL RESEARCH

Observational studies will remain of great value and help provide information on long-term outcomes and define disease subsets, in vasculitis as with most rare diseases. Repositories of data and tissue samples and the "big data" present in electronic health records (EHRs) will continue to provide complementary information derived from better quality (repositories) or greater quantity (EHR). Methods have improved for reducing confounding in observational data to more closely simulate clinical trials.[32] Observational studies will never replace randomized trials for providing definitive data on treatments, but they will be increasingly important for providing hypotheses to test in trials, as the number of hypotheses that can be tested is especially limited in rare diseases.

EHR-based research in the United States offers an opportunity to study vasculitis in populations that form the minority of those affected, which in rare diseases can mean that there is little or no existing literature. Although genetic data to define ancestry will be limited, necessitating the use of self-reported race and ethnicity to define groups, even estimates of incidence and essential objective outcomes would be important additions to knowledge. Examples include AAV in Black/African American and Hispanic/Latino populations, GCA in those groups and also in Asians, and TAK in males. Already, national health records have shown that biopsy-proven GCA is less common but not rare in Black Americans, about 25% to 33% of the incidence in white patients,[33] which contradicts the perception, originating from the cumulative experience of experts practicing in the Northern United States and Europe going back decades that GCA is very rare in Black patients.[34]

Although the humble case series may not require its own heading, it is worth noting that summaries of the experience and ideas of astute clinicians will remain valuable in vasculitis as in other rare diseases and that discoveries such as DADA2,[35,36] VEXAS, rituximab to treat AAV, and tocilizumab to treat GCA all began with single-digit numbers of observations.

CLINICAL TRIALS

Experience with conducting clinical trials in vasculitis has advanced so much in the past 20 years that the standards of evidence required to change practice—whether through official guidelines or individual decision-making—have changed. Unfortunately, trials are expensive and slow, so that few among the many possible options are chosen, and in the end even those trials can be criticized based on dosing, eligibility criteria, and outcome measures, simply because those choices are almost always debatable.

A look at ClinicalTrials.gov will give a good idea about which results to expect in the next 5 years (**Tables 1** and **2** for randomized phase 2/3 trials listed as Recruiting, Active, or Not yet recruiting). In very general terms, we can expect that most trials will continue to involve re-purposing of drugs already approved in other diseases. The choice of drugs being compared will continue to be based on their use in practice and on promising case series. Trials will continue to be designed and sponsored by both medical centers and pharmaceutical companies. Whether the example of avacopan—the first drug that received its first approval for a form of vasculitis rather than a more common inflammatory disease—will be repeated will depend on the financial decisions of drug manufacturers as well as advances in basic science that cannot be predicted. Whether the US Food and Drug Administration will be moved to appropriately consider reduction in glucocorticoid doses or toxicities as a criterion for approval is hard to predict. I will focus further discussion on three areas related to trials: the possibility of paradigm-shifting approaches, an increasing need to study disease subsets, and the mechanics of how trials are conducted.

The Vasculitis Therapies of the Future

I started my research career in tumor immunology, studying the immune response to cancer in mice and trying to come up with ways to make that response effective. After switching to study autoimmune diseases and choosing rheumatology as a specialty, at a time when rapid improvements in treatment of rheumatoid arthritis and psoriasis were being made, I had the opportunity to say into a microphone, "Immunotherapy of cancer is the cancer treatment of the future—and always will be." With that embarrassing history of myopic negativity, I will not be shy about espousing the promise of three additional candidates for "holy grail" in treatment of autoimmune disease.

The prospect of antigen-specific immune-suppression has been a goal ever since diseases started to be linked to autoimmunity against specific antigens. Although vasculitis may not be the first on the list of diseases of interest for the many companies trying to develop the means of eliminating B cells or T cells based on the specificities of their antigen receptors, myeloperoxidase (MPO)-ANCA and PR3-ANCA are particularly appealing targets for antigen-specific B-cell depletion. AAV can be treated effectively with nonspecific depletion of CD20+ B cells, and at least in the case of MPO-ANCA, the autoantibody is probably the direct cause of vasculitis, at least in the kidney.[37] Even though antigen-specific therapy is not yet available for any disease, at some point one or more strategies will work. This is another reason why discovery of autoantigens in other forms of vasculitis is worth pursuing, in addition to the prospect of improved diagnostic testing.

Table 1
Randomized clinical trials in large- and medium-vessel vasculitis in progress as of May, 2022

Ct.gov	Disease	Countries	Sites[a]	Subjects	Treatment
NCT04609397	Behcet's	China	31	252	Hemay005 vs placebo (DB)
NCT03962335	Behcet's	Italy	1	90	Diet: Vegi vs Medi vs Medi + butyrate (CO)
NCT04528082	Behcet's pedi	Euro 7	17	60	Apremilast vs placebo (DB)
NCT04474847	GCA	US	3	78	Abatacept + GC vs placebo + GC (DB)
NCT04930094	GCA	Many	43	240	Secukinumab + GC vs placebo + GC (DB)
NCT04012905	GCA	France	8	150	GC-28 wk vs GC-52 wk
NCT04012905	GCA	France	1	200	Tocilizumab + GC vs MTX + GC
NCT03725202	GCA	Many	174	420	Upadacitinib + GC vs placebo + GC (DB)
NCT03711448	GCA	France	1	38	Ustekinumab + GC vs GC alone
NCT04239196	GCA AION	France	10	58	Tocilizumab + IVGC vs IVGC alone
NCT04888221	GCA stroke	France	1	66	Tocilizumab + GC vs placebo + GC (DB)
NCT01917721	Kawasaki	US	1	50	Doxycycline + IVIG vs placebo + IVIG (DB)
NCT04078568	Kawasaki	China	15	3000	GC + IVIG + ASA vs IVIG + ASA
NCT04656184	Kawasaki-RxR	France	1	84	Anakinra vs IVIG-2ndRx
NCT04972968	PMR	Many	120	160	ABBV1544+GC vs placebo + GC (DB)
NCT04027101	PMR	France	8	34	Baricitinib + GC vs placebo + GC (DB)
NCT03632187	PMR	France	5	34	Abatacept + GC vs placebo + GC (DB)
NCT03576794	PMR	Neth	2	94	Leflunomide + GC vs placebo + GC (DB)
NCT05151848	Takayasu	China	4	100	Adalimumab vs tofacitinib
NCT05102448	Takayasu	China	1	76	MTX vs tofacitinib
NCT04564001	Takayasu	France	1	50	Infliximab vs tocilizumab
NCT04300686	Takayasu	China	1	40	Infliximab vs tocilizumab (CO)
NCT04299971	Takayasu	China	1	130	MTX vs tofacitinib (CO)
NCT04161898	Takayasu	J/K/T	31	54	Upadacitinib + GC vs placebo + GC (DB)
NCT03096275	Takayasu	China	7	138	MMF + MTX + GC vs CYC/AZA + GC

All randomized trials listed as Recruiting, Active not recruiting, or Not yet recruiting are shown.

Abbreviations: AION, anterior ischemic optic neuropathy; ASA, aspirin; AZA, azathioprine; CO, cross-over design; CYC, cyclophosphamide. DB, double-blind; Euro 7, 7 European countries; GC, glucocorticoids; IVGC, intravenous glucocorticoids (high dose); IVIG, intravenous immunoglobulin; J/K/T, Japan, South Korea, and Turkey; many, more than three countries in more than one region; Medi, Mediterranean; MMF, mycophenolate; MTX, methotrexate; Neth, the Netherlands; pedi, pediatric; PMR, polymyalgia rheumatica; RxR, resistant to treatment; Vegi, vegetarian.

ᵃ For trials listing only one site, it is possible that only one contact site is listed for a multi-site study conducted by a consortium.

Table 2
Randomized clinical trials in small-vessel vasculitis in progress as of May, 2022

Ct.gov	Disease	Countries	Sites[a]	Subjects	Treatment
NCT05197842	AAV	China	20	60	BDB001 vs CYC vs GC
NCT03942887	AAV	Netherlands	4	100	RTX + CYC vs RTX, then tailored RTX maint
NCT04316494	AAV	UK	9	76	HCQ vs placebo (DB)
NCT03290456	AAV	France	45	146	GC vs placebo maint (DB)
NCT03323476	AAV-ESRD	France	53	136	Discontinue or continue maint
NCT01940094	AAV-GPA	US/Canada	9	159	GC vs placebo maint
NCT04944524	AAV-GPA	China	1	66	MTX vs tofacitinib maint
NCT02108860	AAV-GPA NS	US/Can/Eur	20	66	Abatacept + GC vs placebo + GC (DB)
NCT04871191	AAV-GPA RxR	France	1	42	RTX vs tocilizumab vs abatacept
NCT03920722	AAV-MPA NS	France	1	106	RTX + GC vs placebo + GC (DB)
NCT03967925	AAV-PR3	UK	6	31	RTX + belimumab + GC vs RTX + GC (DB)
NCT05376319	AAV-PR3	US	2	30	Obinutuzumab vs RTX (DB)
NCT04629144	Cryo non-inf	France	1	48	Belimumab + GC vs placebo + GC (DB)
NCT02939573	Cutaneous	US/Can/Japan	13	90	Colchicine vs dapsone vs AZA
NCT04157348	EGPA	Many	84	140	Benralizumab vs mepolizumab (DB)
NCT03164473	EGPA	France	1	98	RTX vs AZA maint (DB)
NCT05263934	EGPA	US	1	160	Depemokimab vs mepolizumab (DB)
NCT05030155	EGPA sev or NS	France	1	100	Mepo + GC vs CYC + GC or placebo + GC (DB)
NCT05329090	IgAV	France	14	72	RTX + GC vs placebo + GC (DB)
NCT04008316	IgAV skin	France	1	264	Colchicine vs placebo (DB)
NCT04623866	IgAV nephritis	China	1	10	Huaiqihuang vs losartan (DB)
NCT03647852	IgAV pedi	China	3	150	IVGC + GC vs IVIG + GC
NCT01917721	Kawasaki	US	1	50	Doxycycline + IVIG vs placebo + IVIG (DB)
NCT04078568	Kawasaki	China	15	3000	GC + IVIG + ASA vs IVIG + ASA

NCT04656184	Kawasaki RxR	France	1	84	Anakinra vs IVIG-2nd treatment
NCT03482479	Many	US	6	36	LDN vs placebo (DB, CO)
NCT05168475	Many non-AAV	UK	3	140	RTX vs infliximab vs tocilizumab (CO)
NCT04720196	Vasc neurop	Poland	1	24	Transcranial magnetic stim vs sham (CO)

All randomized trials listed as Recruiting, Active not recruiting, or Not yet recruiting are shown.

Abbreviations: ASA, aspirin; AZA, azathioprine; Can, Canada; CO, cross-over design; CYC, cyclophosphamide; DB, double-blind; ESRD, end-stage renal disease; GC, glucocorticoids; HCQ, hydroxychloroquine; IgAV, IgA vasculitis; IVGC, intravenous glucocorticoids (high dose); IVIG, intravenous immunoglobulin; LDN, low-dose naltrexone; maint, maintenance of remission; many, more than three forms of vasculitis including at least two vessel sizes (small, medium, or large); mepo, mepolizumab; MTX, methotrexate; non-inf, non-infectious; NS, non-severe; Pedi, pedi; RTX, rituximab; RxR, resistant to treatment; sev, severe; stim, stimulation; vasc neurop, vasculitic neuropathy.

[a] For trials listing only one site, it is possible that only one contact site is listed for a multi-site study conducted by a consortium.

The microbiome, or at least one of the surface-specific microbiomes, is almost always abnormal when comparing groups of patients with and without different autoimmune inflammatory diseases.[7–11] The question is whether manipulating it with either specific probiotics or nonspecific fecal transplant can reverse or at least reduce the severity of disease that is already established. This is difficult research to conduct, whether due to having to make guesses about key probiotic components or being concerned about transfer of pathogens through fecal transplant, but microbiome-directed trials are in progress in several relatively common inflammatory diseases. If success is ever achieved, vasculitis specialists should mobilize to see whether the dysbiosis at baseline in patients in the successful trial resembles that seen in any group of patients with vasculitis, and then attempt a trial. My own prediction is that diseases that are primarily inflammatory and not driven by antigen-specific autoimmunity are more likely to benefit from manipulation of the microbiome.

Regulatory T cells (Tregs) are one of many mechanisms that evolved to prevent autoimmune disease, but they are the main one that can keep autoimmune T and B cells in check after they have escaped deletion or permanent downregulation (anergy) and have fully matured. Although broad-based stimulation of Tregs carries concern about producing excessive immune suppression and risk of infection or even certain cancers, there is optimism that a range exists where the balance of benefit and harm is more favorable for expansion of Tregs than for immune-suppressive drugs. The example of successful use of low-dose IL-2 to treat refractory cryoglobulinemia[38] should be considered in other vasculitides.

Toward More Personalized Care

I have noted the importance of identifying diseases subtypes and the prospect of using molecular biomarkers and imaging to define such subtypes more accurately. In addition to studying subtypes for differences in short-term and long-term outcomes and responses to different treatments as examined in observational studies (pharmacogenomics), subtypes should be incorporated into clinical trials. This has been done routinely for ANCA specificity for years. The choice of primary versus secondary outcomes in trials also acknowledges how subtypes are expected to respond differently, for example, different trials focused on uveitis or oral ulcers in Behcet's. The diversity of phenotypes in Behcet's, combined with a growing arsenal of treatment options, has led to a call for a "treat to target" approach to that disease, as has been successful in other inflammatory diseases in which excellent control of disease should be the expectation and goal.[39] EGPA is another disease in which subsets defined by ANCA positivity and eosinophilic versus vasculitic manifestations may respond differently to medications that are not as broadly immunosuppressive as glucocorticoids and cytotoxic or antimetabolite drugs. Finally, large-vessel involvement is a key subset to study in randomized trials in GCA. It will be impossible to use every subtype as a stratification variable in trials, and many subtypes will be too uncommon to assess definitively in a single trial. However, pooling results across multiple trials should be feasible, and the mere fact that patients were randomized initially reduces confounding compared with purely observational studies.

Another change that is already well underway is incorporation of patients' perspectives in trials. Patient-reported outcome measures (PROMs) such as the SF-36 summary of health-related quality of life have been the source of secondary outcomes for a wide range of diseases for decades. However, rigorous development and use of PROMs in the vasculitides is a welcome change,[40] as is the recent invitation of patient advocacy groups to contribute to development of outcome measures, trial designs, and guidelines (**Fig. 1**). Personally, I think that patient-reported outcomes

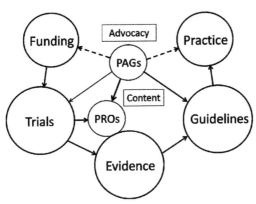

Fig. 1. Role of patients, through patient advocacy groups (PAGs) and patient-reported outcomes (PROs), in vasculitis research and advances in clinical care.

(PROs) should be kept separate as important secondary outcomes rather than including them in omnibus indices that are meant to summarize all aspects of disease, such as the Birmingham Vasculitis Activity Score (BVAS). Summary instruments are necessary for evaluating treatments in trials of any inflammatory disease, but they work best in diseases that either have a dominant organ system of interest (such as rheumatoid arthritis or psoriasis) or have excellent control of all the objective aspects of disease as a goal that can often be achieved (such as all forms of vasculitis).[41] I suspect that incorporating PROs into the descendants of BVAS would result in 0 ("remission") being achieved much less often and for diverse reasons, with resulting confusion among clinicians.

Different Ways of Doing Trials

It is universally acknowledged that clinical trials are too cumbersome and too expensive, slowing the progress of research that promises to save lives and improve quality of life for patients. Much has been written about expanding the use of pragmatic trials, which include features such as unblinded treatments, objective outcomes, and avoidance of collection of tissue samples or study-specific data. Efforts to simplify the process of informed consent have also been made, in particular the use of online signed consent or even oral consent with waiver of requirement for a signature. However, these processes have been greeted with resistance from regulatory authorities, starting at the national level but also trickling down to local institutional review boards (IRBs) or ethics boards. The negative impact of this stance was made particularly clear during the Covid-19 pandemic.[42,43] Where there is prospect for benefit from participation—which there should be even in studies in which there is clinical equipoise—barriers to participation in trials carry an ethical cost that should not be shrugged off.[44]

In considering the ways in which vasculitis care and research in the United States is falling short in "diversity, equity, and inclusion" (DEI), I do not think that the main inequities are derived from race/ethnicity and sex, except when risk for certain diseases is mistakenly thought to be limited to persons of a particular ethnicity or sex. Rather, the main problem is access, and although disability, insurance, and low socioeconomic status must play important roles, I suspect that geography plays an outsized role compared with more common diseases. If European guidelines committees are correct in saying that patients with vasculitis should have specialty referral centers involved in their care,[45,46] quality of care depends on access to a vasculitis center.

In the United States, that usually means at least one rheumatologist, nephrologist, or pulmonologist who specializes in vasculitis, and often colleagues in other specialties who gain more than the typical experience in vasculitis through shared care of patients. Although every large or medium-sized city has medical centers that receive subspecialty referrals for serious or complicated diseases, university centers that participate in clinical trials in vasculitis are concentrated in the East and North, out of proportion to population.

How could access in the United States be improved? For starters, on the purely clinical side, it is going to remain difficult to attract and retain young people to focus on vasculitis as long as caring for a patient with vasculitis earns as much income as caring for a patient with rheumatoid or psoriatic arthritis, at twice the effort (my own guess). Reimbursement for emails with patients and referring MDs would help correct that "inequity," but liberalization of rules for virtual visits, including across state lines, would have a more dramatic benefit to patients and would allow access to patients formerly excluded simply by geography and/or an unacceptable financial burden associated with travel.

Access to care for vasculitis has been linked to access for trials, because in rare diseases, a physician who earns a living primarily through research grants can still develop far greater experience in that rare disease than any generalist despite engaging in clinical care on a very part-time basis. The question then arises whether access to trials could be improved for patients who cannot travel to expert centers, especially for the numbers of visits often scheduled in interventional trials. The "video visit" might be a prerequisite (and therefore produce one of several technology-based inequities…), but at least that technology has been mastered by all US clinicians and many patients during the Covid-19 pandemic. Trials would need to be designed so that eligibility, outcomes, and adverse events could be assessed remotely. Trials focused on PROs are clearly more amenable to being conducted remotely if patients can access secure online reporting tools, but the range of research questions would be limited, and regulatory bodies will be skeptical about any relaxation of requirements for laboratory testing or reporting of adverse events, even with study of widely-used drugs.

Regulatory bodies are skeptical about a lot of things, but they are composed of people who take ethics seriously, and in a time of universal reckoning about DEI, maybe now is the time for a reminder that barriers to participation in trials violate (at least) the E and I components, above and beyond the more abstract point that inefficiency in the advance of medical research carries ethical weight. Advances in technology to facilitate participation—some of the most innovative of which have been deployed in lower- and middle-income countries——may not be enough, so a reconsideration of the concept of "risk" is in order as regards participation in trials.

A colleague and I have argued that for certain decisions about treatment, randomized enrollment into a treatment trial does not confer significant risk beyond what is inherent in normal medical care[44] and that communication about the treatments involved is done more effectively by the treating provider in the course of care than by a researcher who does not know the patient. Examples of trials in which patients could be enrolled without the provider being involved in the research include studies of off-label treatments that are either safe *or* widely used *or* have evidence for benefit in the literature *or* virtually any comparative-effectiveness study of approved treatments. Other proposed characteristics of Embedded, Quantified, Integrated-into-Practice Trials are shown in **Box 1**. Operationally, they are likely to be useful only in health care systems with EHRs. Structurally, a key feature to imitate the way physicians practice is to make the probability of group assignment "adapt" in some way (ideally adaptive randomization) based on the results seen for patients enrolled earlier in the trial.

Box 1
Key features of interventional trials that could be regarded as conferring minimal risk beyond that inherent in everyday life and that do not generate study-specific data

- Embedded: no data collection outside of the EHR, so as to not generate new data for the study
- Adaptive randomization or other assignment method that changes group assignment based on previous outcomes
- Informing patient—much like good clinical practice but noting the research study
- Opt-in, that is, the patient can only be enrolled if permission is given and may decline without adverse consequences
- No financial or other incentive for enrollment, for the provider or patient
- Assessment of eligibility remotely (MD confirms or refutes at the point of care)
- Efficiency bonus if outcomes can be assessed remotely through the EHR
- Efficiency bonus if using one IRB and one coordinating center
- *The key means of improving access, efficiency, and cost: the treating MD should not need to be trained in research, and there should be no need for on-site study staff.*

Abbreviations: EHR, electronic health record; IRB, institutional review board or ethics board.

Adapted from Monach PA, Branch-Elliman W. Reconsidering 'minimal risk' to expand the repertoire of trials with waiver of informed consent for research. *BMJ open.* Sep 14 2021;11(9):e048534.

LIVING DOCUMENTS AND LONG-TERM COLLABORATIONS

Another area of vasculitis care that should adapt based on existing knowledge is guidelines for management of the vasculitides. I was pleased to learn that American College of Rheumatology (ACR)/Vasculitis Foundation (VF) guidelines published recently after several years in development[47–49] are indeed going to be used as "living documents," so that the immense effort and impressive scholarship that went into reviewing all the relevant literature and summarizing the results of each key paper in tabular form will be used as the foundation for assessment of the impact of subsequent studies shortly after they are published. Although the recently published series of guidelines endorsed by the ACR and VF represent a consensus of experts from centers in the United States and Canada, the trend in large-scale vasculitis research has been steady growth of international and multi-continent collaboration, especially in development of classification criteria, outcome measures, and registries, but also in pivotal trials.

CONSENSUS AND SUMMARY

Thus, in contrast to the dark commentary with which I started this manifesto, I am happy to be able to conclude with a prediction that one way or another, vasculitis research aimed at improving care for individual patients will be more and more characterized by collaboration, consensus, and advocacy that cross oceans and national borders. Although paradigm shifts in applied biology are difficult to predict, incremental advances in diagnosis and treatment are responsible for most of the great progress made in vasculitis care and outcomes in the past half-century. Commitment to a shared mission around the world that progresses not only continues but is accelerated by collaboration in application of technological advances.

CLINICS CARE POINTS

- Although the evidence base to support care of patients with vasculitis has grown greatly in the past 20 years, in many patients management decisions must be made without high-quality evidence.
- Although studies in progress give an idea of what experts in the field think are promising treatments, these treatments should not be presumed to be good choices for off-label use if not supported by published early-phase trials or case series.

DISCLOSURE

Dr P.A. Monach reports having performed paid consulting for ChemoCentryx, Kiniksa, Celgene/Bristol-Myers Squibb, and Genentech. He previously served as a site investigator in trials funded in part by ChemoCentryx, Bristol-Myers Squibb, United States, GlaxoSmithKline, United Kingdom, and Genentech, United States, and served as a member of the Board of Directors of the Vasculitis Foundation.

REFERENCES

1. Shochet L, Kitching AR. Animal models of vasculitis. Curr Opin Rheumatol 2022; 34(1):10–7.
2. Jayne DRW, Merkel PA, Schall TJ, et al. Avacopan for the Treatment of ANCA-Associated Vasculitis. N Engl J Med 2021;384(7):599–609.
3. Xia L, Chen M, Zhang H, et al. Genome-wide association study of 7661 Chinese Han individuals and fine-mapping major histocompatibility complex identifies HLA-DRB1 as associated with IgA vasculitis. J Clin Lab Anal 2022;e24457.
4. Koskela M, Nihtila J, Ylinen E, et al. HLA-DQ and HLA-DRB1 alleles associated with Henoch-Schonlein purpura nephritis in Finnish pediatric population: a genome-wide association study. Pediatr Nephrol 2021;36(8):2311–8.
5. Gonzalez-Gay MA, Lopez-Mejias R, Pina T, et al. IgA Vasculitis: Genetics and Clinical and Therapeutic Management. Curr Rheumatol Rep 2018;20(5):24. https://doi.org/10.1007/s11926-018-0735-3.
6. Carmona FD, Mackie SL, Martin JE, et al. A large-scale genetic analysis reveals a strong contribution of the HLA class II region to giant cell arteritis susceptibility. Am J Hum Genet 2015;96(4):565–80.
7. Tariq S, Clifford AH. An update on the microbiome in vasculitis. Curr Opin Rheumatol 2021;33(1):15–23.
8. Ma X, Wang X, Zheng G, et al. Critical Role of Gut Microbiota and Epigenetic Factors in the Pathogenesis of Behcet's Disease. Front Cell Dev Biol 2021;9:719235.
9. Dekkema GJ, Rutgers A, Sanders JS, et al. The Nasal Microbiome in ANCA-Associated Vasculitis: Picking the Nose for Clues on Disease Pathogenesis. Curr Rheumatol Rep 2021;23(7):54.
10. Desbois AC, Ciocan D, Saadoun D, et al. Specific microbiome profile in Takayasu's arteritis and giant cell arteritis. Sci Rep 2021;11(1):5926.
11. Nogueira AR, Shoenfeld Y. Microbiome and autoimmune diseases: cause and effect relationship. Curr Opin Rheumatol 2019;31(5):471–4.
12. Beck DB, Ferrada MA, Sikora KA, et al. Somatic Mutations in UBA1 and Severe Adult-Onset Autoinflammatory Disease. N Engl J Med 2020;383(27):2628–38.
13. Esatoglu SN, Ok AM, Ucar D, et al. Takayasu's arteritis: associated inflammatory diseases. Clin Exp Rheumatol 2020;38(Suppl 124):61–8.

14. Monach PA, Warner RL, Tomasson G, et al. Serum proteins reflecting inflammation, injury and repair as biomarkers of disease activity in ANCA-associated vasculitis. Ann Rheum Dis 2013;72(8):1342–50.

15. Monach PA, Warner RL, Lew R, et al. Serum Biomarkers of Disease Activity in Longitudinal Assessment of Patients with ANCA-Associated Vasculitis. ACR Open Rheumatol 2022;4(2):168–76.

16. Rodriguez-Pla A, Warner RL, Cuthbertson D, et al. Evaluation of Potential Serum Biomarkers of Disease Activity in Diverse Forms of Vasculitis. J Rheumatol 2020; 47(7):1001–10.

17. Moran SM, Monach PA, Zgaga L, et al. Urinary soluble CD163 and monocyte chemoattractant protein-1 in the identification of subtle renal flare in anti-neutrophil cytoplasmic antibody-associated vasculitis. Nephrol Dial Transplant 2020;35(2):283–91.

18. Moran SM, Scott J, Clarkson MR, et al. The Clinical Application of Urine Soluble CD163 in ANCA-Associated Vasculitis. J Am Soc Nephrol 2021;32(11):2920–32.

19. Morris AD, Freitas DLD, Lima KMG, et al. Automated Computational Detection of Disease Activity in ANCA-Associated Glomerulonephritis Using Raman Spectroscopy: A Pilot Study. Molecules 2022;27(7).

20. Pierce ME, Hayes J, Huber BR, et al. Plasma biomarkers associated with deployment trauma and its consequences in post-9/11 era veterans: initial findings from the TRACTS longitudinal cohort. Transl Psychiatry 2022;12(1):80.

21. Jinno S, Monach PA, Nakazawa T. Utility of lower extremity magnetic resonance imaging followed by muscle biopsy for myeloperoxidase-antineutrophil cytoplasmic antibodies positive antineutrophil cytoplasmic antibody-associated vasculitis: a single-centre study. Clin Exp Rheumatol 2022. https://doi.org/10. 55563/clinexprheumatol/eqd0ch.

22. Niu MM, Jiang Q, Ruan JW, et al. Clinical implications of procalcitonin in Kawasaki disease: a useful candidate for differentiating from sepsis and evaluating IVIG responsiveness. Clin Exp Med 2021;21(4):633–43.

23. Mosakowska M, Kania DB, Szamotulska K, et al. Assessment of the correlation of commonly used laboratory tests with clinical activity, renal involvement and treatment of systemic small-vessel vasculitis with the presence of ANCA antibodies. BMC Nephrol 2021;22(1):290.

24. Herrmann K, Schinke S, Csernok E, et al. Diagnostic Value of Procalcitonin in ANCA-Associated Vasculitis (AAV) to Differentiate Between Disease Activity, Infection and Drug Hypersensitivity. Open Rheumatol J 2015;9:71–6.

25. Grayson PC, Carmona-Rivera C, Xu L, et al. Neutrophil-Related Gene Expression and Low-Density Granulocytes Associated With Disease Activity and Response to Treatment in Antineutrophil Cytoplasmic Antibody-Associated Vasculitis. Arthritis Rheumatol 2015;67(7):1922–32. https://doi.org/10.1002/art.39153.

26. King C, Druce KL, Nightingale P, et al. Predicting relapse in anti-neutrophil cytoplasmic antibody-associated vasculitis: a Systematic review and meta-analysis. Rheumatol Adv Pract 2021;5(3):rkab018.

27. Garcia-Martinez A, Hernandez-Rodriguez J, Espigol-Frigole G, et al. Clinical relevance of persistently elevated circulating cytokines (tumor necrosis factor alpha and interleukin-6) in the long-term followup of patients with giant cell arteritis. Arthritis Care Res 2010;62(6):835–41.

28. McKinney EF, Lee JC, Jayne DR, et al. T-cell exhaustion, co-stimulation and clinical outcome in autoimmunity and infection. Nature 2015;523(7562):612–6.

29. Goel R, Gribbons KB, Carette S, et al. Derivation of an angiographically based classification system in Takayasu's arteritis: an observational study from India and North America. Rheumatology 2020;59(5):1118–27.

30. Gribbons KB, Ponte C, Carette S, et al. Patterns of Arterial Disease in Takayasu Arteritis and Giant Cell Arteritis. Arthritis Care Res 2020;72(11):1615–24.

31. Berti A, Warner R, Johnson K, et al. Brief Report: Circulating Cytokine Profiles and Antineutrophil Cytoplasmic Antibody Specificity in Patients With Antineutrophil Cytoplasmic Antibody-Associated Vasculitis. Arthritis Rheumatol 2018;70(7): 1114–21.

32. Hernan MA, Robins JM. Using Big Data to Emulate a Target Trial When a Randomized Trial Is Not Available. Am J Epidemiol 2016;183(8):758–64.

33. Chung SH, Morcos MB, Ng B. Determinants of Positive Temporal Artery Biopsies in the Veterans Health Administration National Database Cohort. Arthritis Care Res 2020;72(5):699–704.

34. Williams JN, Ford CL, Morse M, et al. Racial Disparities in Rheumatology Through the Lens of Critical Race Theory. Rheumatic Diseases Clinics of North America 2020;46(4):605–12.

35. Navon Elkan P, Pierce SB, Segel R, et al. Mutant adenosine deaminase 2 in a polyarteritis nodosa vasculopathy. N Engl J Med 6 2014;370(10):921–31.

36. Zhou Q, Yang D, Ombrello AK, et al. Early-onset stroke and vasculopathy associated with mutations in ADA2. N Engl J Med 2014;370(10):911–20.

37. Xiao H, Heeringa P, Hu P, et al. Antineutrophil cytoplasmic autoantibodies specific for myeloperoxidase cause glomerulonephritis and vasculitis in mice. J Clin Invest 2002;110(7):955–63.

38. Saadoun D, Rosenzwajg M, Joly F, et al. Regulatory T-cell responses to low-dose interleukin-2 in HCV-induced vasculitis. N Engl J Med 2011;365(22):2067–77.

39. Hatemi G. A treat-to-target approach is needed for Behcet's syndrome. Curr Opin Rheumatol 2022;34(1):39–45.

40. Crawshaw H, Wells M, Austin K, et al. Patient reported outcomes in systemic vasculitis. Curr Opin Rheumatol 2022;34(1):33–8.

41. Monach PA. Global versus organ-specific outcome measures in systemic lupus erythematosus: comment on the articles by Furie et al, Nikpour et al, Wallace et al, Burgos et al, and Ramos-Casals et al. Arthritis Care Res 2010;62(4): 580–1, author replies 581-2.

42. Woods P, Flynn M, Monach P, et al. Implementation of documented and written informed consent for clinical trials of communicable diseases: Lessons learned, barriers, solutions, future directions identified during the conduct of a COVID-19 clinical trial. Contemp Clin Trials Commun 2021;23:100804.

43. Branch-Elliman W, Elwy AR, Monach P. Bringing New Meaning to the Term "Adaptive Trial": Challenges of Conducting Clinical Research During the Coronavirus Disease 2019 Pandemic and Implications for Implementation Science. Open Forum Infect Dis 2020;7(11):ofaa490.

44. Monach PA, Branch-Elliman W. Reconsidering 'minimal risk' to expand the repertoire of trials with waiver of informed consent for research. BMJ Open 2021;11(9): e048534.

45. Yates M, Watts RA, Bajema IM, et al. EULAR/ERA-EDTA recommendations for the management of ANCA-associated vasculitis. Annals Of The Rheumatic Diseases 2016;75(9):1583–94.

46. Hellmich B, Agueda A, Monti S, et al. 2018 Update of the EULAR recommendations for the management of large vessel vasculitis. Ann Rheum Dis 2020;79(1): 19–30.

47. Chung SA, Langford CA, Maz M, et al. 2021 American College of Rheumatology/ Vasculitis Foundation Guideline for the Management of Antineutrophil Cytoplasmic Antibody-Associated Vasculitis. Arthritis Rheumatol 2021;73(8):1366–83.
48. Maz M, Chung SA, Abril A, et al. 2021 American College of Rheumatology/Vasculitis Foundation Guideline for the Management of Giant Cell Arteritis and Takayasu Arteritis. Arthritis Rheumatol 2021;73(8):1349–65.
49. Chung SA, Gorelik M, Langford CA, et al. 2021 American College of Rheumatology/Vasculitis Foundation Guideline for the Management of Polyarteritis Nodosa. Arthritis Rheumatol 2021;73(8):1384–93.

Moving?

Make sure your subscription moves with you!

To notify us of your new address, find your **Clinics Account Number** (located on your mailing label above your name), and contact customer service at:

Email: journalscustomerservice-usa@elsevier.com

800-654-2452 (subscribers in the U.S. & Canada)
314-447-8871 (subscribers outside of the U.S. & Canada)

Fax number: 314-447-8029

Elsevier Health Sciences Division
Subscription Customer Service
3251 Riverport Lane
Maryland Heights, MO 63043

*To ensure uninterrupted delivery of your subscription, please notify us at least 4 weeks in advance of move.

Printed and bound by CPI Group (UK) Ltd, Croydon, CR0 4YY

08/05/2025

01864715-0001